"*In* Naked Calories *the Caltons explore micronutrient sufficiency as a meaningful way to prevent chronic disease and achieve optimal health.*"

—**Bruce N. Ames, Ph.D.,** Senior Scientist, Children's Hospital Oakland Research Institute Nutrition and Metabolism Center and Professor of the Graduate School, University of California–Berkeley

"Naked Calories *deserves to become a classic on par with Dr. Weston Price's* Nutrition and Physical Degeneration. *The Caltons' six-year expedition to more than 100 countries confirmed once again how modern diets and lifestyle changes sabotage health, leading to the consumption of 'naked calories' or foodless-foods, devoid of life-giving minerals and enzymes. If there is any book you need to read this season,* Naked Calories *is it!*"

—**Ann Louise Gittleman, Ph.D., CNS,** *New York Times* award-winning author of more than thirty books on health and healing

"Naked Calories *provides a beacon of hope for anyone looking to lose weight or reverse a chronic illness. It is a must-read!*"

—**Laurentine ten Bosch,** director and producer of the documentaries *Food Matters* and *Hungry For Change*

"*I've always said the internal workout is as important as the external, what you eat determines your energy, weight control, and that's just the start.* Naked Calories *gives a clear idea on all these topics and more. This is a must-read!*"

—**Dolvett Quince,** trainer, NBC's *Biggest Loser*

"*The Caltons are true pioneers. Their personal story is mesmerizing and inspiring, their information impeccable and their message is important. One of the best books I've seen on the micronutrient-deficiency epidemic. I highly recommend this book to everyone!*"

—**Jonny Bowden, Ph.D., CNS,** aka "The Rogue Nutritionist"™, board-certified nutritionist and bestselling author of *Living Low Carb, The 150 Healthiest Foods on Earth,* and *The Great Cholesterol Myth*

"*The Caltons are pioneers in the field of nutrition, relentless in the pursuit of maximal micronutrient absorption, and dedicated to unlocking the doors to preventing disease and increasing overall health and well-being.*"

—**Dr. John Demartini,** coauthor of the *New York Times* bestseller *The Secret* and bestselling author of *Inspired Destiny*

"*In my own life and on ABC's* The Chew, *I highlight choosing organic, pasture-grazed, and non-GM ingredients wherever possible, but we all know budget can get in the way of even the best health intentions. With* Naked Calories, *the Caltons give us a winning strategy for micronutrient sufficiency as they teach us how to boost the nutritional content of the meals we love and avoid common, micronutrient-depleting lifestyle habits—all without costing a penny extra!*"

—**Daphne Oz,** cohost of ABC's *The Chew* and author of
the national bestseller *The Dorm Room Diet* and *Relish*

"Naked Calories *is a D-lightful exposé that brings into focus the adage, 'You are what you eat.' Mira and Jayson skillfully take the reader on a whirlwind global tour exploring how traditional diets and Westernized diets have influenced the health and well-being of children and adults. A common denominator for the increased incidence of chronic diseases and obesity is micronutrient deficiency . . .* Naked Calories *provides the reader, in an easily digestible fashion, a road map for how to accomplish fulfilling this prescription for good health.*"

—**Michael Holick, M.D., Ph.D.,** Director of the Vitamin D,
Skin and Bone Research Laboratory, Boston University
Medical Center, and author of *The Vitamin D Solution*

"*Despite alarmingly high obesity rates around the world, we have a 'hunger' crisis on our hands. But it's not a hunger for calories but rather a 'hidden hunger' borne out of a deep-seeded desire your body has for adequate micronutrients. Jayson and Mira Calton have put their finger on an all-but-ignored aspect of human nutrition—it's really not about calories as much as it is the vitamins, minerals, and other essential elements of optimal health that are found in real food. While much of the dietary focus in the past few decades has been placed on macronutrients—fat, protein, and carbohydrates—perhaps this forgotten part of the modern-day diet is the missing element in rectifying the out-of-control epidemics of heart disease, diabetes, obesity, chronic fatigue, depression, and cancer.* Naked Calories *arms you with solid information about how to insure you are maximizing your intake of these all-important micronutrients.*"

—**Jimmy Moore,** Livin' La Vida Low-Carb™ blog & podcast

"Naked Calories *changes the way you think about food, exercise, and your lifestyle. It's a wake-up call to put your best foot forward. The good news is anyone can turn around and make healthy changes in their everyday lives. As former Biggest Losers, we would highly recommend this book to anyone who is looking for a fresh start to a better life!*"

—**Dan and Jackie Evans,** former *Biggest Loser* contestants, Kid Fit Foundation

"*In this easy-to-read exposé, the Caltons reveal America's hidden epidemic. Take the book's personal assessment and find out how, without even knowing it, you may be causing your own micronutrient depletion and subsequent ill health! The life you save may be your own—and your family's.*"

—**Hyla Cass, M.D.,** author of *8 Weeks to Vibrant Health* (www.cassmd.com)

"*With all the recent emphasis on the macronutrient breakdown of our diet (fats, proteins, and carbohydrates), many of us seem to have ignored the critical role that micronutrients (vitamins, minerals, and related phytochemicals) play in helping us achieve optimal health. In* Naked Calories, *the Caltons have done a super job of explaining—in easily understood terms—exactly why we need these micronutrients, why we're probably not getting enough of many of them, and how we can easily address the problem. I highly recommend this book for anyone intent on achieving the maximum level of health possible.*"

—**Mark Sisson,** author of *The Primal Blueprint* and publisher of the blog Mark's Daily Apple (www.marksdailyapple.com)

"*In a word—Amazing! I totally agree with the Caltons. The modern diet and our stressed-out society has brought about the reality of micronutrient deficiency and our need for supplementation. Run, don't walk, to buy* Naked Calories— *your health may depend on it!*"

—**J.J. Virgin, Ph.D., CNS, CHFS,** celebrity nutrition expert, and *New York Times* bestselling author of *Six Weeks to Sleeveless and Sexy* and *The Virgin Diet*

“*The Caltons' passion is infectious as they guide the reader through the modern reality of micronutrient deficiency in their important work. Micronutrients are absolutely necessary co-factors for all metabolic processes in the body. Simply put, without proper micronutrient nourishment the body can't properly function.*”

—**Carolyn Dean M.D., N.D.,** author of *The Magnesium Miracle* and creator of the “Completement Now!” wellness program (www.drcarolyndean.com)

“Naked Calories *is the perfect book for anyone looking to improve their health or the health of their child. As an Olympian, optimal health and the ability to compete against the world's most elite athletes are a must. To achieve this I follow a strict program that includes a lot of different vitamins and minerals. In* Naked Calories, *Jayson and Mira have opened my eyes to ways even I can improve my nutrition program and perform at an even higher level. I am proud to be working alongside the Caltons in the fight against childhood obesity. I believe* Naked Calories *is an invaluable tool for parents to improve not only their own health, but to learn ways to incorporate healthier, micronutrient-rich options in their child's diet.*”

—**Carol Rodriguez,** Olympic athlete, Track & Field

“*As a physician and sports medicine surgeon, the Caltons' work on micronutrient deficiency has been an invaluable resource for both me and my patients. Through their groundbreaking work in* Naked Calories, *they have demonstrated that they are the industry leaders in their field. Their work is an important and indispensable resource for those of all ages and activity levels.*”

—**Dr. Robert Nicoletta, M.D.,** Chief of Orthopedic Surgery and Sports Medicine, St. Elizabeth's Medical Center, and Assistant Professor in Orthopedic Surgery, Tufts University

“*The science behind the benefits of micronutrients is extremely compelling. Mira and Jayson Calton clearly and concisely explain how micronutrients increase energy, improve the immune system, and enhance brain function. By following their philosophy, you will be able to rebalance your hormones and decrease your cravings for the wrong foods that are causing illness and disease in the first place. If you want to feel and look good for a lifetime,* Naked Calories *is a must-read.*”

—**Tony Horton,** celebrity trainer and creator of P90X

NAKED
CALORIES

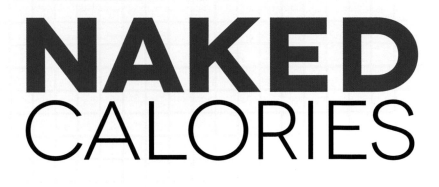

THE CALTONS'
SIMPLE 3-STEP PLAN
TO MICRONUTRIENT SUFFICIENCY

MAXIMIZE WEIGHT LOSS,
PREVENT DISEASE, AND
LIVE YOUR OPTIMAL LIFE

JAYSON CALTON, PhD, AND MIRA CALTON, CN

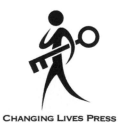

CHANGING LIVES PRESS

The information contained in this book is based upon the research and personal and professional experiences of the authors. It is not intended as a substitute for consulting with your physician or other healthcare provider. Any attempt to diagnose and treat an illness should be done under the direction of a healthcare professional.

The publisher does not advocate the use of any particular healthcare protocol but believes the information in this book should be available to the public. The publisher and authors are not responsible for any adverse effects or consequences resulting from the use of the suggestions, preparations, or procedures discussed in this book. Should the reader have any questions concerning the appropriateness of any procedures or preparation mentioned, the authors and the publisher strongly suggest consulting a professional healthcare advisor.

Mention of specific companies, organizations, or authorities in this book does not imply endorsement by the authors or publisher, nor does mention of specific companies, organizations, or authorities imply that they endorse this book, its authors, or the publisher.

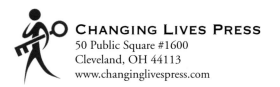

CHANGING LIVES PRESS
50 Public Square #1600
Cleveland, OH 44113
www.changinglivespress.com

Library of Congress Cataloging-in-Publication Data is available through the Library of Congress.

ISBN: 978-0-9894529-0-8

Editor: Michele Matrisciani
Cover design: Mira and Jayson Calton
Photos of Mira and Jayson Calton on Cover, flaps, pages 1, 2, and 3 by Sara Hanna Photography.
Back cover photo by Sara Hanna Photography
All other photos copyright © Mira and Jayson Calton

Printed in the United States of America

10 9 8 7 6 5 4 3 2 1

Contents

Chapter Eight The Obesity Puzzle:

Chapter Nine The ABCs of Optimal Supplementation:

Chapter Ten The Web of Competition and the Dynamic Duos of Synergy:

Chapter Eleven The Hypothesis of Health:

WE DEDICATE THIS BOOK *To my father, Burton Kozel, who taught me to not be afraid of hard work and long hours. You are still my biggest cheerleader, even if you are not here to share this with me today.*

—MIRA CALTON

To my grandparents, Bernard and Frances Jensen, who were always there to listen to my dreams and aspirations, no matter how radical or grand. They taught me to believe in myself, to "give 'em hell," and that anything is possible!

—JAYSON CALTON

Foreword

● ●

I was introduced to Mira and Jayson Calton when I received a review copy of the first version of *Naked Calories*. As a Certified Nutrition Consultant who is constantly out to learn the most cutting-edge information on ways to optimize health, I immediately devoured the content. I flipped through page after page, nodding my head and thought to myself, "This book is something everyone who thinks they're eating a healthy diet needs to read." As much as I loved the book, I was in the midst of working on *my own* first book, so I was quick to cast its contents from my memory while I was nose to the grindstone writing and didn't want outside information to influence my own work. This was my first "run-in" with the Caltons.

Several weeks later, I interviewed Mira and Jayson for my weekly radio show, *The Balanced Bites Podcast,* and learned, in short order, that these two were serious about their *micronutrient-sufficiency-for-all* mission. The couple exuded passion about exactly how much a modern lifestyle—and, of course, most modern food choices—contribute to a state of suboptimal health for the vast majority of us. This was my second "run-in" with the Caltons.

A few months later, I was lucky enough to be a part of the Low Carb Cruise where I finally met Mira and Jayson in person. The week turned into the beginning of a fantastic friendship between us. Our friendship, which has lasted far beyond that week, is just part of the reason why I was honored when they asked me to write the foreword for this re-release of *Naked Calories*. They say the third time's a charm, right? On this third "run-in" with the Caltons, I knew that their message was something I needed to bring into my own work.

I began to weave the concept of micronutrient sufficiency into my teachings more and more—whether in simple replies to Tweets or Facebook posts, or in large-scale topics covered in my full-day seminars. Light bulbs began to turn on for folks in the audience, whether in person or over the Internet. "Wow, so it isn't just about how much protein, fat, and carbs I'm eating, but about the nutrient-density—the *micro*nutrient density—of those foods?!" People would have this reaction over and over—and things just started to *click* for them.

Now it was all making so much more sense! Sure, some people may need to eat different ratios of *macro*nutrients, but it's the *micro*nutrients that are doing the most richly important work. Whether we consistently eat foods rich in these micronutrients and avoid depleting them as much as possible or not became a bigger issue that touched more and more people.

The Caltons possess a unique perspective on the concept of micronutrient sufficiency based both on their own self-experimentation and experience as well as their travels around the globe visiting tribe after tribe of indigenous people. Much like Weston A. Price did in the 1930s, the Caltons collected information and observations about the kinds of foods eaten and how people lived in each location.

This type of observational information is some of the most critical, in my estimation. It's in this way that we begin to recognize not only the vast differences in what tribes eat from one to the other, but also finding common ground in what foods are avoided, how they live, and how these diet and lifestyle factors work in synchrony to promote optimal health.

The comparison of modern-day indigenous tribes eating as closely to their ancestral roots as possible to those of us pounding the pavement, heads-down texting on our iPhones is quite powerful. The Caltons worked to bridge the gap between what research "shows" was eaten by tribes for thousands of years and what these tribes of people are actually doing right now. They present their findings to us here, in *Naked Calories*, in a very tangible way so that we can understand what it all means for us and what we can do to improve our own lives based on their findings.

I was thrilled to write this foreword because, amidst the massive amounts of information swirling in the Paleo and Primal nutrition communities about *macro*nutrients, there was this little-discussed-topic that it seemed many were ignoring—or just not enlightened to completely yet! Sure, people talked about eating enough omega 3-rich foods, or getting vitamin D from sunshine, but the vast majority haven't been focused on micronutrients as critical to their optimal health. The Caltons revised the book to include a whole new section that compares popular diets and their micronutrient values, not the least of which are a Paleo and Primal diets. As a *New York Times* bestselling author of a book based upon the Paleo diet, clearly I took an interest in how this way of eating stacks up!

It's extremely important that folks not hold dogma around their way of eating while also acknowledging the shortcomings of nearly *any* modern diet and lifestyle. It's quite difficult to get everything we need from our food, even if we know what we need and where to get it. However, there are often other limiting factors including time, ease of preparation, the quality of our soils, and the everyday micronutrient-depleting activities we participate in regularly.

Naked Calories is the tool we all need to understand exactly why and how we're affecting our own micronutrient-sufficiency status and how to optimize it to achieve the best health we possibly can.

Diane Sanfilippo, BS, NC
Certified Nutrition Consultant
New York Times bestselling author, *Practical Paleo*

Acknowledgments

● ●

We would first like to thank Beth Davey, our visionary agent, who saw the potential in our early work and without whom this book would never have seen the light of day. We are grateful to our publishers at Changing Lives Press, Francesca Minerva and Ellen Ratner, who have changed our lives and allowed us the opportunity to change the lives of many others. We are excited about continuing this journey together. We look forward to many more Friday-night business phone calls with Francesca, who shares in our passion as well as our drive. We'd also like to offer a special thank-you to the artistic Michele Matrisciani, our editor. Thank you for not changing our words, but molding them. To Lisa, who masterfully placed our words on the page and gave the images life—the book looks fantastic. To the meticulous Shari Johnson, who not only gave us the gift of kind words when we needed them most, but also allowed us to share her "scoop." To Sara Hanna, whose photo made the cover come to life—we love you, Red. Additionally, we'd like to thank Mike "the caveman" Kuhns for helping with research and Lindy Stoler for teaching us to *tell tales* and *ask questions.*

We would also like to acknowledge our families. Jeanne, thank you for believing in the project from the beginning and reading the work until you knew it by heart; and Chad, thanks for always being there. To Elaine, Lisa, Michelle, and Danielle, thank you for your unfailing support. You have endured our excitement like true champions. Diana, we could not have done this without you. Thank you for reading and rereading, and for all the positive feedback along the way.

We would also like to acknowledge the thousands of people who made the Calton Project possible. To those who opened their homes to us and shared their cultures, the memories we created together will forever be remembered as our "colorful days." We would be remiss to forget our floating family aboard *The World,* both staff and residents. You met us at the beginning of this journey as young newlyweds. We miss you and will return home soon.

Finally, we must recognize all of the nutritional visionaries who have come before us. Your work has inspired and guided us. This book would not be the same without all of the works from the gifted nutritionists, researchers, professors, doctors, and scientists we have quoted. Your words have breathed life into this book, and we are humbled that you have allowed us to use them. A very special thanks to Diane Sanfilippo for writing the foreword, and to all of the phenomenal individuals who took time out of their busy schedules to read our work and offer such kind words in support—you will never be forgotten.

Introduction

What Is a Naked Calorie?

My name is Mira Calton.

BY THE TIME I WAS THIRTY YEARS OLD I had the bone density of an eighty-year-old woman. I have the DEXA scan to prove it. My doctor's official diagnosis was advanced osteoporosis, and he prescribed a host of medications with detrimental side effects that I would be married to for the rest of my life.

I was stunned. Initially I went to the doctor to take care of a nagging back pain that had plagued me for more than a year—it was getting almost impossible for me to walk. Like many other busy women, I blamed the intermittent bouts of discomfort on my hectic lifestyle and long hours in stilettos running my own public relations firm in Manhattan. For five years I had been working almost nonstop, filling my days with writing press releases, contacting magazine editors, and visiting television and film sets throughout the city to generate much-deserved press for the young fashion designers I represented.

In the evenings I attended glamorous restaurant openings and film premiers. To those around me it seemed as if I had it all, but that lifestyle would soon come to a screeching halt. I began to reflect on my way of living: how it contributed to my losing control of my health and what needed to be done to regain it. *Why was this happening to me? What could have possibly caused my bones to become so frail so early in my life? Was there a way to stop or even reverse my advanced osteoporosis without medication?*

After much soul searching, I decided not to follow the advice of my physician and I chose not to take the medication. Instead, I took my health into my own hands and began a search for an alternative natural treatment.

In this pursuit, I left behind my public relations firm and everything I had worked so hard to build. I moved to Florida to be closer to my family and pledged to be more active, eat healthier, and find alternate theories on the reversal of osteoporosis. After several years of trying unsuccessfully to reverse the condition on my own, fate stepped in. My search for answers led me to a nutritional theorist with more than fourteen years of clinical experience working with people who had chronic health conditions and lifestyle diseases just like mine.

My name is Dr. Jayson Calton.

HAVING FIRST MET MIRA through a chance social encounter, I was shocked to find out that a young vibrant woman was suffering from such an advanced form of osteoporosis. Upon learning that she was actively looking for an alternative natural treatment for her condition, I was immediately intrigued.

I informed Mira that over the previous fourteen years I had worked in the field of nutritional medicine and that my diet programs, which focused on whole foods and supplementation with micronutrients (vitamins and minerals), had helped thousands of clients suffering from a wide variety of health conditions and diseases.

Although many of my early clients had come to me simply to lose weight, once in a while a client would report back to me that the program lowered their high cholesterol or that their chronic headaches were gone. By the time I met Mira I had been successful in alleviating or reversing more than twenty different health conditions beyond weight loss. Because of this, I believed I could be of help to her in finding a way to reverse her condition.

Although my successful diet and exercise programs were part of my recommendations, I thought that micronutrient deficiencies could have played a central role in Mira's condition, and this forced us to take a much deeper look at the essential micronutrients themselves.

Together we pinpointed specific lifestyle habits that may have contributed to her disease. Her life in the big city, like many other urban dwellers, had been filled with stress, excessive caffeine and alcohol consumption, carbon monoxide inhalation, and frequent dieting. As we suspected, Mira's diet and lifestyle had caused her to become micronutrient deficient.

Her diet consisted of foods filled with what we call "naked calories." Her food choices had been stripped of their essential, health-promoting vitamins and minerals, and were therefore "naked." Mira's lifestyle and environment further contributed to the sabotage of her body's ability to absorb the necessary micronutrients for health and vibrancy.

We changed Mira's eating habits to replace her prepackaged processed foods and reheated takeout with more nutrient-rich alternatives. We added vitamin and mineral supplementation, eliminated many poor lifestyle habits, and began a program of weight-bearing exercise. Slowly Mira began to feel better. However, we knew that only a new DEXA scan would give us the information and the proof we were looking for. I joined Mira on her return visit to her doctor's office to hear the test results. The news couldn't have been better. Within two years, Mira's advanced osteoporosis was completely reversed.

Together we are the Caltons—Jayson and Mira.

AFTER WORKING SIDE BY SIDE BUILDING a solid nutritional program that addresses micronutrient deficiency and its main causative factor, naked calories, we became bonded through our common desire to help others uncover the mysteries as to the sources of their disease and help them gain power over their health.

We spent months digging through scientific research on the roles that nutrition and lifestyle habits had in the causation, prevention, and reversal of disease. We devoured studies conducted at acclaimed universities, including Duke, Harvard, Tufts, Cornell, and Johns Hopkins, and scrutinized research papers from well-established foundations and government agencies such as the American Heart Association, the World Health Organization, and the Centers for Disease Control and Prevention. We discovered extensive evidence that pointed less often to genetic components and more toward nutritional and lifestyle factors as the culprits of disease prevalence in modernized societies. We also discovered something else during those long months of research: our mutual respect for one another had blossomed into love.

Working as a couple and inspired by our success in reversing Mira's osteoporosis, we further investigated the combination of naked calories and lifestyle habits and their collective effect on Mira's health. *Could what we accomplished with Mira's health play a role in the prevention or reversal of other conditions as well? Can a person really take herself from a frail-boned individual living in pain and limited by her disease, to a pain-free, strong-boned individual through proper nutrition and supplementation alone? Is it possible to slow down, stop, or even reverse advanced stages of disease without medications?* This search for answers on micronutrient deficiency and naked calories became our passion, and this passion took us to places we had never imagined.

• • • • • • • • • • • • • • • •

The Calton Project

IN 2005, WE WERE MARRIED and said goodbye to our families and friends and set off on a six-year, around-the-world research expedition with one particular goal in mind: to study the effects of modernization on the lifestyle and nutrition habits of people and to determine whether there was a correlation between modernization and disease. In order to get an accurate reading on modernization, we needed to observe people from vastly different regions in remote, semi-remote, and urban settings. We would compare the habits of communities as remote as those that still existed without electricity or running water with "in-between" cultures that had advanced to some modern conveniences (such as motorized canoes and occasional packaged foods), and the most fast-paced urban societies that were fully dependent on cell-phone towers and fuel.

We called this quest for a global perspective on nutrition the Calton Project. From Tibet and Tunisia to Peru and Papua New Guinea to Australia and the Amazon, we sat with, ate with, and interviewed people from diverse cultures. Our travels to more than 100 countries on all seven continents led us to a new understanding of nutrition.

A large portion of our time was spent with primitive groups who, for the most part, were still living as their ancestors had for thousands of years. We found them deep in the Amazon forest living along the ancient river; high in the Andes Mountains of Ecuador and Peru; in remote rarely traveled areas of China, India, and Tibet; and on the mysterious islands of Papua New Guinea. These isolated areas were only accessible by foot, long bumpy truck rides, hand-paddled canoes, or single-engine planes.

We were able to uncover several universal commonalities in the routines that promoted health in the everyday lives of the people living in these remote areas. The first of these similarities was the fact that these remote groups had little or no contact with the outside world. For these people, the tribe or clan was everything. It was the foundation for their happiness, survival, love, and spirituality. It bound them, held them, and nourished their physical and emotional health. Everything they did, they did for the betterment of that immediate group.

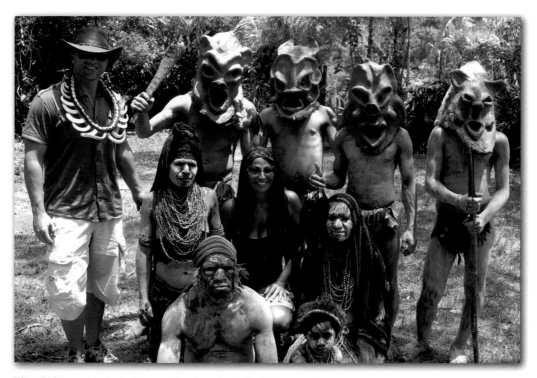

The Caltons spend time with the close-knit Asaro Mudmen, indigenous to the highlands of Papua New Guinea.

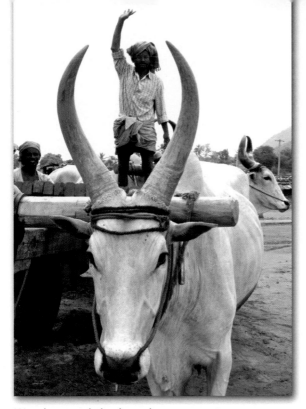

Due to the lack of refrigeration and electricity in these regions, the food was always fresh and never factory-processed. Tribe members ate only what was available to them through hunting, fishing, farming, foraging, or trading with surrounding tribes. Seasonal eating patterns were also evident. If the tribe lived in an area that experienced a season change, the tribe would be forced to change its eating patterns to accommodate the available food choices.

For example, a community might plant certain crops along the river and enjoy the fruits of this labor until the river rose, covering their crops, and forcing them to live off a diet consisting almost exclusively of fish.

We observed the long hours spent working the land in Southern India.

Although the variety of food would be considered limited by "developed" standards, the ingredients were always fresh and natural. Many communities fished daily, while others scavenged for turtle or chicken eggs for their fats and proteins. In some communities, such as in the Andes, it was the responsibility of the men to hunt and farm, while on the Sepik River, in Papua New Guinea, it was the responsibility of the women to catch enough fish for their families early every morning.

Regardless of their cultural and ancestral beliefs and traditions, life depended on daily success in gathering and farming and/or hunting and fishing. This meant that physical labor was prevalent. Life in these remote tribal villages usually involved quite a bit of walking or canoeing from one place to another. It was not uncommon to see people working or gathering food for several hours every day.

Women in the highlands of Papua New Guinea teaching us how to cook sweet potatoes and greens for our dinner.

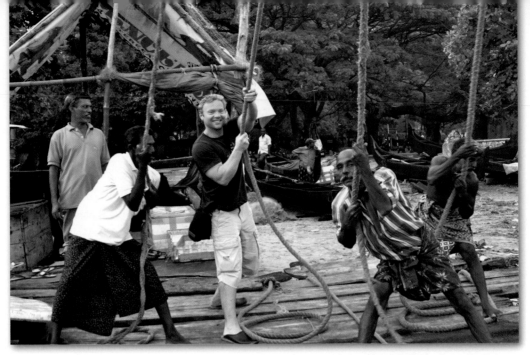

Jayson bringing in the fishing nets with the villagers of Kerala, India.

Of the thousands of children we encountered, not one was overweight or obese. This was also the case for the adult males, whose fit bodies looked decades younger than their actual ages. Another interesting observation was that in the remote tribes there was little or no tooth decay and most often, their teeth were straight and white. Tribes that primarily consumed protein and fat through hunting or fishing were leaner and taller than those who received their protein mainly through a plant-based diet.

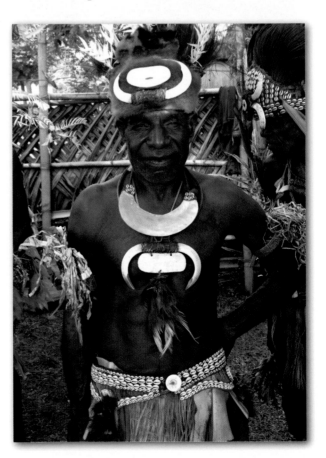

We observed the lean, strong body of a nearly seventy-year-old man living on the Sepik River in Papua New Guinea.

Our next stop was to the "places in between," where the introduction of modernization and the infiltration of Westernization were just beginning to take hold. Some of these places, dotted along long stretches of lonely road all throughout India, China, and Africa, were so small that we were through them almost as soon as we arrived. Others were large, vast areas like Lhasa, Tibet, that were steeped in history, but fundamentally torn concerning their traditions and their place in our ever-changing world. For the people living in these semi-remote areas it's an exciting time. From their perspective, their lives are becoming easier as they become connected to the modern world around them.

Electricity is most often available, as is running water. We found that almost immediately upon modernization a little store opens, selling the much sought-after, brightly packaged

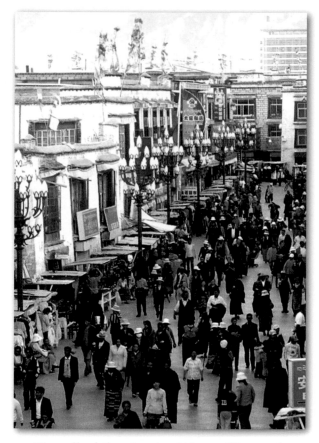

We walked the streets of Lhasa, Tibet—where modernization met with ancient traditions.

soft drinks, candies, and chips. These factory-processed, sugar-laden, energy (calorie) dense, and nutritionally poor foods immediately hook the community, beginning with the children and spreading like wildfire. Oftentimes we found these products as part of the government subsidization programs at schools.

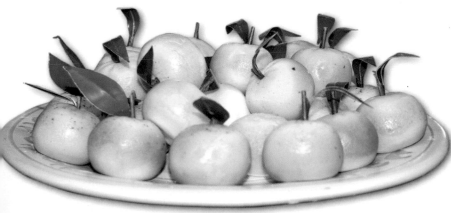

Candied apples? It was hard for us to believe that these sweet treats weren't fresh-picked apples, but candies made of pure sugar.

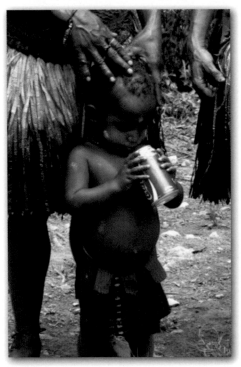

We watched the men making rolls with refined white flour in the highlands of Papua New Guinea.

These new foods drastically alter the eating profile of the children. Instead of fresh fruit, the children are given processed treats with ingredients never before ingested by their ancestors. We also observed the Huli tribesmen from the Tari region of Papua New Guinea, whose breakfast now consisted of what appeared to be big white dinner rolls and soda. When we inquired about the unusual meal, our guides explained that about two years earlier refined white flour became available and since that time many of the village people began their day with a breakfast of several freshly baked white rolls and a can or two of Coke.

Our guides revealed even more about the new foods of these Tari tribesmen when they told us that it was also about two years before when the first signs of obesity and mouth cancer were reported in their area. After putting two and two together, we asked them if they had any idea of what these foods were doing to their health. *Were they aware that these new foods had any effect on their health at all?* They told us they had noticed that these new foods caused them to gain belly fat; however, they were completely unaware that food could cause any kind of health condition or disease.

The potential health and financial implications that these "new" foods have on the semi-remote areas we visited are among the biggest problems they face. Modernization is costing the people of Papua New Guinea in other ways too. Already, the cell-phone companies are aggressively giving away free cell phones in order to sell prepaid phone cards. One guide proudly pulled from his pocket a stack of them. He carried them, like many of the men we encountered, as a sign of status. That year alone he had spent half of his total salary on phone cards to call people living no more

We were saddened to discover that even the youngest children are not immune to the Western influence.

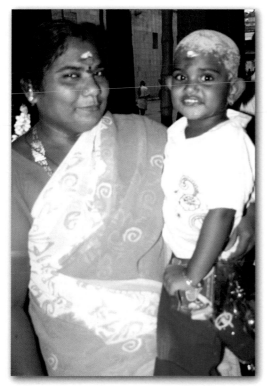

A Huli Wigman proudly demonstrating his cell phone to us—an expensive sign of status in Papua New Guinea.

than a stone's throw away. He no longer needed to walk the mile to confer with clansmen—now he could just pick up his cell and make a call.

We also witnessed many other examples of how modernization brought about a reduction in physical activity. Even as we traveled down the Ecuadorian Amazon River, we could see that the villages closest to civilization were adopting modern conveniences. New machine-fabricated metal canoes powered by small gas-guzzling engines replaced the wooden canoes that were typically rowed by two men. These modern monstrosities left behind a cloud of black smoke as they sped out of sight with a deafening roar.

The changes in the men's physiques were immediately apparent. Loose skin and protruding bellies replaced tight, well-muscled bodies. Many of the villages we visited were trying to stay self-sufficient. People, whether scientist, nutritionist, or tourist, had warned a few of these "in-between" groups that it was in their best interest to maintain their old nutritional ways. While many were experimenting with ways to somehow grow or raise enough food for their villagers as their ancestors had before them, there seemed to be more villagers than ever before.

With the help of the missionaries far fewer were dying of avoidable diseases such as malaria, and tribal warfare was at an all-time low. The increased life expectancy naturally caused an increased demand for food—food that most villages were not equipped to grow or raise on their own. Some communities started trout farms or raised cuy (pronounced kwee), a type of guinea pig, to provide a constant source of proteins and fats for their people. However, most communities were quickly becoming dependent on the prepackaged foods delivered by strangers.

In many of these semi-remote areas tooth decay was already becoming rampant, and

We witnessed obesity on the rise in India.

diabetes, obesity, heart disease, and cancer were all starting to rear their ugly heads. Areas that just a generation ago had no knowledge of these devastating conditions were now beginning to suffer from them. The modern imported diet of these semi-remote people is always the same—consisting of high amounts of processed carbohydrates and fewer essential fats and proteins.

Our last stop was to visit the buzzing hubs of the most urban and modern cities. Here, obesity, heart disease, osteoporosis, diabetes, and cancer, among other diseases, are rampant. These urban dwellers have become intimately familiar with these conditions, and most are on one or more prescription medications. However, the medications are not helping. More people are dying of cancer and heart disease and being diagnosed with diabetes and obesity despite pharmaceuticals.

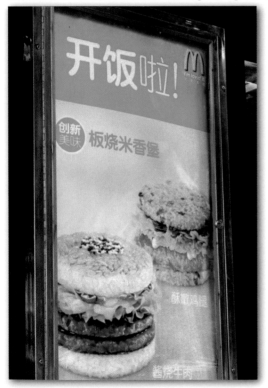

We saw how McDonald's in China lures patrons with burger buns made of white rice.

Throughout our years of travel, we began to note the many similarities these otherwise vastly different cities of the world had in common. We wanted to see if we were able to identify what exactly had brought about the explosion of disease across these communities. *How did it happen? What was the cause of the increased disease rates? Could there be a way to reverse these trends?* Many of the urban dwellers shared similarities in how they ate, what they ate, and how they lived their lives. And ultimately those nutritional and lifestyle habits noticeably affected their overall health.

From New York to Shanghai we found overworked, undernourished, sick, medicated, disease-ridden, outwardly happy, productive, smiling people. While their faces and actions tell one story, their disease-ridden, medicated bodies tell a completely different one. Through our observations, we were able to conclude that there were two basic factors that all of the urban areas and emerging modern communities seemed to share. The first was that, thanks to the processing of food, pasteurizing of milk, the time and distance food traveled to the table, plus modern food production and preparation techniques, people in these areas consumed far fewer micronutrients (essential vitamins and minerals) than their more remote-dwelling counterparts.

The second common factor was that all of these people were actively participating in their own micronutrient depletion. They were consciously making choices to consume alcohol, sugar, refined flour, high fructose corn syrup, and high levels of caffeine. In turn, they also stressed more, exercised less, skipped meals, smoked, and took medications. All of which further depleted their already insufficient level of micronutrients.

The Calton Project coupled with our continuous painstaking research of mainstream scientific studies and reports have led us to one final truth: There exists a preventable "hidden" pandemic, which is a primary causative factor in almost every one of today's most debilitating health conditions and diseases. Diseases like heart disease, cancer, diabetes, high blood pressure, high cholesterol, and obesity, to name a few. It was this same pandemic that made Mira sick and caused her severe osteoporosis. It is called micronutrient deficiency. We refer to its primary causative factor as "naked calories" because our foods have been stripped of their life-giving vitamins and minerals and are therefore naked.

THE "WESTERN" INFLUENCE

The more modern the society, the more prevalent are the following in their culture:

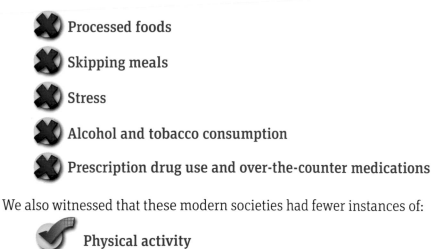

Processed foods

Skipping meals

Stress

Alcohol and tobacco consumption

Prescription drug use and over-the-counter medications

We also witnessed that these modern societies had fewer instances of:

Physical activity

Community gatherings

Are naked calories making you sick? Are they killing someone you love? Do the effects of modernization threaten your health every day? Fear not. Just as it led to our identification of the true culprit in our decrease in overall health and well-being, the Calton Project brought about some pretty remarkable discoveries about what to eat, how to live, and where to turn in order to become micronutrient *sufficient* to prevent and reverse the dangerous and widespread effects of naked calories. These discoveries became the foundation for our three-step plan to achieving micronutrient sufficiency you will be learning about as you read this book. They worked for Mira, and they can work for you. Our experience tells us this is true.

Read on.

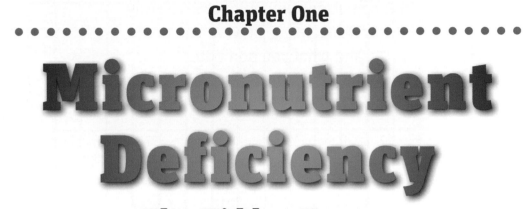

Chapter One

Micronutrient Deficiency

The Hidden Hunger

Vitamins CoQ10

Minerals

quercetin

Antioxidants alpha lipoic acid

> **"**Your health is not something
> you biologically lose as you age.
> It is something you build or give away
> a little each day, in what you do,
> and what you don't do.**"**
> —Dr. Jayson Calton

Micronutrient deficiency is the most widespread and dangerous health condition of the 21st century. It is at the heart of many of today's most common and life-threatening health conditions and diseases. Think of the word *micronutrient* as an all-encompassing term for all of the "good stuff" found in food. Different from carbohydrates, fats, and proteins, micronutrients are needed in small, or micro, quantities by the body to keep it healthy and strong. They include things you may have heard of like vitamins, minerals, and antioxidants, as well as other things you may not have heard of such as CoQ_{10}, quercetin, and alpha lipoic acid. Micronutrient deficiency occurs when even one micronutrient is not available when the body needs it.

"Vitamin and mineral [micronutrients] deficiency is the source of the most massive 'hidden hunger' and malnutrition in the world today," says Kul C. Gautam, former deputy executive director of UNICEF. There are two types of hunger the body can experience. The first, which we are all familiar with, occurs when we do not eat enough food or have not eaten for a long period of time. Stomach grumbling and slight discomfort typically signal this *obvious hunger*. However, eating food can easily curb this hunger. The second kind of hunger, the "hidden hunger" that Mr. Gautam refers to, occurs when one or more of the essential micronutrients the body needs are not available. Hidden hunger caused by a micronutrient deficiency is not always as obvious as its counterpart. Unlike obvious hunger, eating more food will not necessarily reverse hidden hunger because many of today's foods have become increasingly devoid of essential micronutrients.

There are several reasons for this; soil depletion, global distribution, factory farming, food packaging, and preparation methods are all responsible for leaving our food lacking in these essential vitamins and minerals. For instance, over-farming due to excessive planting to accommodate the world's growing population affects the vegetables on your plate. The manner in which your food is prepared can also determine the micronutrient density of your dinner. With our food stripped of micronutrients we are left with little more than a plateful of naked calories. To make matters worse, there is an abundance of everyday actions, many of which you may take part in, that deplete or block the absorption of essential micronutrients from your body before they can be used.

Do you drink alcohol, smoke, take prescription medications, or exercise? Have you contemplated how these common habits and many other lifestyle choices affect your micronutrient

Traditional healthy cooking techniques are changing in India.

sufficiency? Unlike our ability to immediately recognize an obvious hunger, most of us will go years without ever knowing that we are experiencing hidden hunger due to a deficiency in one or more essential micronutrients.

In Mira's case, her deficiencies didn't become obvious until they revealed themselves as the advanced stage of osteoporosis. Mira didn't realize that her lack of dietary calcium-rich products and her constant reheating of Chinese take-out that contained processed white rice and overcooked vegetables were robbing her of the essential micronutrients required for her bones to stay healthy. What are the chances that your body is experiencing a hidden hunger from a micronutrient deficiency? Perhaps you, like Mira, have bone-density issues, or maybe you have cardiovascular disease, high blood pressure, diabetes, or suffer from depression. Perhaps your weight has increased as you've aged or migraine headaches are paralyzing your life. Have you ever stopped to consider whether your health conditions or those of your children, spouse, or friends could be intrinsically linked to micronutrient deficiency?

Could the heart conditions of Toni Braxton, Bill Clinton, Barbara Walters, or David Letterman have been outward manifestations of micronutrient deficiencies lurking inside them? Could Jim Carrey's depression, which required him to take Prozac for years, have been caused by a hidden hunger as well? Consider Farrah Fawcett, Audrey Hepburn, and Steve Jobs. Could all of their cancers have been caused, influenced, or rooted in this same global pandemic?

While many of today's devastating diseases may be undetectable to the naked eye until it's too late, there is one health condition that is immediately evident, prevalent, and spreading globally at a staggering rate—obesity. According to Thomas Frieden, M.D., MPH, director of the

Centers for Disease Control and Prevention, "The big picture is that over the past several decades, obesity has increased faster than anyone could have imagined it would . . . Obesity has doubled in adults and tripled in children." Obesity is now a very real threat to all of us worldwide. While we have been led to believe that diet and exercise are the answers to the obesity epidemic, what if they aren't? What if they are actually contributing to the overall problem? Have you ever considered the fact that as you restrict calories by dieting and increase calorie expenditure through exercise, you may actually be causing serious vitamin and mineral deficiencies?

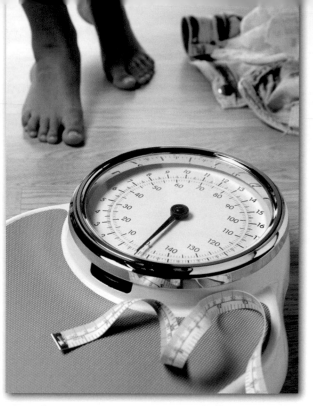

Are you on a diet right now, or are you considering starting one? Most people don't know that many of the menus prescribed by popular diet plans have been found to be substandard in providing even the minimum amounts of essential micronutrients recommended to maintain health. One of the many things that we will share with you in this book is Dr. Jayson Calton's shocking research on the prevalence of micronutrient deficiencies in today's most popular diet plans. Even more alarming are the truths we expose showing that these deficiencies can actually cause increased hunger, weight gain, and ultimately obesity. Yes, you read that right. Your "healthy diet" may be causing micronutrient deficiencies that are starving you into obesity and disease.

Your "healthy diet" may be causing micronutrient deficiencies, which are starving you into obesity and disease.

While some people may choose to look at the looming micronutrient-deficiency pandemic as yet another depressing, overwhelming reality facing the global population, we would like everyone to see it for what it can be. It just may be the best news of the century. If we understand that suboptimal levels (a deficiency) of essential micronutrients is a causative factor in the majority of today's lifestyle conditions and diseases, then optimal levels (a sufficiency) of these same vitamins and minerals would logically lead to the suppression or reversal of these same conditions and diseases.

According to Drs. Robert Fletcher and Kathleen Fairfield of Harvard University, "Inadequate intake or subtle deficiencies in several vitamins are risk factors for chronic diseases such as cardiovascular disease, cancer, and osteoporosis." In the Dietary Supplement Health and Education Act of 1994, the U.S. 103rd Congress passed public law 103-417 that states, "There is a link between the ingestion of certain nutrients or dietary supplements and the prevention of chronic disease such as cancer, heart disease, and osteoporosis." Additionally, Bruce N. Ames, Ph.D., one of the world's leading experts on cancer and anti-aging states that "remedying micronutrient deficiencies is likely to lead to a major improvement in health and an increase in longevity at low cost."

These experts are in agreement with our exciting hypothesis and clearly state that our hidden hungers caused by micronutrient deficiencies are linked to disease and that an inexpensive remedying of these same deficiencies would improve health and longevity.

Our personal experience indicates this is very much the case. As mentioned in the Introduction, we increased the micronutrient values of Mira's foods and gave her better-quality supplementation to create a micronutrient sufficient regimen. Coupling good nutrition and supplementation with changing lifestyle habits that were further contributing to Mira's deficiency, such as lowering her stress level, led us to understand that micronutrient deficiency was the primary causative factor of Mira's osteoporosis and many other diseases.

After extensive academic and field research and more than twenty years of direct clinical experience working with thousands of international clients, it has become clear to us that micronutrient deficiency is a primary causative factor of numerous globally devastating diseases. It is our belief that a policy of micronutrient sufficiency could prevent disease and lead to a savings of trillions of health-care dollars and an age of unparalleled health.

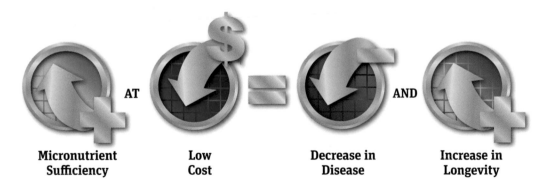

| Micronutrient Sufficiency | AT | Low Cost | = | Decrease in Disease | AND | Increase in Longevity |

If osteoporosis can be prevented or reversed through a sufficiency of specific bone-building micronutrients such as calcium, magnesium, vitamin D, and vitamin K, would it not hold true that the world's largest killer, cardiovascular disease—often referred to as the CoQ_{10} deficiency disease—would be reduced by a sufficiency in CoQ_{10}?

If reduced levels of selenium and folic acid were found to increase chances of heart disease, then could we not presume that sufficiency in these same micronutrients could reduce the occurrence of this disease that currently claims 17.1 million lives a year?

If chromium, biotin, vitamin D, and niacin have been scientifically shown to influence insulin sensitivity, and diabetes is a disease caused by the inability to control insulin levels, then would it not make sense to suggest these micronutrients as treatment for diabetes?

Can we afford to ignore Tufts University's 2010 statement, "Vitamin D and calcium may be as essential to cancer protection as they are to bone formation"?

By now you should have a pretty good idea of just how powerful the information you are about to discover in this book can be toward transforming your life and increasing your chances of achieving optimal health. Even if you don't currently suffer from a serious health condition or disease, learning how to increase micronutrient sufficiency can have a plethora of outstanding results for you as well.

Did You Know

Here is just a short list of the incredible health benefits—those above and beyond disease prevention—that are made possible through micronutrient sufficiency.

- Increased natural energy
- Decreased depression and mood swings
- Anti-aging
- Balanced hormones
- Improved sleep patterns and fewer leg cramps
- Superior immunity
- Better brain function, memory, and clarity
- Weight loss and decreased appetite and cravings
- Improved athletic performance and rapid recovery from intense activity
- Youthful skin, hair, and nails
- Improved vision
- Enhanced dental health
- Improved fertility
- Increased longevity

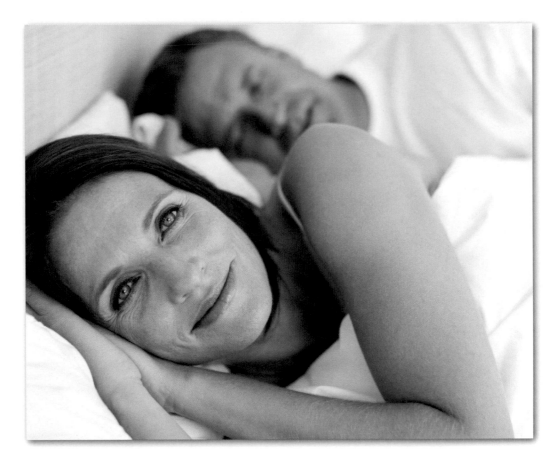

For example, did you know that vitamins and minerals are essential in creating hormone balance? Are you aware that there are at least eight micronutrients that contribute to a good night's sleep? Have you considered the fact that healthy skin, nails, and hair begins on the inside of your body? Even athletic performance can be greatly enhanced through a sufficiency of specific micronutrients that include sodium and potassium (electrolytes), as well as calcium, iron, and zinc.

Are you aware that there are at least eight micronutrients that contribute to a good night's sleep?

Regardless of your circumstance, whether it is a serious, chronic health condition or simply a desire for a better complexion, the first step toward reaching your goal is the same: You must first determine the prevalence of micronutrient deficiency in your own life by evaluating your personal micronutrient-sufficiency level. You can begin by taking our quick-and-easy personal sufficiency profile quiz in Chapter 2, which we created to help you identify the micronutrient-depleting factors hiding in your life. Your score will help you establish a baseline that reflects your current sufficiency based on your present dietary and lifestyle choices. This original score is in no way set in stone. As you make changes in your life, you can retake the quiz as often as you like to see how these changes are affecting your overall sufficiency.

By using our simple three-step plan, you will have the ability to dramatically improve your sufficiency score and thus increase your chances of better health in the years to come. We are confident that at the end of our journey together you will look at your food, your lifestyle, and your multivitamin in an entirely new way.

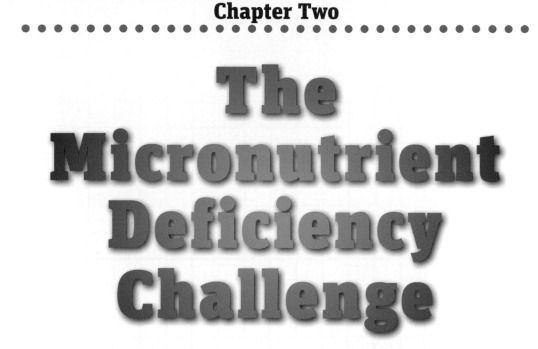

Chapter Two

The Micronutrient Deficiency Challenge

Your Personal Assessment

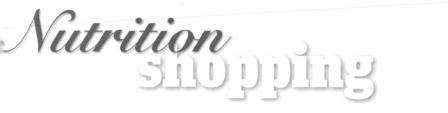

Nutrition shopping *Stress* preparation *Activity* techniques

> **"Knowledge is power."**
> —Sir Francis Bacon

Before you delve into all that this book has to offer, we invite you to test your personal micronutrient-sufficiency level. Statistics cited by the United States Department of Agriculture indicate the likelihood that you are deficient in one or more of the essential micronutrients. This is largely due to the reality that you unavoidably consume food that has been grown or produced in over-farmed, nutrient-depleted soil and take part in a variety of common micronutrient-depleting lifestyle factors. To help you take stock of what you can readily do to gain more control over your nutrition and overall lifestyle by identifying (and then disarming) the naked calories and micronutrient-depleting habits in your life, we created the Micronutrient Deficiency Challenge.

This quiz considers all the aspects of your life, including nutrition, activity, stress level, food shopping and preparation preferences, and cooking techniques. By the time you complete the challenge you will know whether naked calories are present in your life. Don't worry, there is no passing or failing grade—just the knowledge you will obtain about yourself—and the more you learn about yourself and your micronutrient levels, the better equipped you will be to improve your micronutrient intake, your lifestyle, and to prevent or reverse disease.

Take the electronic version of this quiz at www.caltonnutrition.com. *We even do the math for you!*

This assessment highlights the areas in your life where you are willfully losing micronutrients. That's right! You may be actively participating in your own micronutrient depletion.

Answer the following statements as honestly as you can. Don't worry about your initial score. What ultimately matters is that you use the breakthrough research, eye-opening information, and pragmatic advice offered in this book to influence and control your personal micronutrient-sufficiency level.

ARE YOU MICRONUTRIENT DEFICIENT?

	OFTEN	SOMETIMES	NEVER
1. I eat locally grown foods.	☐	☐	☐
2. I eat organically grown foods.	☐	☐	☐
3. I eat my foods raw.	☐	☐	☐
4. I buy the majority of my food from a chain grocery store.	☐	☐	☐
5. I peel my fruits and/or vegetables.	☐	☐	☐
6. Fruits, vegetables, cheeses, and meats may sit in my refrigerator or the grocery store refrigerator for a few days before being used.	☐	☐	☐
7. I eat out at restaurants more than two times a week.	☐	☐	☐
8. I eat grain-fed beef and store-bought cheese, eggs, and butter.	☐	☐	☐
9. I use canned or frozen vegetables.	☐	☐	☐
10. I eat potato chips, French fries, tortilla chips, nuts, or other salty snacks.	☐	☐	☐
11. I eat candy (gummy, hard, or anything else made of sugar).	☐	☐	☐
12. I take home and eat leftovers.	☐	☐	☐
13. I eat white bread, rolls, or bagels, and/or traditional pasta.	☐	☐	☐
14. I drink carbonated sodas.	☐	☐	☐
15. I use products containing high fructose corn syrup (including salad dressing and ketchup).	☐	☐	☐
16. I eat dessert-like baked goods (muffins, croissants, cakes, biscuits, crepes, quiche).	☐	☐	☐
17. I eat spinach, collard greens, sweet potatoes, rhubarb, or beans.	☐	☐	☐
18. I eat whole-grain breads, corn, beans, grains (including cereal), or soy isolates.	☐	☐	☐

	OFTEN	SOMETIMES	NEVER
19. I eat nuts, apples, carrots, seeds (including flaxseeds), or oats.	☐	☐	☐
20. I drink pasteurized (grocery store–bought) milk.	☐	☐	☐
21. I drink alcohol (beer, wine, or spirits).	☐	☐	☐
22. I drink coffee, tea, or coffee drinks.	☐	☐	☐
23. I drink caffeinated sodas or energy drinks.	☐	☐	☐
24. I drink fruit juices or sports drinks sweetened with sugar or enhanced with high fructose corn syrup.	☐	☐	☐
25. I have stress in my life.	☐	☐	☐
26. I take prescription medication, birth control, or medication for erectile dysfunction.	☐	☐	☐
27. I take aspirin or other over-the-counter pain and fever reducers (including acetaminophen and ibuprofen).	☐	☐	☐
28. I take antacids.	☐	☐	☐
29. I smoke cigarettes, cigars, or a pipe, or live with (or spend a large amount of time with) someone who does.	☐	☐	☐
30. I purchase conventional moisturizers, toothpaste, shampoo, or household cleaning products at the local grocery store.	☐	☐	☐
31. I live in a large city.	☐	☐	☐
32. I am physically active in a gym, at home, and or outdoors (walking, bike riding, swimming).	☐	☐	☐
33. I skip meals.	☐	☐	☐
34. I follow a low-carbohydrate, low-fat, paleo, Primal, Mediterranean, medically founded, or calorie-restricting diet.	☐	☐	☐
35. I take fat burners, diuretics, and/or appetite suppressants.	☐	☐	☐

	OFTEN	SOMETIMES	NEVER
36. I have had surgery to help me lose weight. (Check never for no, often for yes.)	☐	☐	☐
37. I eat vegetarian, vegan, and/or gluten free.	☐	☐	☐
38. I prepare meals ahead of time, and refrigerate or freeze them to be eaten at a later date.	☐	☐	☐
39. I feel lethargic.	☐	☐	☐
40. I suffer from type 2 diabetes or have been diagnosed as pre-diabetic. (Check never for no, often for yes.)	☐	☐	☐
41. My physician has warned me about my elevated cholesterol levels. (Check never for no, often for yes.)	☐	☐	☐
42. My blood pressure is too high. (Check never for no, often for yes.)	☐	☐	☐
43. I feel depressed and/or anxious.	☐	☐	☐
44. I have been diagnosed with low bone density or have been told I am at risk for it. (Check never for no, often for yes.)	☐	☐	☐
45. I eat at least 27,575 calories a day.*	☐	☐	☐
46. I eat five servings of fruit and five servings of vegetables every day.	☐	☐	☐
47. I am currently overweight or obese. (Check never for no, often for yes.)	☐	☐	☐
48. I am currently underweight. (Check never for no, often for yes.)	☐	☐	☐
49. I take a daily multivitamin and mineral in a pill or capsule form.	☐	☐	☐
50. I take a liquid multivitamin supplement that is labeled to include Anti-Competition Technology.	☐	☐	☐

*Twenty-seven thousand five hundred and seventy-five calories. That's no typo! We'll tell you why in Chapter 7.

It's Time to Tabulate!

Scoring
Tabulate the scores for each step separately. We will combine the totals of each step at the end.

STEP 1: Look at statements 1, 2, and 3. If you answered often, give yourself a round of applause and **add 10 points** for each often answered. **Add 5 points** for each time you answered sometimes. Don't add any points if you answered never. **TOTAL** _____

STEP 2: For statements 4 through 44 **deduct 5 points** for every time you answered often. **Deduct 3 points** for every time you answered sometimes. Don't deduct any points if you answered never. **TOTAL** _____

STEP 3: Look at statement 45. If you answered often to statement 45, **add 100 points**. If you answered sometimes, **add 50 points**. Don't do anything if you answered never. **TOTAL** _____

STEP 4: Look at statement 46. If you answered often, **add 10 points**. If you answered sometimes, **add 5 points**. Don't do anything if you answered never. **TOTAL** _____

STEP 5: Look at statements 47 and 48. If you answered never or no, do nothing. If you answered often or yes to either question, **deduct 20 points**. **TOTAL** _____

STEP 6: Look at statement 49. If you answered often, **add 10 points**. **Add 5 points** if you sometimes remember to take a multivitamin in pill or capsule form. **Deduct 10 points** if you answered never. **TOTAL** _____

STEP 7: If you answered often to statement 50, then bravo! **Add 100 points** to your score. You must be one very informed supplement consumer. And we'll tell you why in Chapter 9. If you answered sometimes, **add 50 points** and try to remember to take it more often. Do nothing if you answered never. **TOTAL** _____

STEP 8: Add up all the totals from Step 1 through Step 7. **GRAND TOTAL** _____

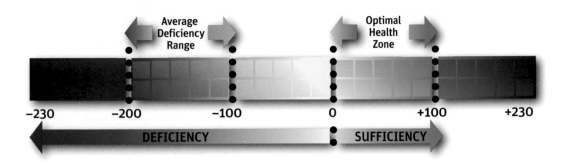

What does your score reveal about you?

BASED ON YOUR SCORE, you have probably come to the conclusion that we are fans of "the trick question." (Enter sinister laugh here.) Did some of the questions seem like good, "healthy" choices? Did you deduct points from your score for things you have always been told are good for you, as in questions 17 through 20? Some statements in the quiz may appear to be about "healthy" habits, but as you will learn throughout this book, even "healthy habits" can have some very unhealthy side effects where micronutrient depletion is concerned.

Each chapter explains in detail every question asked on the quiz. The chapters are cumulative, building on one another to offer you the big picture on naked calories and how (and why) they impact your personal micronutrient-sufficiency level—and ultimately, your health.

You can see on the previous chart that the highest possible score is 230. However, you should also notice that we indicate you should strive to be in the "Optimal Health Zone," which falls anywhere between 0 and 100. You may be wondering why the highest score of 230 does not represent optimal health. Well, it goes back to the trick questions. While some of the "healthier" habits actually contribute to a lower level of micronutrient sufficiency, the truth is that we don't want you to give up all of these habits. You will learn as you read on that while many of these lifestyle choices deplete micronutrients, they also offer health benefits that should not be overlooked.

For example, when Mira needed to rebuild her bones she began an exercise program that included both cardiovascular and weight-bearing exercises. As you will later learn, exercise is a micronutrient depleter; however, the benefits of this type of program were necessary in the reversal of her osteoporosis. This is precisely why your score should never reach the highest limits. If you removed all the micronutrient depleters from your life, you would also be removing some fantastic and essential benefits of these foods and activities.

The importance of recognizing a depleter, even if it's a beneficial one like exercise—which we will ultimately advise you to keep doing—is to make you aware that your lifestyle requires that you compensate for the existence of the depleter. It is all about awareness. Your body needs each and every one of the essential micronutrients, and it is essential to your health that you become aware of all of the healthy and unhealthy depleters robbing you of them. Even awareness of the healthy habits will require replenishment of micronutrients. We will discuss the smartest ways to do this later, in Chapter 9.

As you examine your score, remember that no one is perfect. We applaud you for all the fantastic decisions—small or large—you are making (or are about to make) in your life. If you received a score between 0 and 100, you are in the "Optimal Health Zone," and we salute you. You are making great decisions to consume high-quality micronutrient-rich foods, eliminate a few micronutrient-robbing lifestyle habits, and supplement with the highest quality products on the market. You may not even know what things you have done right or why you scored so high. This book will reveal the habits that got you here, so that you can be sure to continue them.

Don't worry if you have a low score, or even a really low score. In fact, there is a good chance you have a negative number. If this is the case, get excited because the lower your score, the more you can improve by the end of your journey. Your mission, as you move along chapter by chapter, is to learn all of the essential facts needed to create optimal health. And it's our mission to teach you. For now, simply record your score in the space provided so you won't forget it. When you finish this book and incorporate our three-step plan into your life, we encourage you to take the test again; this time with all the knowledge you have accumulated along the way. We think you will be amazed at your new score and how much control you actually have over your personal micronutrient-sufficiency profile.

Chapter Three

Nutrition 101

Understanding Nutrients

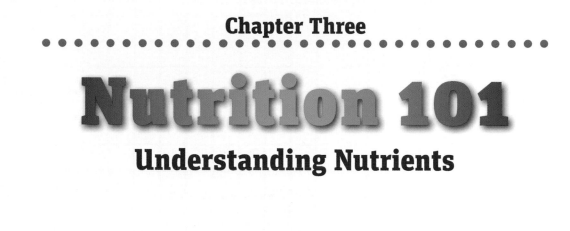

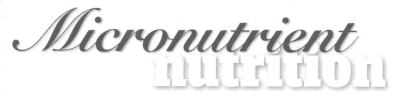

Micronutrient

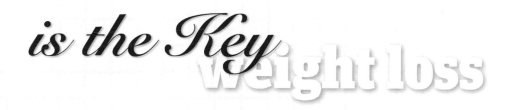

Sufficiency

is the Key

> **"**The beginning is the most important
> part of the work.**"**
> —Plato

We wouldn't expect Pavarotti to perform an opera without learning the music or Kobe Bryant to top the NBA's payroll without first learning to dribble. And we never met a parent who ever felt comfortable throwing their four-year-old onto a bicycle without a little training-wheel action! Becoming micronutrient sufficient requires the same criterion—preparation. Consider this the training-wheel portion of your nutrition Tour de France. The more you know and understand about how nutrition fuels you (or fouls you), the more adept you will be at achieving micronutrient sufficiency.

Whether you are currently on a diet or wellness program, or are considering starting one, micronutrient sufficiency should be at its core. As we already shared with you, micronutrient deficiency contributed to Mira's osteoporosis, but being micronutrient deficient can also cause your body to malfunction in a multitude of other ways: high cholesterol, high triglycerides, and high blood pressure have all been found to be negatively affected by micronutrient deficiency. Additionally, micronutrient deficiency may also cause you to have heightened appetite, more frequent food cravings, and poor fat metabolization—the same culprits that are at the root of many failed weight-loss programs. Regardless of age, micronutrients found in your food and your multivitamins are affecting your health in ways you may have never imagined.

For some of you "Nutrition 101" is a refresher course, while for others it is a building block to understanding how to make beneficial nutritional decisions. Although we have already supplied you with some simplified nutrition definitions in Chapter 1, we would like to help you become acquainted with some scientific definitions so you can fully understand micronutrient deficiency. Away we go!

● ● ● ● ● ● ● ● ● ● ● ● ● ● ●

Nutrients

IN ORDER FOR OUR BODIES to live and grow, we require nutrients. A nutrient is a chemical or any substance that nourishes us. As humans, we take in our nutrients through the everyday actions of eating and drinking. The nutrients in our food regulate body processes, build and repair tissue, supply energy, and regulate body temperature. Nutrients can be broken down into two equally important and life-sustaining components: *macronutrients* and *micronutrients*. Since "macro" means large, macronutrients refer to nutrients needed in large quantities by the body. There are three macronutrients: carbohydrates, fats, and proteins. Their main purpose is to provide calories, which supply the human body with energy.

Micronutrients, in contrast to macronutrients, are the second type of nutrients found in food and are needed in "micro" or small quantities by the body. Micronutrients, for our purposes of discussion in this book and in the interest of scientific simplification, will be narrowed to include vitamins, minerals, essential fatty acids (EFAs), and accessory micronutrients.

While micronutrients contain relatively no caloric value, they are equally as important as macronutrients because their job is to produce hormones, enzymes, and other substances essential for proper growth and development. Most authors of health-based books focus on macronutrients; in *Naked Calories,* we will focus on the overall health benefits of micronutrients.

Micronutrients are categorized as *essential* and *nonessential.* The terms "essential" and "nonessential" are tricky, because you would normally believe that when something is "nonessential," it is not required—such as a basket-weaving elective in college. But in the case of micronutrients, the terms refer to whether or not your body naturally produces or "synthesizes" the nutrient on its own, or if your body needs to find a source (food/drink) from which to take it.

An essential micronutrient is scientifically defined as a substance that must be consumed by an organism from its environment because it is unable to be synthesized internally—either at all, or in sufficient quantities to provide health. So, you need to have it, but you can't make it, so it is *essential* that you take it in from an outside source. Almost all of the vitamins, minerals, and EFAs that you have heard of are considered essential, including, but not limited to, vitamins A, C, E, calcium, magnesium, zinc, omega-3, and omega-6. (A list is provided in Table 3.2 at the end of this chapter.)

Now, again, nonessential does not mean that you do not need a specific micronutrient. In fact, in the case of micronutrients, nonessentials have significant impact on your overall health. Just as the school credits from that basket-weaving course count toward earning your diploma, nonessential micronutrients work toward your overall health. The term *nonessential* refers to the fact that your body can, under normal circumstances, create or derive this micronutrient on its own; it is *nonessential* for you to take it in from the environment. However, as you will soon learn, many lifestyle habits can deplete these nonessential micronutrients from your body. This creates conditions where you must take in these nonessential micronutrients from an outside source in order to sustain basic health. Let's imagine it this way: Under normal circumstances your body does not need to take in blood; it can create it on its own. However, after experiencing a large amount of blood loss, perhaps due to a car accident, your body no longer has the ability to create the large volume of blood necessary to keep you alive. You must get a transfusion and take it in from an outside source. While blood was once *nonessential* (no need to take it in from an outside source), in this circumstance it became essential to do so. Perhaps this example illustrates just how important these nonessential micronutrients really are.

In *Naked Calories,* we don't differentiate between essential and nonessential micronutrients; we mentioned the two categories above only so you will understand that some micronutrients are synthesized by the body while others must be taken in from the environment. Moving forward, when we refer to all micronutrients as "essential," we are qualifying them as a necessary contribution to the achievement of optimal health.

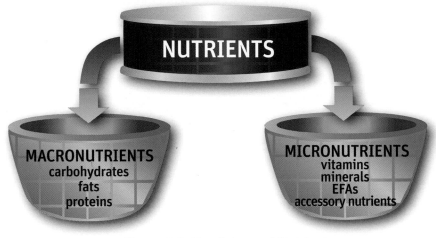

Figure 3.1. Breakdown of Nutrients

Vitamins and Minerals

SO IF VITAMINS AND MINERALS are both micronutrients, then what's the difference? Good question! *Minerals* are found in the earth's soil and water. Our most direct connection to them is through the plants we eat. However, plants don't create minerals; they must extract them from the soil as they grow. If the soil in which the plant is growing is devoid of minerals, the plant will be devoid of minerals as well. We can also obtain minerals by eating animals that have eaten these plants, or by eating animals that have eaten other animals that have eaten mineral-laden plants. Minerals can be subdivided into two categories: *macrominerals,* of which we require greater than 100 mg daily, and *trace minerals,* of which we require less than 100 mg daily.

Vitamins, on the other hand, are not found in soil or water. Instead, they are produced by the plants and animals we consume. Vitamins can be either fat-soluble or water-soluble. The fat-soluble vitamins A, D, E, and K are absorbed with the help of bile acids and can be stored in significant amounts in your body fat and liver until they are needed. All of the other vitamins are water-soluble, which means they cannot be stored in the body in significant amounts (B_{12} is an exception). Instead, water-soluble vitamins travel through the bloodstream, and if the body does not utilize them, they are eliminated through urination; they are not readily stored for a rainy day, as are fat-soluble vitamins.

A Little Bit About EFAs

WHEN WE FIRST DEFINED MICRONUTRIENTS, we mentioned vitamins, minerals, and accessory micronutrients, as well as something called essential fatty acids—or as we in the biz like to call them, EFAs. These aren't the bad fats that clog your arteries. No, EFAs are "good fats"—fats that can save your life. They are essential for every cell in every system of your body to function properly. EFAs are found in both plant and animal sources, and are split into two families: omega-3 and omega-6.

As is the case with most families, finding a harmonious balance can be a bit tricky. Omega-3, which is underconsumed in the Western diet, has a calming or anti-inflammatory effect, and has been proven to strengthen the immune system, promote brain development, improve cardiovascular function, reduce anxiety, alleviate arthritis pain, and burn excess body fat. While you may have heard about many of these health benefits, what you may not know is that these benefits are largely due to the EPA (eicosapentaenoic acid) and DHA (docosahexaenoic acid) found only in animal-source omega-3, like fish.

Plant-source omega-3, like canola oil or flax oil, does not naturally contain EPA or DHA. It contains something called ALA (alpha-linolenic acid), which can be converted within the body to EPA, which can then convert to DHA. The problem is that the body only converts plant-source omega-3 to EPA and then to DHA at an efficiency of approximately 5 to 10 percent and 2 to 5 percent, respectively. Animal-source omega-3, on the other hand, naturally contains both EPA and DHA, so there's no conversion process necessary, and they can be directly absorbed. This means that consuming animal-source omega-3s may offer greater health benefits. However, DHA and, to a lesser extent, EPA have recently been derived from algae, which can be an exciting discovery if you are a vegan or vegetarian. In Chapter 6, we will further discuss the impact diet lifestyles like veganism and vegetarianism can have on micronutrient intake.

In contrast to omega-3, omega-6 is extremely prevalent in the Western diet and can be found in foods like whole grains, corn, avocado, nuts, and vegetable oils, including olive oil. Just as plant-source omega-3 converts into EPA and EPA into DHA, both plant- and animal-source omega-6 converts to GLA (gamma-linolenic acid), DGLA (dihomo-gamma-linolenic acid), AA (arachidonic acid), and finally DA (docosa tetraenoic acid). While omega-3 has a calming or anti-inflammatory effect, omega-6 has a stimulating effect and tends to increase inflammation, which is essential for blood clotting, cell proliferation, and a normal immune system.

Increasing omega-3 intake and reducing omega-6 intake would help create a more balanced essential fatty acid family.

The typical Western diet can have an omega-6 to omega-3 ratio as high as 30 to 1. It is thought that a ratio closer to 1 to 1 is optimal for the promotion of health. Medical studies suggest that this excessively unbalanced ratio of omega-6 to omega-3 is a probable cause of depression and numerous diseases associated with inflammation, including Alzheimer's disease, heart disease, diabetes, cancer, and arthritis.

Accessory Micronutrients

OUR FINAL MEMBER OF THE MICRONUTRIENT FAMILY is a group that we will name our *accessory micronutrients*. The items in this category are also vital to the human body, even though there are no government intake guidelines for them. They work hand in hand with our primary vitamins and minerals to help us on our mission toward optimal health. They include *vitamin-like substances, bioflavanoids, polyphenols, and antioxidants*, just to name a few. As you see names such as alpha lipoic acid, coenzyme Q_{10}, quercetin, and grape seed extract popping up in studies, just remember that these items in this catch-all category of accessory micronutrients are important to maintaining your health.

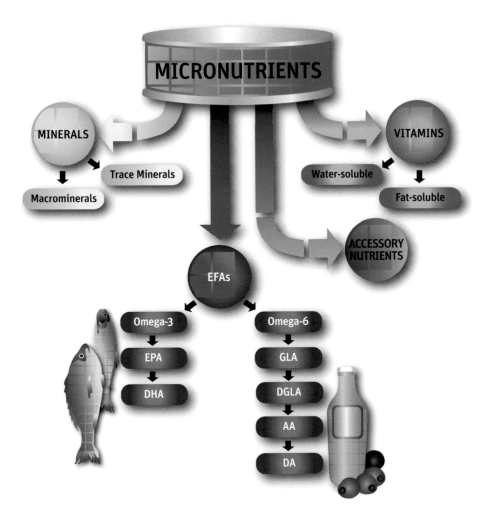

Figure 3.2. Breakdown of Micronutrients

Connecting the Dots

NOW THAT WE HAVE GIVEN YOU all of the technical terms you will need for our journey, we should take a step back and examine how your macronutrients and micronutrients work together as a team. There's a lot to keep track of, and we appreciate that, so here's an easy way to visualize all that we have taught you in Nutrition 101. We call it the House of Optimal Health.

As with every new construction, the House of Optimal Health starts out as an empty lot. In order to begin construction you will need flooring, roofing, concrete, and many other building materials. In building our House of Optimal Health, these building materials are represented by macronutrients—fats, carbohydrates, and proteins. They are delivered to the empty lot through the food we eat every day, and as they say, "You are what you eat."

For example, if you eat a salad topped with chicken, balsamic vinegar, and olive oil, you have an assortment of quality-building materials to utilize (fats, proteins, and carbohydrates). However, if you skip a meal and have a bag of chips instead, the variety of your materials is limited and the quality will be poor (fats and carbohydrates with no protein). A quality house needs a wide variety of quality materials. High-quality fats, proteins, and carbohydrates can only be received from the foods you ingest. When these macronutrients, or raw materials, are supplied through food, they arrive at an empty lot. Obviously, the house cannot build itself. This is where micronutrients come in.

The micronutrients—vitamins, minerals, EFAs, and accessory micronutrients—represent the workers who show up to the lot to manipulate those "macronutrient" materials. As with macronutrients, the micronutrients that arrive are also dependent on your food choices. High-quality choices deliver a plentiful supply of vitamins, minerals, EFAs, and accessory micronutrients, each of which has a unique job to perform on the construction site.

Vitamins act as the handymen (and women) who perform a multitude of tasks, while essential fatty acids

The micronutrients— vitamins, minerals, EFAs, and accessory micronutrients—represent the workers who show up to the lot to manipulate those "macronutrient" materials.

(EFAs) are highly skilled independent contractors; accessory micronutrients act as assistants in the construction process. They are all vital in building a sound structure. However, the construction team isn't complete yet. What most people don't know is that while EFAs and accessory micronutrients perform tasks independently, vitamins are useless without minerals. That's right! Without minerals, vitamins would have no idea what they are building. Your minerals are the architects and foremen in this analogy and need to be plentiful and available in the foods you choose to eat. Minerals design the structure, organize the building plan, and allocate tasks for the individual vitamins to perform.

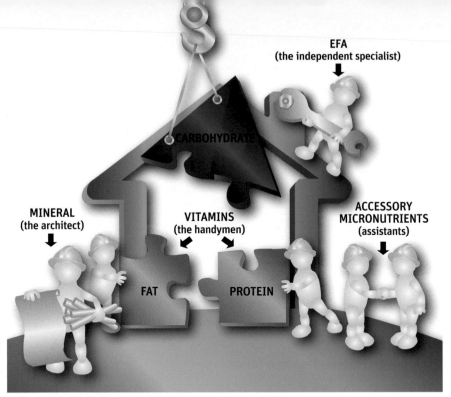

EFA
(the independent specialist)

CARBOHYDRATE

MINERAL
(the architect)

VITAMINS
(the handymen)

ACCESSORY
MICRONUTRIENTS
(assistants)

FAT

PROTEIN

Figure 3.3. Can you see how all of these different macronutrients and micronutrients are working together to build the House of Optimal Health?

Can you see how a sound structure would be created if a wide variety of quality-building materials arrived (macronutrients), along with a complete team of workers, contractors, assistants, and foremen (micronutrients)? Your body is this House of Optimal Health, and it will be kept healthy and strong when high-quality macronutrients are accompanied by micronutrients in sufficient quantities.

• • • • • • • • • • • • • • •

Micronutrients: Friends and Foes

EACH MICRONUTRIENT, WHETHER VITAMIN, MINERAL, EFA, or accessory, differs in form, function, and amount needed by the body to produce or maintain our individual health. They are absorbed by the body by attaching to receptor sites, or absorption pathways, which act as docking locations for specific micronutrients. These receptor sites are found throughout the entire gastrointestinal tract. For the most part, the majority of micronutrients are absorbed in the small intestine. However, the process of absorption can be more like an epic battle scene than a harmonious event.

This display of combative behavior between micronutrients is one of the topics most commonly omitted from nutritional education. It is called micronutrient competition. Just as David Letterman and Jay Leno vie for audience ratings, the New York Giants and Dallas Cowboys battle for a division championship, and only one person can be elected president, certain micronutrients compete with one another for absorption pathways (receptor sites) in your body. But someone has to win. Only Jay or Dave can get more Nielsen ratings, only one football team can take the title, and only one candidate can sit in the Oval Office. Similarly, certain micronutrients will duke it out for domination of the receptor site, resulting in the absorption of one at the expense of the other. For example, it has recently been discovered that lutein and beta-carotene compete for the same absorption receptor site. Copper and zinc also compete for the same receptor site, as do vitamin B5 and vitamin B7 . . . and the list goes on.

In contrast, if we think of micronutrient competition as the "villain" in our story that is plotting to decrease micronutrient absorption, then our "hero" could be the synergistic relationships between specific micronutrients that enhance absorption.

Imagine Fred Astaire and Ginger Rogers. Each was uniquely talented, but together they elevated each other to stardom. How about Sherlock Holmes and Dr. Watson? They needed to work as a team to solve difficult cases, harnessing Holmes's intellectual prowess and Dr. Watson's scientific background. What do these famous people have in common? They are synergistic pairs, who, like synergistic micronutrients, work best when they work together. While micronutrient competition can completely block the benefits of competing micronutrients, micronutrient synergy can increase the absorption of certain micronutrients by as much as 200 percent! To put it metaphorically (haven't you noticed that we love to?) consider Lennon and McCartney. Both had iconic solo careers, but together they made history. The same is true in the case of making the right micronutrients match. Alone, micronutrients are important, but if you get the right connection, they can make nutritional magic.

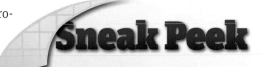

Sneak Peek

While the number of studies revealing the competitions and synergies between micronutrients is increasing, very little attention has been paid concerning how these relationships may affect overall micronutrient absorption and, ultimately, your health. Later, in Chapter 10, we will discuss these competitions and discover just how many of the micronutrients in the typical multivitamin may not be able to be absorbed. You will learn that the method and combination in which your micronutrients are delivered is just as important as the decision to take a multivitamin in the first place.

WARNING: If at any time while you are reading this book you feel the urge to put it down to run and buy a multivitamin—STOP! Make sure you read the ABCs of Optimal Supplementation guidelines in Chapter 10 first. You'll be glad you did.

Now that we've covered the different relationships between micronutrients, we need to focus on how they are measured. Many people find the numerous dietary guideline reference intake acronyms and abbreviations confusing. There are EARs, RDIs, DVs, AIs, DRIs, and ULs (more acronyms of the biz!), so we are providing you a handy table defining what those terms mean. As you read them, we want you to notice something: look closely at the EAR in comparison to the RDI.

Notice that the RDI recommends micronutrient intake levels considered sufficient to meet the requirements of nearly all healthy individuals (97 to 98 percent), while the EAR recommends a level expected to satisfy the needs of only 50 percent of the population. While at first this may seem inconsequential, let's look at how this affects actual intake recommendations for a specific micronutrient.

TABLE 3.1. A GUIDE TO UNDERSTANDING INTAKE ACRONYMS

EAR (Estimated Average Requirement)	The amount of a micronutrient that would be expected to satisfy the requirement needs of 50 percent of the people in that age group.
RDI (Reference Daily Intake)	The RDI replaces the RDA and is the daily dietary intake level of a micronutrient designed to be sufficient to prevent micronutrient deficiency diseases by meeting the requirements of nearly all (97 to 98 percent) healthy individuals in each life-stage and sex group.
DV (Daily Value)	The RDI is used to determine the Daily Value (DV) of foods, which is printed on nutrition facts labels in the United States. The DV tells you what percentage of the RDI is delivered in a specific food or supplement.
AI (Adequate Intake)	The daily dietary intake of a micronutrient when no RDI has been established. These amounts are somewhat less firmly believed to be accurate or adequate for everyone in the demographic group.
DRI (Dietary Reference Intake)	The Dietary Reference Intake (DRI) is the most recent set of dietary recommendations as determined by a non-governmental American organization. They may be the basis for eventually updating the RDIs.
UL (Upper Level of Tolerable Intake)	This is the highest level of continuing daily micronutrient intake that is likely to pose no risk of adverse health effects in almost all individuals in the specified life-stage group.

The EAR for vitamin B12 is 2 mcg. This means that 2 mcg of B12 are required daily to make 50 percent of the population's intake sufficient. However, the RDI for vitamin B12 is 6 mcg. This means that 6 mcg of B12 are required to make 97 to 98 percent of the population's intake sufficient. Notice that the amount to achieve EAR sufficiency is far lower than that for RDI sufficiency. This information will become important in the next chapter as we delve deeper into micronutrient deficiencies. However, for now we will use this information to create the very first **Naked Fact.**

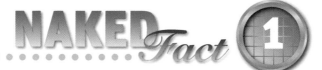

The RDIs are daily micronutrient intake levels considered sufficient to meet the requirements of nearly all (97 to 98 percent) healthy individuals in each life-stage and gender group, while the EAR is ONLY the amount expected to satisfy the micronutrient requirements of 50 percent of the population.

There is another level of intake that we, as well as many reputable nutrition experts, believe is even more important than those listed in Table 3.1. It is referred to as Optimal Daily Dose (ODD). Optimal Daily Doses are the amount of essential micronutrients needed to produce optimal health and are often several times higher than the RDI, which, as you remember, are only absolute minimums for the majority of people to prevent micronutrient-deficiency diseases. We will discuss ODD further in Chapter 9 when we explore how to choose a quality supplement using the ABCs of Optimal Supplementation.

ODD = Optimal

RDI = minimal

TABLE 3.2. THE STANDARD ESSENTIAL VITAMINS AND MINERALS ALONG WITH THEIR REFERENCE DAILY INTAKE (RDI)

ESSENTIAL VITAMINS	RDI
Vitamin A (Retinol/Beta-Carotene)	5,000 IU
Vitamin B$_1$ (Thiamine)	1.5 mg
Vitamin B$_2$ (Riboflavin)	1.7 mg
Vitamin B$_3$ (Niacin)	20 mg
Vitamin B$_5$ (Pantothenic Acid)	10 mg
Vitamin B$_6$ (Pyridoxine)	2 mg
Vitamin B$_7$ (Biotin)	300 mcg
Vitamin B$_9$ (Folic Acid)	400 mcg
Vitamin B$_{12}$ (Cobalamin)	6 mcg
Vitamin C (Ascorbic Acid)	60 mg
Vitamin D (Calciferol)	400 IU
Vitamin E (Tocopherol)	30 IU
Vitamin K (Phylloquinone)	80 mcg
Choline (considered essential in 1998)	AI 550 mg

ESSENTIAL MACROMINERALS	RDI
Calcium	1,000 mg
Chloride	3,400 mg
Magnesium	400 mg
Phosphorus	1,000 mg
Potassium	4,700 mg
Sodium	2,400 mg

ESSENTIAL TRACE MINERALS	RDI
Chromium*	120 mcg
Copper	2 mg
Iodine	150 mcg
Iron	18 mg
Manganese	2 mg
Molybdenum	75 mcg
Selenium	70 mcg
Zinc	15 mg

ESSENTIAL FATTY ACIDS	RDI
Linolenic Acid (Omega-3)	1.6 gm
Linoleic Acid (Omega-6)	17 gm

* Not considered essential

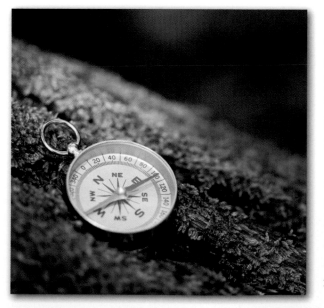

Well, that's it. That wasn't so hard, was it? You now have the basic information you need to continue your journey to micronutrient sufficiency. While the word *micronutrient* can, at first glance, look quite complicated, it's really pretty simple.

In the next chapter, you will be introduced to the biggest question in nutrition today, learn about the prevalence of micronutrient deficiency, and discover just how serious things can get when . . . **the minerals go missing.**

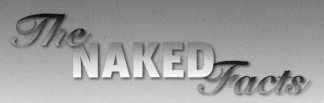

The RDIs are daily micronutrient intake levels considered sufficient to meet the requirements of nearly all (97 to 98 percent) healthy individuals in each life-stage and gender group, while the EAR is ONLY the amount expected to satisfy the micronutrient requirements of 50 percent of the population.

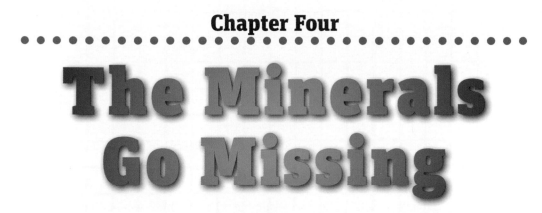

The Minerals Go Missing

Micronutrient Depletion Begins

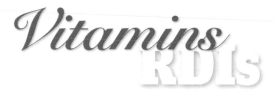

Vitamins RDIs

Minerals

nutrition

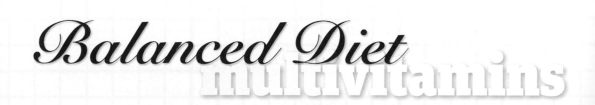

Balanced Diet multivitamins

> **"** A nation that destroys its soils
> destroys itself. **"**
> —Franklin D. Roosevelt

D avid had heard about our work on micronutrient deficiency and tried to learn as much as he could about it all evening. Between sips of champagne and the canapés that were passed around, David had been listening intently to our stories about our recent research expedition, the Calton Project. By the time we got around to having dinner we could anticipate the question simmering just below the surface. David was a Ph.D.—a real-life rocket scientist—and he was about to ask one of the most debated and important questions of our time. He sat back, wiped his mouth, and said, "So tell me this. . . . Can I get all the essential micronutrients I need from a balanced diet or do I need to take a multivitamin?"

Without fail, we have been asked this same question in every city and in every country we have visited. So, what is the answer? When a staff of trained nutrition professionals working for the United States Department of Agriculture's (USDA) website, www.nutrition.gov, was asked a similar question, the answer was, "It is true that healthy individuals can get all of the vitamins and minerals they need from a well balanced diet."

However, many other well-known and well-respected nutritional academics disagree. The late Shari Lieberman, Ph.D., a certified nutrition specialist, professor of human nutrition, and author of *The Real Vitamin & Mineral Book,* had a different opinion: "It is virtually impossible to meet the RDIs (Reference Daily Intakes) by eating the food available to us today."

Walter Willett, M.D., Chairman of the Department of Nutrition at the Harvard School of Public Health, believes that even the individuals eating the healthiest diets may still be deficient in specific micronutrients. Dr. Willett recommends a daily multivitamin as a good insurance policy for overall health.

So, who is right? How can one group of nutrition professionals state that a well-balanced diet is sufficient to meet the RDIs, while another group tells us that our calories are virtually stripped naked of vitamins and minerals, and that meeting the RDI of essential micronutrients through a balanced diet is virtually impossible? Welcome to the biggest face-off in nutritional history. Hanging in the balance is your health.

If the first group is right, then we will all be just fine. Maybe we need to clean up our diets a bit, but the ability to be micronutrient sufficient and prevent deficiency-based health conditions and diseases is just a balanced meal away. However, if the second group is right, without proper supplementation millions of people worldwide will have a multitude of micronutrient deficiencies.

The research we collected through the Calton Project confirmed our deeply held belief that eating fresh, natural foods such as fruits, vegetables, meats, dairy products, eggs, nuts, seeds, fish, legumes, oils, and whole grains is the best and most efficient way to receive the essential micronutrients your body needs on a daily basis. There is no doubt in our minds of the superiority of natural foods over that of nutritional supplements, prescription nutrients/drugs, or fortified foods.

Our ancestors survived and thrived by simply eating the foods nature provided and allowing nature, in her infinite wisdom, to nourish and sustain them. We would like nothing more than to be able to write a book showing research indicating sustained or increased levels of essential micronutrients in our food. We would love to be the ones to reveal to you that a typical modern diet alone could provide your body with even the minimum RDI of each essential micronutrient. Instead, we must face the fact that for a large majority of people everywhere, the reality of achieving essential micronutrient sufficiency through food alone is all but impossible.

Our ancestors survived and thrived by simply eating the foods nature provided and allowing nature, in her infinite wisdom, to nourish and sustain them.

> "In the future, we will not be able to rely anymore on our premise that the consumption of a varied balanced diet will provide all the essential trace elements, because such a diet will be very difficult to obtain for millions of people."
> —Dr. Walter Mertz, U.S. Department of Agriculture,
> remarks to Congress, 1977

• • • • • • • • • • • • • •

Digging for Answers

WHAT WOULD CAUSE Dr. Walter Mertz, the former director of the USDA Human Nutrition Research Center, to warn Congress that millions of people would be unable to receive their essential nutrients through a balanced diet? We begin digging for this answer in the soil.

Mineral deficiency begins in the soil. If minerals are not available in the soil, then they won't be available in the food we eat—and over the past 100 years the level of minerals in soil throughout the world has been on the decline. While many people are unaware of this, it isn't breaking news. In fact, we found sentiments that support this statement in an article presented to Congress in 1936 in U.S. Senate Document 264, presented by Senator Duncan Fletcher:

> The alarming fact is that foods, fruits, vegetables, and grains now being raised on millions of acres of land no longer contain enough certain needed minerals and are starving us, no matter how much of them we eat . . . Ninety-nine percent of the American people are deficient in minerals, and that a marked deficiency in any one of the more important minerals actually results in disease. We know that vitamins are complex chemical substances, which are indispensable to nutrition, and that each of them is important for the normal function of some special structure of the body. Disorder and disease result from any vitamin deficiency. It is not commonly realized, however, that vitamins control the body's appropriation of minerals, and that in the absence of minerals they have no function to perform. Lacking vitamins, the system can make some use of minerals, but lacking minerals, vitamins are useless.

Does it surprise you that micronutrient-deficient soil has been a concern in America since as far back as 1936? What you may find even more alarming is just how deficient our soil, and the soil of the world, has continued to become since then. At the United Nations Conference on Environment and Development in 1992, it was revealed in the Earth Summit Report that in the past 100 years, farmlands in North America, South America, Asia, Africa, Europe, and Australia have become mineral depleted on an alarming scale. While Australia's farms showed the least depletion, with a 55 percent reduction in mineral content, America's farm and rangeland showed the greatest amount, with a startling average mineral depletion of 85 percent.

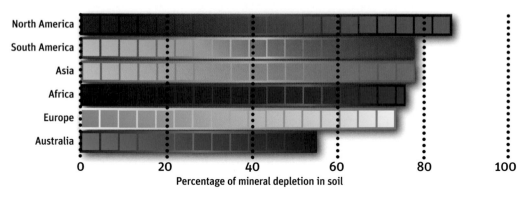

Figure 4.1. Percentage of Mineral Depletion in Soil in 100 Years
Source: Statistics from the 1992 Earth Summit Report

Our review of history gives us a timeline that looks like this:

1936 Congress puts information on record that reveals the land is lacking in micronutrients causing more than 99 percent of the American people to be deficient in essential minerals.

1977 Dr. Walter Mertz warns Congress that due to soil depletion, a balanced diet will not provide the majority of Americans with all of the essential trace elements.

1992 The United Nations Conference on Environment and Development reveals that the situation had become worse. Even after the initial warning in 1936, the land had become more devoid of essential minerals.

2011 The micronutrient content of harvested food continues to decline. According to the article "Dirt Poor" in April 2011's *Scientific American,* "Fruits and vegetables grown decades ago were much richer in vitamins and minerals than the varieties most of us get today. The main culprit in this disturbing nutritional trend is soil depletion."

The Birth of the Naked Calorie

WHILE WE MAY ALL BE BORN NAKED, it is not the way we want our food! Crops grown in soils stripped of essential minerals produce foods that are also stripped of essential micronutrients. Essentially, when our soil is naked, our food is naked. Which ultimately means the calories we consume are . . . naked calories.

The bottom line is that naked calories are calories that have had their micronutrients stripped in one way or another. Chronically consuming naked calories can lead to micronutrient deficiencies—the cause of "hidden hunger." However, naked soil is not the only cause of naked calories. What you have just read is only the beginning of the story—the conception of the naked calorie.

We are not suggesting a conspiracy theory that farmers or government agencies are purposely depleting our soil in order to make us sick. This is not what we believe. What we do know is that farmers are being paid to produce maximum yield per acre, not maximum nutritional value. That's why in the 1930s, corn yields of 50 bushels an acre were considered quite good, but today, some farmers are pushing their land and are producing corn yields greater than 200 bushels an acre. Farmers are forced, for economic reasons, to grow crops faster and are not financially rewarded for increasing a crop's micronutrient value.

In fact, the USDA limits its produce standards to size, shape, and color only, and has no set standards that address nutritional values. We assure you that the farmers we interviewed while conducting the Calton Project shared with us that they would love to grow the most nutritious, healthy food they could. However, until food is sold at a cost that considers its nutritional value instead of only its size, shape, and color, farmers cannot afford to grow their crops with the nutritional benefit of the consumer in mind.

While the advances in farming have allowed for new crops to grow bigger, more rapidly, and more resilient to pests and climate, they have not taken into consideration the plants' ability to both derive and produce micronutrients. Because of this, the micronutrient value of our food is on a steady decline.

In a 2006 article for the Nutrition Security Institute titled "Human Health, the Nutritional Quality of Harvested Food and Sustainable Farming Systems," John B. Marler and Jeanne R. Wallin examine an additional aspect of mineral-depleted soil: soil erosion. They state:

> In the United States and throughout the world much of the world's inventory of arable [capable of producing crops] topsoil has been lost due to erosion, overuse of inorganic nitrogen fertilizers, and other farming practices that leave the soil depleted. The depletion of soil nutrients and soil microorganisms contributes to soil erosion and the loss of arable topsoil. The Earth is losing arable topsoil at a rate of 75 to 100 gross tons per year. If soil loss continues at present rates, it is estimated that there is only another 48 years of topsoil left. In the United States soil is eroding at a rate that

is ten times faster than the rate at which it is being replenished . . . Without adequate nutrition from food, we become susceptible to disease. Simply stated . . . a lack of nutrients leads to malnutrition . . . malnutrition leads to disease.

TABLE 4.1. EIGHTY-YEAR DECLINE IN MINERAL CONTENT OF ONE MEDIUM APPLE RAW, WITH SKIN

MINERAL	1914	1963	1992	% CHANGE (1914–1992)
Calcium	13.5 mg	7.0 mg	7.00 mg	−48.15%
Phosphorus	45.2 mg	10.0 mg	7.00 mg	−84.51%
Iron	4.6 mg	0.3 mg	0.18 mg	−96.09%
Potassium	117.0 mg	110.0 mg	115.00 mg	−1.71%
Magnesium	28.9 mg	8.0 mg	5.00 mg	−82.7%

The saying, "An apple a day keeps the doctor away" comes from an old English adage, "To eat an apple before going to bed, will make the doctor beg his bread."

TABLE 4.2. CHANGES IN MICRONUTRIENT CONTENT OF BEEF AND CHICKEN PER 100 GRAMS

MICRONUTRIENT	FOR GROUND BEEF			FOR CHICKEN		
	1963	1992	% CHANGE	1963	1992	% CHANGE
Calcium	10.00 mg	8.00 mg	−20%	12.00 mg	10.00 mg	−16.67%
Iron	2.70 mg	1.73 mg	−35.93%	1.30 mg	1.03 mg	−20.77%
Magnesium	17.00 mg	16.00 mg	−5.88%	23.00 mg	23.00 mg	0.00%
Phosphorus	156.00 mg	130.00 mg	−16.67%	203.00 mg	198.00 mg	−2.46%
Potassium	236.00 mg	228.00 mg	−3.39%	285.00 mg	238.00 mg	−16.49%
Vitamin A	40.00 IU	0.00 IU	−100%	150.00 IU	45.00 IU	−70%
Thiamine	0.08 mg	0.038 mg	−52.5%	0.100 mg	0.069 mg	−31%
Riboflavin	0.16 mg	0.151 mg	−5.63%	0.120 mg	0.134 mg	+11.67%
Niacin	4.30 mg	4.48 mg	+4.19 %	7.70 mg	7.87 mg	+2.21%

Source: USDA, 1963 and 1997

Don't Take Our Word for It!

Research conducted at major universities and government agencies offer compelling findings of a "growing" micronutrient-deficiency condition in the world's food supply.

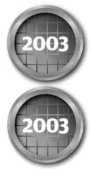

The Journal of Nutrition and Health. U.S. and UK government statistics show a sharp decline in the trace minerals in both fruits and vegetables of up to 76 percent over the period 1940 to 1991.

News Canada. Data from the U.S. Department of Agriculture involving vegetable quality was examined, and it was concluded that vegetables were found to contain far fewer micronutrients than they did fifty years ago. In fact, average mineral content in lettuce, tomatoes, cabbage, and spinach declined from 400 mg to less than 50 mg, and potatoes had lost 100 percent of vitamin A content, 57 percent of vitamin C and iron, and 28 percent of calcium.

The Journal of the American College of Nutrition. Donald Davis, Ph.D., a senior researcher at the University of Texas, performed research into the disappearing nutrients in food. Forty-three crops were examined for changes in food composition between 1950 and 1999. When comparing the USDA food composition tables, they found statistically "reliable declines" for six nutrients: protein, calcium, phosphorus, iron, riboflavin, and vitamin C. Davis and his colleagues concluded that this nutritional decline was due to agricultural practices designed to improve size, growth rate, and pest resistance, rather than nutrition.

Food Magazine, **published by the United Kingdom's Food Commission, "Britain's leading independent watchdog on food issues,"** analyzed food quality changes in the UK over the period 1940 to 2002 and revealed that milk's iron content had decreased 62 percent. Further, magnesium had fallen 21 percent and copper content had perished completely. Parmesan cheese had a 70

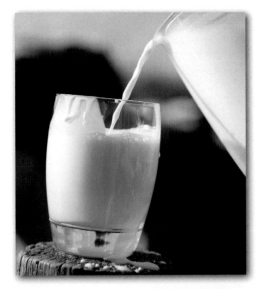

percent reduction in magnesium. Both the calcium and iron contents of all the foods examined were reduced dramatically.

Washington State University. Professor Stephen Jones, Ph.D., and researcher Kevin Murphy conducted research that revealed today's wheat has less nutritional value. They concluded, "You would have to eat twice as many slices of modern bread as you would of the older variety to get the same nutritional value."

When you put together all of the evidence you just read, a clear picture emerges. We will make the results of this research the basis for our **Naked Fact #2.**

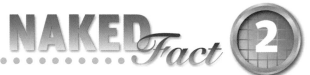

Soil and food have been studied and a micronutrient-depletion trend has been established.

Sick Soil? Then What?

SO FAR, WE HAVE ESTABLISHED the fact that micronutrient levels in soil and food are dramatically depleted, but how does this soil depletion affect you? How does it affect your children, your parents, or your friends? Can micronutrient-depleted soil make you sick? The fact is, depleted soil only leads to one thing—depleted people.

> "Sick soil mean sick plants,
> sick animals, and sick people."
> —U.S. Senate Document 264

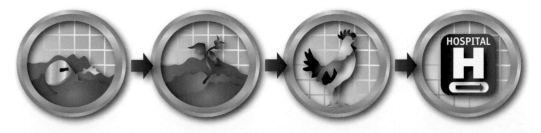

Okay, so sick soil ultimately means sick people, but how sick? People get sick all the time. What kind of health conditions are we talking about? Are we talking about a resurgence of obscure diseases like scurvy, pellagra, and beriberi? Or are we talking about sicknesses that threaten most of us today like diabetes, cancer, high blood pressure, and obesity? The answer is, all of these diseases and many more, including:

- Atherosclerosis
- Osteoporosis
- Increased risk of heart disease
- Anemia
- Chronic bronchitis
- Hair loss
- Asthma
- Arthritis
- High blood cholesterol
- Aneurysms
- Cataracts
- Bone deformities
- Age spots
- Tinnitus
- Multiple sclerosis

The list goes on. In fact, there is an affiliated sickness or disease associated with the deficiency of every one of the essential vitamins and minerals listed in Table 3.2 in Chapter 3. If a micronutrient is not provided through diet or supplementation in the minimum amount needed to produce health, then a related health condition or disease will follow. It is simply a matter of cause and effect.

The length of time and level of deficiency are major factors in determining the seriousness of the potential health condition or disease. Biochemical individuality also plays a role. For one person, a small deficiency may not manifest itself for years, or it could reveal itself as a lack of energy or feelings of depression. For others the same amount of deficiency might mean sleepless nights or unexplainable hunger. However, a greater level of deficiency for an extended period, spanning multiple years or decades, might eventually contribute to the formation of a much more serious condition, such as cancer. Each micronutrient deficiency can manifest itself differently in each person and can become more serious with time.

Established medical and scientific communities accept the fact that a deficiency in one or more of the essential micronutrients has a high potential of causing a related health condition or disease. To provide proof of this, we first share with you an abstract on a study published in 1999 out of the University of California at Berkeley.

The length of time and level of deficiency are major factors in determining the seriousness of the potential health condition or disease.

MICRONUTRIENTS PREVENT CANCER AND DELAY AGING

Abstract by Bruce N. Ames, Ph.D.

Approximately forty micronutrients are required in the human diet. Deficiency of vitamins B_{12}, folic acid, B_6, niacin, C or E, or iron or zinc, appears to mimic radiation in damaging DNA . . . half of the population may be deficient in at least one of these micronutrients. . . . Folate deficiency causes extensive incorporation of uracil into human DNA leading to chromosomal breaks. This mechanism is the likely cause of the increased cancer risk, and perhaps the cognitive defects associated with low folate intake. Some evidence and mechanistic considerations suggest that vitamin B_{12} and B_6 deficiencies also cause high uracil and chromosome breaks.

Micronutrient deficiency may explain, in good part, why the quarter of the population that eats the fewest fruits and vegetables (five portions a day is advised) has approximately double the cancer rate for most types of cancer when compared to the quarter with the highest intake. Eighty percent of American children and adolescents and 68 percent of adults do not eat five portions a day. Common micronutrient deficiencies are likely to damage DNA by the same mechanism as radiation and many chemicals appear to be orders of magnitude more important, and should be compared for perspective. Remedying micronutrient deficiencies is likely to lead to a major improvement in health and an increase in longevity at low cost.

● ● ● ● ● ● ● ● ● ● ● ● ● ●

The idea of micronutrient deficiency potentially causing a variety of common diseases is clearly accepted in this study—and there are countless others. In fact, according to Robert H. Fletcher, M.D., M.Sc., and Kathleen M. Fairfield, M.D., of Harvard Medical School and the Harvard School of Public Health, and writers of the guidelines for the *Journal of American Medical Association* (JAMA), ". . . insufficient vitamin intake is apparently a cause of chronic diseases."

In their *JAMA* article, "Vitamins for Chronic Disease Prevention in Adults," Drs. Fletcher and Fairfield further state that "recent evidence has shown that suboptimal [below standard] levels of vitamins, even well above those causing deficiency syndromes, are risk factors for chronic diseases such as cardiovascular disease, cancer, and osteoporosis. A large proportion of the general population is apparently at increased risk for this reason."

It is no secret that our soil and food are micronutrient depleted and that micronutrient deficiency is an established risk factor in a multitude of health conditions and diseases. In fact, in a study published in the *Proceedings of the National Academy of Science,* researchers concluded that congestive heart failure (from a wide variety of causes) has been strongly correlated with significantly low blood and tissue levels of the accessory micronutrient CoQ_{10}. The study determined that the severity of heart disease correlates with the severity of CoQ_{10} deficiency and concluded "CoQ_{10} deficiency might be a major, if not the sole cause of cardiomyopathy (heart disease) . . ."

At the University of Texas Southwestern Medical Center, researchers analyzed data from 3,300 subjects in a Dallas heart study. The results proved a strong correlation between potassium deficiency and the likelihood of high blood pressure. "The lower the potassium in the urine, hence the lower the potassium in the diet, the higher the blood pressure," reported the study's lead author Saghar Hedayati, M.D., Assistant Professor of Internal Medicine.

> *Individuals with elevated homocysteine levels caused by vitamin B_{12} deficiency had more than twice the risk of developing Alzheimer's disease.*

Further, it was concluded in the *European Journal of Neurology* that individuals with elevated homocysteine levels caused by vitamin B_{12} deficiency had more than twice the risk of developing Alzheimer's disease.

Guy Abraham, M.D., former clinical professor of obstetrics and gynecology at University of California, Los Angeles, tested twenty-six sufferers of premenstrual syndrome (PMS), which is estimated to affect more than 75 percent of women, and discovered his subjects were deficient in their levels of magnesium. An additional study performed by researchers from the University of Massachusetts, Harvard, and the University of Iowa, indicates that higher intakes of the B vitamins thiamine and riboflavin may reduce the incidence of PMS by about 35 percent.

According to Micheal Holick, M.D., of Boston University School of Medicine, women who are vitamin D deficient have a 253 percent increased risk for developing colorectal cancer and a 222 percent increased risk for developing breast cancer. He suggests that the blood levels of vitamin D at the time of diagnosis of breast cancer accurately predict a woman's survival. Additionally, studies out of Mt. Sinai Hospital in Toronto, Canada, showed that women with low levels of vitamin D at diagnosis are 94 percent more likely to have the cancer metastasize and 73 percent more likely to die within ten years of diagnosis.

Still another study out of Purdue University found that boys diagnosed with attention deficit hyperactivity disorder (ADHD) had lower levels of the omega-3 essential fatty acid DHA. Additional studies have determined that 95 percent of ADHD children tested were deficient in magnesium, and that ADHD children had zinc levels that were only two-thirds the level of those without ADHD.

The scientific data collected overwhelmingly reveals micronutrient deficiency to be a causative factor in today's most prevalent health conditions and diseases. However, for some of you, research might not be as interesting as it is to us, so we include below some of the most apt quotes from popular experts to help further underscore the position we support.

"I do think vitamin D is one of the most promising nutrients for prevention of cardiac disease and cancer, and I believe in it strongly."

—JoAnn Manson, M.D., D.PH.,
Professor, Harvard School of Public Health

"This low-nutrient diet establishes a favorable cellular environment for disease (like cancer, heart disease, and dementia) to flourish."

—Joel Fuhrman, M.D.,
New York Times bestselling author of *Eat to Live*

"Although obese people may appear well fed, they often lack essential nutrients, leading to poor health and disease."

—The United Nations Food and Agriculture Organization

"This is like the holy grail of cancer medicine; vitamin D produced a drop in cancer rates greater than that for quitting smoking, or indeed any other countermeasure in existence."

—Dennis Mangan, Ph.D., National Institute of Health,
Office of Research on Women's Health

"They [the eight members of the vitamin B family] can help you lose weight, because they stimulate your metabolism, they help prevent heart disease and cancer, and they promote healthy nerves and muscle and function."

—Mehmet Oz, M.D., *The Dr. Oz Show*

"(Today) vitamin deficiency does not cause acute diseases such as scurvy or rickets, but they do cause what have been called 'long-latency deficiency diseases.' These include conditions like blindness, osteoporosis, heart disease, cancer, diabetes, dementia, and more."

—Mark Hyman, M.D.,
Chairman of the Institute for Functional Medicine

> **"**Deficiencies in micronutrients such as iron, iodine, vitamin A, folate and zinc affect nearly one-third of the world's population, and the consequences can be devastating.**"**
> —Centers for Disease Control and Prevention

You have now been presented with the opinions and research of well-respected medical professionals and scientists supporting the fact that micronutrient deficiency is a potential gateway to much more serious conditions and diseases. You have reviewed scientific data identifying that numerous micronutrient deficiencies increase disease risks and rates. Finally, you read quotes from trustworthy sources on the devastating effects of such deficiencies. We are now ready to present our **Naked Fact #3.**

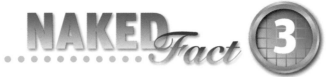

A deficiency in one or more of the essential micronutrients can ultimately cause health-related conditions or diseases.

Naked Fact #3 makes sense when you think about it. After all, if sufficiency causes health, then one would expect deficiency eventually to cause illness. Take a moment to examine Table 4.3; it clearly outlines each of the essential micronutrients that has an established RDI and several of its associated deficiency conditions/diseases.

TABLE 4.3. A SAMPLING OF NUTRIENTS AND SOME OF THEIR ASSOCIATED DEFICIENCY CONDITIONS

ESSENTIAL VITAMINS	ASSOCIATED CONDITIONS OF DEFICIENCY
Vitamin A	Night blindness, defective teeth, stunted growth in children
Vitamin C	Coronary heart disease, delayed blood clotting, cancer
Vitamin D	Decreased immunity, high blood pressure, rickets, osteomalacia
Vitamin E	Cataracts, Alzheimer's disease, cardiovascular disease, cancer
Vitamin K	Impaired blood clotting, easy bruising, osteoporosis
Vitamin B_1 (Thiamine)	Beriberi, cataracts, Alzheimer's disease, congestive heart failure

Vitamin B$_2$ (Riboflavin)	Sore throat, preeclampsia, cataracts, stress
Vitamin B$_3$ (Niacin)	Gastrointestinal disorders, dementia, dermatitis
Vitamin B$_5$ (Pantothenic Acid)	Insomnia, fatigue, intestinal disturbances, high cholesterol
Vitamin B$_6$	Impaired immune system, Alzheimer's disease, kidney stones
Vitamin B$_7$ (Biotin)	Hair loss, rash, depression, numbness and tingling in extremities
Vitamin B$_9$ (Folic Acid)	Megaloblastic anemia, neural tube defects, cardiovascular disease
Vitamin B$_{12}$	Gastritis, peptic ulcer, anemia, dementia, tingling in limbs, constipation
Choline	Fatty liver, cancer, Alzheimer's disease, neural tube defects

ESSENTIAL MACROMINERALS	ASSOCIATED CONDITIONS OF DEFICIENCY
Potassium	Stroke, osteoporosis, kidney stones, hypertension
Sodium Chloride	Osteoporosis, hypertension, kidney stones, dehydration
Calcium	Osteoporosis, colorectal cancer, high blood pressure, PMS
Phosphorus	Loss of appetite, anemia, bone pain, rickets, osteomalacia
Magnesium	Hypertension, coronary heart disease, osteoporosis, asthma

ESSENTIAL TRACE MINERALS	ASSOCIATED CONDITIONS OF DEFICIENCY
Manganese	Abnormal skeletal development, diabetes, seizures, impaired reproduction
Copper	Lowered HDL (good) cholesterol, binge eating, anemia
Iodine	Brain damage, goiter, hyperparathyroidism
Selenium	Impaired immunity, cancer, cardiovascular disease, thyroid disease
Molybdenum	Inability to eliminate toxic substances
Zinc	Impaired neuropsychological development, lowered immunity, dwarfism, diabetes

Iron	Anemia, heart palpitations, lead poisoning, restless leg syndrome
Chromium*	Diabetes, obesity, hypoglycemia

*Not considered essential.

ESSENTIAL FATTY ACIDS	ASSOCIATED CONDITIONS OF DEFICIENCY
Linolenic Acid (omega-3) and Linoleic Acid (omega-6)	Diabetes, poor visual and neurological development, coronary heart disease, stroke, high triglycerides, Alzheimer's disease, arthritis, asthma

Source: Linus Pauling Institute at Oregon State University, Micronutrient Research for Optimum Health.

Thus far we've gathered three facts:

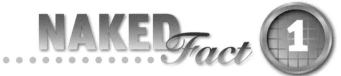

The RDIs are daily micronutrient intake levels considered sufficient to meet the requirements of nearly all (97 to 98 percent) healthy individuals in each life-stage and gender group, while the EAR is ONLY the amount expected to satisfy the micro-nutrient requirements of 50 percent of the population.

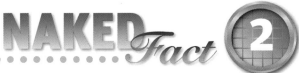

Soil and food have been studied and a micronutrient-depletion trend has been established.

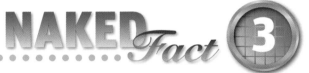

A deficiency in one or more of the essential micronutrients can ultimately cause health-related conditions or diseases.

You may have noticed that in the report by Drs. Fletcher and Fairfield of Harvard University, suboptimal levels of vitamins are risk factors for chronic diseases such as cardiovascular disease, cancer, and osteoporosis. However, they also said, "A large proportion of the general population is apparently at increased risk for this reason." *What did they mean? Are a large proportion of people deficient in vitamins? Could widespread micronutrient deficiency really be a problem? Have studies been published showing the worldwide population deficient in essential micronutrients?*

The answer is yes to all of the above. Many reports and studies have been published showing deficiencies in numerous essential micronutrients in countries throughout the world. What may surprise you is how widespread and severe these deficiencies are. For example, according to the Centers for Disease Control and Prevention, more than half of the general population in the United States is vitamin D deficient, regardless of age. About 70 percent of elderly Americans and 90 percent of Americans of color are vitamin D deficient. Additionally, magnesium expert Carolyn Dean, M.D., N.D., states that "Up to 80 percent of the U.S. population is suffering from a magnesium deficiency." Finally, according to the USDA, Americans typically lack a sufficient amount of the minerals calcium, magnesium, and potassium, and the vitamins A, C, and E.

Let's take this step by step. First, we will examine the findings on one specific micronutrient—vitamin E. Below you will find the USDA's report on the percentage of the population in each state over two years old that receives the adequate intake of vitamin E.

TABLE 4.4. PERCENTAGE OF POPULATION PER STATE TWO YEARS OLD AND OVER WITH ADEQUATE INTAKES FOR VITAMIN E FROM FOOD SOURCES

STATE	PERCENTAGE	STATE	PERCENTAGE
Alabama	10.0	Florida	11.4
Alaska	16.2	Georgia	9.6
Arizona	15.0	Hawaii	16.2
Arkansas	12.9	Idaho	14.6
California	15.8	Illinois	12.0
Colorado	12.2	Indiana	14.7
Connecticut	14.3	Iowa	16.1
Delaware	12.6	Kansas	16.1
District of Columbia	13.3	Kentucky	10.0

STATE	PERCENTAGE	STATE	PERCENTAGE
Louisiana	11.2	Ohio	11.9
Maine	14.3	Oklahoma	11.4
Maryland	14.1	Oregon	16.2
Massachusetts	14.3	Pennsylvania	13.4
Michigan	14.0	Rhode Island	14.3
Minnesota	18.3	South Carolina	15.0
Mississippi	10.2	South Dakota	16.1
Missouri	13.8	Tennessee	9.9
Montana	14.6	Texas	14.1
Nebraska	16.1	Utah	15.3
Nevada	14.6	Vermont	14.3
New Hampshire	14.3	Virginia	14.0
New Jersey	12.6	Washington	18.7
New Mexico	18.7	West Virginia	12.6
New York	12.0	Wisconsin	12.0
North Carolina	18.7	Wyoming	14.6
North Dakota	16.1		

Source: www.ars.usda.gov/services/docs.htm?docid=15791

HOW IS THIS DATA COLLECTED AND WHERE CAN I FIND IT?

The data in Table 4.4 came from measuring intake of foods without supplementation. It is reflective of how much vitamin E was in the foods that a person ate. These included pre-made food items as well as fortified foods. For a homemade meal, one would take the individual ingredients, measure their micronutrient contents, and then figure the micronutrients in the total meal per individual serving size. The formula with which this data is collected and analyzed can be found on the USDA website, www.ars.usda.gov/services/docs.htm?docid=15791

Did you notice how low the adequacy rates were? Is America really this deficient in vitamin E? Why doesn't everyone know about this? According to the data, the highest percentage of sufficiency can be found in North Carolina, and they had a sufficiency rate of only 18.7 percent. You have probably already realized that an 18.7 percent sufficiency equals an 81.3 percent deficiency rate. Last we checked, if this were a test, a score of 18.7 percent would be failing. And this was the highest adequacy rate in America!

The fact that the nationwide average for vitamin E adequacy is only 13.6 percent means that almost nine out of ten individuals living in America, according to the USDA, are deficient in the essential micronutrient vitamin E. To reiterate, nearly nine out of ten people age two and older do not get the adequate amount of vitamin E from their diets to maintain basic health. In Table 4.3, you have just seen that a deficiency in vitamin E was shown to be associated with cardiovascular disease, cancer, Alzheimer's disease, and cataracts.

Nearly nine out of ten people age two and older do not get the adequate amount of vitamin E from their diets to maintain basic health.

Did you know that according to the American Heart Association, an American dies of cardiovascular disease every 39 seconds, or that cancer causes one out of every four deaths in America, and global cancer rates are expected to increase by 50 percent by the year 2020? What about the fact that 5.4 million Americans have Alzheimer's disease or that it is the sixth leading cause of death? In the United States, cataracts will affect 22 million people, and 400,000 new cases are reported each year. Could vitamin E deficiency really be at the root of these widespread health conditions? One thing is for sure: when almost 90 percent of a population is affected by anything, one word comes to mind.

ep•i•dem•ic [ep-i-**dem**-ik] – noun. An occurrence of a condition in a population at a frequency higher than that expected; extremely prevalent; widespread.

An epidemic is defined as something that is extremely prevalent or widespread. We just examined published U.S. government documents showing that nearly 90 percent of the U.S. population is deficient at achieving an adequate intake of the essential micronutrient vitamin E. This alone should be enough to cause grave concern for us all, especially as we start to understand the potential health conditions associated with this single deficiency.

Based on the data from the USDA report and the definition of "epidemic," we must conclude that there is a vitamin E deficiency epidemic going on right now in America. This means that out of an estimated 300 million people living in the United States, approximately 260 million are deficient in this one micronutrient. What you are about to discover is that this deficiency epidemic does not end with vitamin E. The fact is it goes far deeper than most of us had ever imagined. Are you ready to continue digging?

Digging Deeper

TAKE A LOOK at Table 4.5 below, the USDA's adequacy rates for sixteen more essential micronutrients.

TABLE 4.5. PERCENTAGE OF POPULATION IN U.S. OF TWO YEARS OLD AND OVER WITH ADEQUATE INTAKES BASED ON AVERAGE REQUIREMENT

MICRONUTRIENT	PERCENTAGE	MICRONUTRIENT	PERCENTAGE
Vitamin A	46.0	Phosphorus	87.2
Vitamin C	51.0	Magnesium	43.0
Vitamin E	13.6	Iron	89.5
Thiamine	81.6	Selenium	91.5
Riboflavin	89.1	Zinc	70.8
Niacin	87.2	Copper	84.2
Vitamin B_6	73.9	Calcium	30.9
Folate	59.7	Potassium	7.6
Vitamin B_{12}	79.7		

Source: www.ars.usda.gov/services/docs.htm?docid=15656

So, what do you think? I bet there are a few of you out there who, at first glance, are a little bit surprised to see that the adequacy rates for many of the listed micronutrients were not as bad as you might have thought. However, upon closer examination we can see that only 7.6 percent of the population has an adequate intake of potassium, a deficiency associated with stroke, osteoporosis, kidney stones, and hypertension. This means that in addition to the nearly nine out of ten Americans who are deficient in vitamin E, more than nine out of ten are deficient in potassium. The data also states that more than seven out of ten are deficient in calcium, and approximately five out of ten are deficient in vitamin A, vitamin C, and magnesium. In fact, of the seventeen essential micronutrients studied by the USDA, all showed a deficiency rate of some kind. However, in order to uncover the real deficiency rates, we'll need to take a closer look.

Consider the following scenario: One morning an interesting story caught our attention on the TV news. The reporter announced the new USDA adequacy rates for seventeen essential vitamins and minerals. As this is our field of study, we were surprised at how high some of the adequacy rates were reported to be and decided to investigate the findings. After a half hour of searching the Internet for the story's source, Jayson found the information in Table 4.5 on the USDA's website. However, still conflicted by the data he encountered, Jayson decided to dig a little deeper and read the "documentation" section to find out how these adequacy rates were actually calculated. It was here Jayson found the pertinent piece of information that we have not yet shared with you, which sent him fuming into his office.

What did Jayson find that made him so angry? Through his online research, he found a heading in the "documentation" section of the USDA website titled "Selected Populations." It was within these documents that he discovered that the adequacy rates he had just been looking at, and that were announced on the TV news program, were figured in the following way:

> **"**The estimates are based on Estimated Average Requirements (EARs).**"**

> **"**Adequate Intakes (AIs) are used for nutrients that do not have EAR values.**"**

What does this mean? Do you remember Table 3.1, a guide to understanding intake acronyms, outlining the differences between the RDIs and EARs? It clearly states that the estimated average requirements (EARs) are the amounts of micronutrients that would be expected to satisfy the micronutrient requirements of **only 50 percent** of the population. This was the basis for our Naked Fact #1. This means that the adequacy rates you just reviewed on that government study were calculated on an amount that **only creates adequacy for 50 percent of the population.** What about the other 50 percent?

What do you think would happen to the adequacy rates if the USDA used the RDIs as the baseline? Remember that the RDI is an amount **considered sufficient to meet the requirements of nearly all (97 to 98 percent) healthy individuals.** Needless to say, the adequacy rates would be much different. To see just how important this piece of information is, let's do a quick experiment.

Look back at the EAR sufficiency rate for B_{12} in Table 4.5. We are going to round it up from 79.7 percent to 80 percent to make things as easy as possible. You will need three key pieces of information to conduct this experiment. First, you will need to know that the amount of B_{12} an individual would have had to ingest to reach EAR sufficiency is 2 mcg. Next, you need to know that the amount an individual would have had to ingest to reach RDI sufficiency is 6 mcg. It seems obvious now that if only 80 percent of the population ingested 2 mcg or more of vitamin B_{12} (the amount needed to make half the population sufficient—EAR), that a much smaller percentage of people would have ingested 6 mcg (the amount needed for RDI sufficiency). Finally, you will need to know that the mean, or average, level of B_{12} ingested by the study participants was approximately 5.1 mcg. Let's continue our experiment using the diagrams in Figure 4.2.

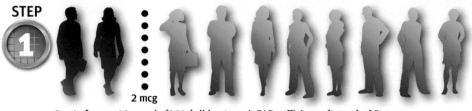

STEP 1

2 mcg

2 out of every 10 people (20%) did not reach EAR sufficiency (2 mcg) of B₁₂.

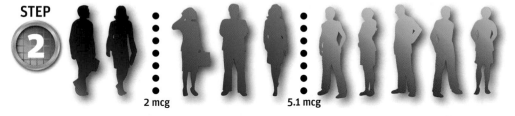

STEP 2

2 mcg   5.1 mcg

The mean, or average, level of B₁₂ ingested by the study participants was 5.1 mcg. We can see that, given even distribution, approximately 5 of the 10 people ingested less than 5.1 mcg of B₁₂.

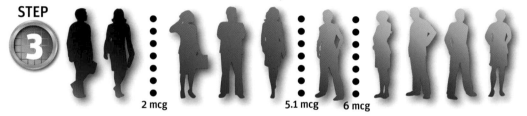

STEP 3

2 mcg   5.1 mcg   6 mcg

If 2 out of every 10 of the study participants were deficient at meeting the 2 mcg EAR requirement for B₁₂, then when we adjust the diagram to include the 6 mcg requirement of the RDI, we can see that 6 out of the 10 people (60%) would not meet RDI sufficiency (6 mcg) of B₁₂. This would leave only 4 of 10 individuals (40%) of the U.S. population sufficient in B₁₂.

Figure 4.2. Vitamin B₁₂ Sufficiency: EAR versus RDI

Is this starting to make sense? While we are in no way suggesting anyone can determine actual sufficiency rates without more information, we believe these numbers are a fair estimate. In truth, since the RDI only refers to 97 to 98 percent of the population, the adequacy rates could be a few percentage points worse. Even with as much as a 10 to 20 percent margin of error, we can see that the adequacy rates when using RDIs would be disturbingly low.

Let's examine what we just learned in our experiment. These numbers shed some much-needed light on just how many people may actually be living with a B₁₂ deficiency based on the RDI.

B₁₂ Adequacy Rate using the EAR	80%
B₁₂ Adequacy Rate using the RDI	40%
Adequacy Rate Accounting for a 10–20% Margin of Error using the RDI	32–48%

Remember, saying "adequate" is just the USDA's way of saying "sufficient." What do we know about sufficiency? It is the opposite of deficiency. If we flip the information around and examine it from a different perspective, we may begin to get a more complete picture.

B_{12} Deficiency Rate using the EAR	20%
B_{12} Deficiency Rate using the RDI	60%
Deficiency Rate Accounting for a 10–20% Margin of Error using the RDI	52–78%

Can you see why Jayson was so angry? We started out the morning watching a televised report that 80 percent of Americans were sufficient in B_{12}. Of course, no one bothered to mention that this sufficiency rate was based on the EAR, making it, in reality, 80 percent of 50 percent of the population. We are not blaming the television network or the news reporter; chances are that even if they had mentioned that the reports statistics were based on EAR adequacy rates, most of us would not have knowledge of that term or how it affects actual sufficiency levels.

● ● ● ● ● ● ● ● ● ● ● ● ● ● ● ●

How Sufficiency Should Be Measured

AFTER WORKING OUT THE NUMBERS in our experiment, we can clearly see that the 80 percent adequacy rate for B_{12} quickly decreases to a rate closer to a mere 40 percent when we use the RDI and include 97 to 98 percent of the whole population. Now the good news is that two of the micronutrients will not be affected, because they were calculated in AI and not in EAR. In these two cases, the AI intake requirements were the same as the RDI requirements. The bad news is that they are calcium and potassium, which both had exceedingly low levels of adequacy to begin with—30.9 percent and 7.6 percent, respectively. We also want you to notice that we chose B_{12} to use in our experiment for a good reason: B_{12} had one of the highest adequacy rates of all of the vitamins and minerals listed. Obviously, those micronutrients that had lower adequacy rates on the USDA report using the EARs would be reduced to far smaller percentages using RDI requirements.

We think that sufficiency rates based on the RDI would be a more accurate and honest way to present such important information that ultimately affects the overall health of every one of us. After all, if we don't know something is broken, why would we think to fix it?

This USDA data is misleading in another way. While it may be telling us that 30.9 percent of us are sufficient in calcium, 7.6 percent are sufficient in potassium, and 80 percent are sufficient in B_{12}, where does it tell us what percentage of us are sufficient in all three of these micronutrients? Better yet, where can I find out the percentage of the population that is sufficient in all of the essential micronutrients? That information is not included.

One would have to think that the odds go way down. According to four-time *New York Times* bestselling author Mark Hyman, M.D., "A whopping 92 percent of us are deficient in one or more nutrients at the Recommended Daily Allowance (RDA) level . . . The RDA standards do not necessarily outline the amount needed for optimal health."

Mehmet Oz, M.D., chooses these sad statistics in reporting on the prevalence of micronutrient deficiency: "A study of 3 million people revealed that less than 1 percent of the participants got enough essential vitamins from diet alone. That's why you must take a multivitamin; it also helps prevent heart disease, breast cancer, and colon cancer."

The fact is that no matter how you look at it, whether you choose to focus on the adequacy rates based on the EAR or the RDI, or if you prefer to listen to the statistics of today's most trusted physicians, millions of Americans are living with a micronutrient-deficiency condition. The USDA's report makes this fact quite clear.

Did You Know

The U.S. Food and Drug Administration (FDA) is considering changing the way our food and supplements are labeled. The Daily Value (DV) on these labels tells us how much of a specific micronutrient is delivered per serving. However, while the current DV is based on the Reference Daily Intake (RDI), the FDA is trying to change the DV to be based on the Estimated Average Requirements (EAR). As we have just learned, using the EAR can be misleading. For example, a product that now touts 100% DV of vitamin A, *without changing anything other than the label,* would miraculously contain 333% DV if the FDA makes this change. This means that our food and supplements would appear to be more micronutrient-rich than they actually are.

• • • • • • • • • • • • • • • •

Micronutrient Deficiency Around the World

AMERICA LEADS THE DEFICIENCY pack among developed countries; however, the world at large shares similar statistics. In the National Diet and Nutrition Survey, carried out in Great Britain on behalf of their Food Standards Agency, UK residents were observed to determine if they were taking in enough micronutrients from food alone to maintain basic health. It was determined that every person was at risk for micronutrient deficiency to some degree.

For example, the average intake of selenium, a micronutrient important for proper immune function, was only at 50 percent of the reference nutrient intake (RNI)—the UK's equivalent to the U.S. RDI. Subjects were also found to be 60 percent deficient in zinc and 30 percent deficient in calcium. Women were 51 percent deficient in folic acid. Teenage females showed the greatest deficiencies: calcium (76 percent), magnesium (97 percent), zinc (72 percent), and folic acid (52 percent).

In Canada, approximately 40 percent of adults are deficient in reaching *even the EAR* for vitamin A and magnesium, and you know how EAR deficiency rates skyrocket when converted to RDI.

In 1987, the World Health Organization (WHO) estimated that vitamin A deficiency affected only 39 countries. In 2005, it stated that estimates indicate that 122 countries had vitamin A deficiency of public health significance. This means that even while more countries became developed, the number of countries affected by vitamin A deficiency nearly tripled between 1987 and 2005.

It's obvious we're all in this together. We can clearly see that America is not alone in this micronutrient-deficiency epidemic. In fact, micronutrient deficiency is spreading at a hastened rate. Perhaps a new word comes to mind.

Pan•dem•ic (pan-**dem**-ik) – noun. An epidemic that is spreading through human populations across a large region; for instance multiple continents, or even worldwide.

We will base our **Naked Fact #4** on USDA research data, the UK National Diet and Nutrition Survey, World Health Organization statistics, global deficiency studies, and our accepted definition of the term *pandemic*.

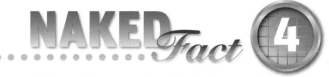

NAKED *Fact* **4**

Collected data reveals a global micronutrient-deficiency pandemic.

We have come a long way in this chapter. We've examined the soil and discovered it is becoming increasingly devoid of the minerals that are needed to produce micronutrient-rich foods. A diet rich in naked calories can lead to a "hidden hunger," or deficiency, in one or more of the essential micronutrients, which may ultimately cause a related health condition or disease in the human body.

We have determined that there exists a micronutrient-deficiency pandemic. We've determined this pandemic is spread through the naked calorie and that one of the causes of naked calories is depleted, "sick," or "naked" soil. *But how many other causes are there? In what other ways can* 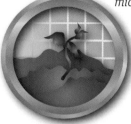 *micronutrients be stripped from our foods? How are our foods being robbed? What might you be doing that causes micronutrients to be further depleted? Are there changes that you could make to limit further stripping from taking place?* In the next chapter we will begin to answer these questions as you identify the culprits causing your body's micronutrient bank account to go bust.

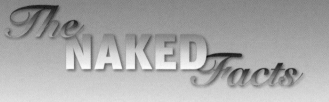

The **NAKED** Facts

- Soil and food have been studied and a micronutrient-depletion trend has been established.

- A deficiency in one or more of the essential micronutrients can ultimately cause health-related conditions or diseases.

- Collected data reveals a global micronutrient-deficiency pandemic.

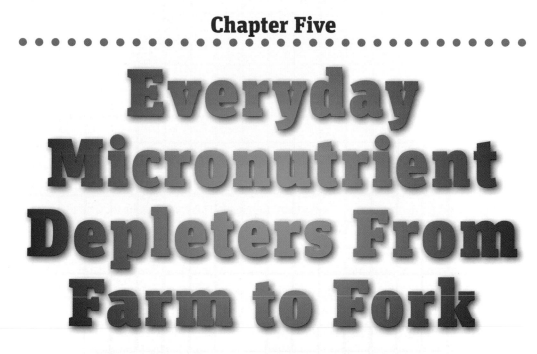

Chapter Five

Everyday Micronutrient Depleters From Farm to Fork

The Bank Account Goes Bust

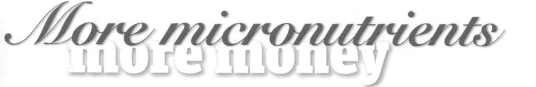

More micronutrients more money

Fewer micronutrients less money

> **"**Let us not look back in anger or forward in fear,
> but around in awareness.**"**
>
> —James Thurber, Illustrator, *The New Yorker*

He opened the envelope with great anticipation. It was Rob's first paycheck, and he already knew exactly how he was going to spend it. His new job would finally allow him to purchase the large flat-screen television he had dreamed of throughout college. His fingers ripped off the perforated perimeter that enclosed the check. *This can't be it,* he thought to himself. Where had all of the money gone? Had he been robbed? Did they give him the wrong check? Rob's pay was much smaller than he had expected.

He frantically turned to the itemized deduction section to review. There he discovered some unexpected deductions, things he had not taken into account when he was first budgeting for his flat screen. Fees for a training course and a new uniform had been subtracted. He let go a sigh; luckily these were only one-time deductions. There were steps he could take, like keeping his uniforms neat and clean, that could help him avoid these reductions again. Then there was another set of deductions: health insurance and 401K contributions and, of course, taxes.

Taxes were an unavoidable reduction in wage, and Rob considered his health insurance and 401K equally unavoidable. Deflated, Rob buried his dream of the flat screen with a new knowledge: Whether avoidable or unavoidable, there would be deductions taken from every paycheck, and now he'd plan appropriately for this reality.

Nutritionally, the foods we eat are like paychecks. Some foods contain more micronutrients (more money), while other foods contain fewer micronutrients (less money). Eating foods that are micronutrient rich every day can lead to a sizable "bank account," bringing you closer to a healthy micronutrient-*sufficient* state; whereas frequently eating foods that are micronutrient poor can leave your body's bank account "overdrawn," making you vulnerable to an unhealthy micronutrient-*deficient* state.

The objective of eating food is to supply your body energy (macronutrients) as well as to fill the requirements of essential micronutrients your body must have in order to function correctly. If you are successful at this task, then your body can perform well and keep you healthy. However, if you are not, and a large majority of what you eat is micronutrient-poor food, then your body must choose which functions it can perform with the micronutrients available to it.

Can you see how your body's micronutrient bank account may be more important than you previously thought? Like your personal bank account, your body holds the micronutrients you deposit so that they are available to "pay the bills," or run your bodily functions when they are needed. The foods you eat, whether a muffin for breakfast, a fresh salad for lunch, or a steak for dinner, carry the micronutrients that are deposited in your body's bank account. But what if the micronutrients you expect to be in these foods aren't really there at all? What if somehow, as in Rob's story, they are being deducted without your knowledge—before you get a chance to deposit them into your body's bank account?

From this point forward we will refer to the causes of these deductions, or depletions, as Everyday Micronutrient Depleters, or EMDs, which is another way your food can be stripped of vital micronutrients and contribute in the creation of naked calories. Everyday Micronutrient Depleters can be divided into two groups, based on when you will come into contact with them. The first group you will encounter *before* you eat your food, while those in the second group will occur *after*. In this chapter we focus on the first group of EMDs; the ones that occur directly to our food—from farm to fork—*before* you eat it.

Like the deductions from Rob's paycheck *before* being deposited, EMDs cause the foods you eat to be depleted of micronutrients. While they greatly affect your micronutrient-sufficiency level, EMDs can often go undetected, overlooked, or ignored. There are some EMDs that are avoidable and/or preventable, such as an additional uniform for Rob, while others, like taxes, are unavoidable and will inevitably cause the loss of essential micronutrients.

Your individual choices concerning each EMD have the potential to affect your micronutrient-sufficiency level and ultimately your health. However, we are not telling you to change *everything* in your life. For some of you, some of these changes might not even be possible. Our objective is solely to increase your *awareness* of the impact that EMDs can have on micronutrient sufficiency.

Let's begin by focusing on the EMDs that can happen directly to our food *before* we eat it. In Chapter 4 we discovered that decreased levels of minerals in the soil equates to decreased levels of micronutrients in food. We also reviewed the USDA report and numerous international studies and identified a global micronutrient-deficiency pandemic. What we haven't yet accounted for is a little thing called *life.*

Do you shop for produce at your local supermarket once a week? Do you peel your vegetables before serving them to remove the harmful pes-

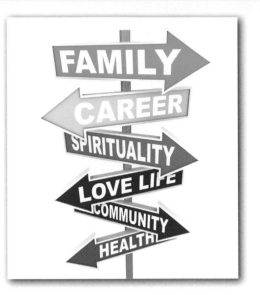

ticides? Do processed, frozen, or canned foods help you save time? Do you take home doggie bags from restaurants? Have you shopped at the local gourmet grocer and purchased precooked culinary creations for your family's dinner? Do you reheat any of these foods in the oven or microwave? Have you ever stopped to think how any of these actions could affect your personal micronutrient-sufficiency level?

As a society moves away from its traditional roots and begins its journey toward modernization, its population naturally increases. A larger population leads to greater food demands and a switch from local, natural farming, to large-scale, high-tech farming methods designed to increase crop yields to levels high enough to feed a nation. As we mentioned in the Introduction to this book, while conducting the Calton Project we observed that as modernization became more prevalent in a society, micronutrient deficiency increased, and with it, so did health problems and chronic disease. Our goal was to take what we observed and use that information to rethink how we eat here, in America, and throughout the world. In this section we examine five of today's most common food distribution and production practices: global distribution; factory-farming methods; and food packaging, preparation, and processing—to evaluate just how many essential micronutrients we lose when we choose modern methods over time-honored, traditional methods.

 GLOBAL DISTRIBUTION

For many people, eating locally grown foods may seem like a new concept, but it's our current global distribution system—importing and exporting foods across countries and continents—that is a rather recent development. Every minute of every mile that your food travels matters, because as fresh food is exposed to environmental elements—temperature, light, and air—it loses micronutrients. Our first EMD encountered due to modern global distribution practices is travel time and storage, and it affects all fresh foods across the board from carrots to chicken, apples to spinach.

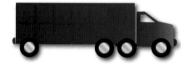

Travel Time and Storage

Many conventional farmers harvest produce early, prior to its reaching peak ripeness, in order for it to withstand mechanical harvesting and long-distance travel without damage. This may be detrimental to a food's overall micronutrient value. According to Harvard Medical School's Center for Health and the Global Environment, "While full color may be achieved after harvest, nutritional quality may not." Tomatoes, for example, will have some increase in vitamin C after being prematurely harvested; however, they will never reach the micronutrient levels of those that ripen on the vine. This is particularly important, as tomatoes make up one-quarter of Americans' total vegetable consumption!

Let's look at research conducted at Penn State University on the ability of spinach to retain micronutrients. According to Luke LaBorde, Ph.D., Associate Professor of Food Science, "If the spinach is coming from the other side of the country, then the produce might be kept at a warm temperature in a shipping truck for an extended period of time. By the time the spinach reaches the dinner table, much of the nutrient content might already be gone."

In fact, the study showed that it only took four days for spinach to lose 47 percent of its folate (folic acid) and carotenoid content when stored at 68 degrees. As we can imagine, the back of a container truck can get much hotter than that, and the hotter it is, the faster micronutrient loss occurs. It is not only heat that robs foods of their micronutrients; exposure to light (UVs) and exposure to air (oxidation) are also culprits. Even fresh foods in a refrigerator averaging 39 degrees Fahrenheit, perhaps similar to your local grocery store or restaurant cooler, lose micronutrients. Penn State researchers found that after eight days spinach lost an average of 53 percent of its folate and carotenoid content, despite its being stored at a cool 39 degrees. Additionally, vitamin E loss can occur when food is overexposed to air or light. Vitamin C is even less stable, as it is vulnerable to all three elements—air, light, and heat exposure.

According to Joel Salatin, featured in *Food Inc.*, and *Omnivore's Dilemma,* "In 1945, 40 percent of all vegetables consumed in the United States were grown in backyards." This is in sharp contrast to today, where according to the Leopold Center for Sustainable Agriculture at Iowa State University, the average potato has traveled 1,155 miles before it reaches your dinner table. Similarly, a tomato travels 1,569 miles, and a carrot travels an exhausting, micronutrient-depleting 1,838 miles prior to being served. Choosing naturally ripened, locally grown produce can greatly impact your total micronutrient intake.

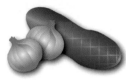

Hometown Heroes

Do exotic fruits and vegetables make your mouth water? Have you tried dragon fruit, rambutan, guava, or lychee? Don't you just love shopping in the produce section at your grocery store? Mega stores have dramatically expanded these areas, presenting us with a plethora of beautiful fruits and vegetables. Numerous exotic varieties await our discovery. While these faraway favorites are a fantastic feast for the eyes, we must remember that the micronutrient loss is most often proportional to the distance the food has traveled.

The USDA Economic Research Service database reveals that the amount of imported produce consumed by Americans has been rising since 1970. An increasing proportion of what Americans eat is produced in other countries, including an estimated 39 percent of fruits, 12 percent of vegetables, 40 percent of lamb, and 78 percent of fish and shellfish. The typical American meal contains, on average, ingredients from at least five countries *outside* U.S. borders.

How might this affect the micronutrient content of your food? Let's consider a spinach salad. Perhaps the spinach in the salad wasn't local and sat in a truck for hundreds of miles to get to your town; then it was stored in the grocery store's refrigeration area for several days before being displayed for sale. Finally, you purchased the spinach, but left it in your refrigerator for a few more days before you made your "fresh" spinach salad. We won't turn this into a math problem, but you can see how the micronutrient values in fresh food can decline rapidly. Imagine the potential impact the EMD of travel time and storage would have on your personal micronutrient-sufficiency levels.

The movement to avoid the depletion caused by travel time and storage by reverting to more traditional local food consumption has grown so popular that today we call those supporting it *locavores.*

Locavores believe that locally grown foods are more beneficial to their health due to their superior micronutrient value, and they attempt to eat only foods grown or raised within a one hundred mile radius. However, this is only one of the reasons that millions are joining this movement. Here are a few others:

- Produce picked and eaten fresh tastes better.
- With 80 percent of Americans nervous about food safety, locavores say they feel safer knowing who is growing their food.
- If they have questions regarding pesticides, locavores can visit the farm themselves.
- Buying locally grown produce and dairy keeps money in the community and sustains the local economy.
- While conventional farming rapidly depletes topsoil fertility, most local growers use practices that protect soil, air, and water resources.
- Buying locally grown foods reduces our "carbon footprint" by decreasing our dependence

on petroleum, a nonrenewable energy source. Agriculture consumes one-fifth of all the petroleum in the U.S.; not only does local food conserve energy by not relying on petroleum-derived fertilizers, it conserves energy at the distribution level.

- Shopping at local farmers' markets can equal serious cash savings. Grocery stores factor the high cost of fuel into food prices; local farmers pass this savings on to their customers.

The bottom line is, buying locally grown or raised foods decreases the micronutrients lost in transport and storage, and therefore decreases the intake of naked calories.

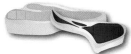

Benefits of Organics

While there is no arguing the benefits of eating locally grown foods, purchasing organic foods can exponentially increase these benefits. For produce to be considered organic in the United States, it must comply with certain USDA standards, which include omitting synthetic pesticides and fertilizers and genetically modified organisms (GMOs)—seeds that have been genetically altered to create an abundance of larger, more pest-resistant produce.

Organic livestock must have regular access to pasture and must be raised without the routine use of genetically modified feed, growth hormones, or antibiotics. No organic foods can be processed using irradiation, chemical food additives, or industrial solvents. While the term *organic* may have only just started popping up in supermarkets, organic farming is the traditional type of agriculture that has been practiced for thousands of years. Since the 1940s, modern, conventional farming's reliance on synthetic fertilizers to increase crop yields and growth hormones to produce larger livestock in less time has caused us to create foods that are depleted of their essential goodness. While the benefits of organically grown, chemical-free foods may seem obvious, what is less obvious is their ability to *increase* micronutrient intake.

One research report published as a "State of Science Review" by the Organic Center (TOC), found organic food to have higher micronutrient values over conventional food. The authors state, "We identified all peer-reviewed studies published in the scientific literature appearing since 1980 comparing the nutrient levels in organic and conventional foods . . . From ninety-seven published studies, we identified 236 scientifically valid 'matched pairs' of measurements that include an organic and a conventional sample of a given food."

The report compared eleven nutrients and found organic foods to be nutritionally superior in 145 matched pairs, or in 61 percent of the cases. Additionally, organic foods contained higher concentrations of antioxidants in 75 percent of the cases.

Organic food supporters also point to another study conducted in Spain and published in 2008 in the *Journal of the Science of Food and Agriculture.* A team of scientists grew conventional and organic mandarin oranges on the same farm, using the same irrigation methods and tree variety. Interestingly, the study found few differences between the conventional and organic oranges at the time of picking, although the organic fruit was marginally smaller in size and contained 13 percent more vitamin C.

The study found, however, that these organically grown mandarin oranges produce juice that is more intensely colored, has a superior aroma and taste, contains higher levels of all eight minerals studied (in three cases by 50 percent or more), and has a 40 percent higher concentration of vitamin A (beta-carotene). While these studies illuminate the increased micronutrient contents of organic foods, some scientists are still skeptical as to their micronutrient superiority and only recognize organic foods for their omission of harmful toxic substances.

• • • • • • • • • • • • • • • •

The Fab 14 and the Terrible 20

WE OFTEN HEAR FROM OUR CLIENTS that purchasing organic foods is just too expensive. When deciding where to allocate your hard-earned dollars, it can be helpful to know which foods contain the most dangerous amounts of pesticides; you can then identify which foods are most important to buy organic.

To help make this decision easier, we offer you our very own produce list to convey which fruits and vegetables are safe to buy conventionally (the Fab Fourteen) and which ones you should never buy conventionally (the Terrible Twenty).

In creating our list, we first took the Environmental Working Group's yearly compilation of the cleanest and dirtiest produce in terms of pesticide residue. This protected us from toxins but didn't take into account GMOs. So, next we asked Jeffrey Smith, executive director of the Institute for Responsible Technology, for his recommendations on how to best avoid GMO produce.

By utilizing this easy-to-use produce guide, you can reduce your pesticide exposure by 80 percent and avoid GMO produce 100 percent of the time! If you cannot find a particular fruit or vegetable on the list, that means it fell in the middle somewhere or was not ranked. In these cases, use your best judgment. If you can get it organic without paying too much more, do so; if not, buy it conventionally.

Photocopy the page, or download your free wallet-size version of the following list from the Calton Nutrition Rich Food Resource Center online and bring it with you to the grocery store to pick safe produce that doesn't break the bank.

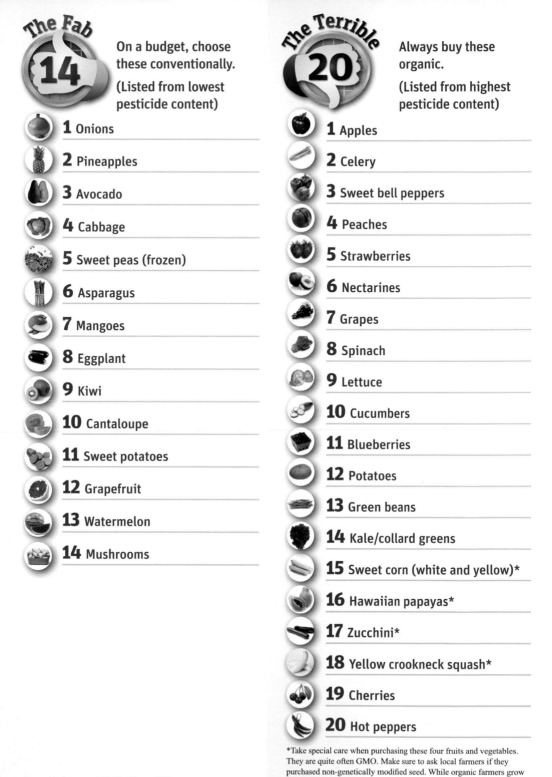

The Fab 14

On a budget, choose these conventionally.

(Listed from lowest pesticide content)

1 Onions
2 Pineapples
3 Avocado
4 Cabbage
5 Sweet peas (frozen)
6 Asparagus
7 Mangoes
8 Eggplant
9 Kiwi
10 Cantaloupe
11 Sweet potatoes
12 Grapefruit
13 Watermelon
14 Mushrooms

The Terrible 20

Always buy these organic.

(Listed from highest pesticide content)

1 Apples
2 Celery
3 Sweet bell peppers
4 Peaches
5 Strawberries
6 Nectarines
7 Grapes
8 Spinach
9 Lettuce
10 Cucumbers
11 Blueberries
12 Potatoes
13 Green beans
14 Kale/collard greens
15 Sweet corn (white and yellow)*
16 Hawaiian papayas*
17 Zucchini*
18 Yellow crookneck squash*
19 Cherries
20 Hot peppers

*Take special care when purchasing these four fruits and vegetables. They are quite often GMO. Make sure to ask local farmers if they purchased non-genetically modified seed. While organic farmers grow organically, some might not yet realize that these seeds are often GMO.

Source: Environmental Working Group, 2011

Figure 5.1. The Fab 14 and the Terrible 20

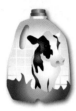

Moo-ve Over to Organic Milk

Another organic food worth the splurge is milk. The cost may be up to one-and-a-half times greater per gallon, but the increase in micronutrient content is just as impressive. A study done by Newcastle University in Great Britain reported that organic milk contained 67 percent more antioxidants than conventional milk. According to Cynthia Sass, MPH, R.D., New York–based nutritionist, bestselling author, and contributor to *Shape* magazine, when compared to non-organic milk, organic milk contains 75 percent more beta-carotene and two to three times more of the powerful antioxidants lutein and zeaxanthin.

Organic milk also supplies 50 percent more vitamin E and about 70 percent more omega-3 fatty acids, which are thought to reduce the risks of cancer and cardiovascular disease.

Organic milk supplies 50 percent more vitamin E and about 70 percent more omega-3 fatty acids

Ultimately, it is our belief that purchasing locally grown organic food is the healthiest, safest, and most environmentally responsible choice. These foods may not only contain higher micronutrient density, they also guarantee to protect us from dangerous pesticides, toxins, antibiotics, and GMOs.

2 FACTORY FARMING

While our examination of local and organic produce touched briefly on milk, we must investigate even further beyond the greens of our gardens. Our choices when purchasing beef, fish, chicken, eggs, and dairy products can also greatly affect the amount of micronutrients brought to the table.

In the last chapter we learned that micronutrient-depleted soil led to micronutrient-depleted animals. However, there is another new and disturbing trend depleting vitamins and minerals from our meat and dairy products. In our modern age of mass-produced food, we feed and raise our commercial protein sources in a way completely foreign and unnatural to their nurturing. Cattle, once allowed to roam the plains grazing on fresh grass, are now kept in large feedlots, fattening themselves with grains. Fish, once caught wild in our waters, many of which are carnivores, are now confined and fed a constant diet of pellets filled with cornmeal, soy, and canola oil. Chicken no longer see the light of day and live their lives with no physical exercise.

While these treatments are obviously inhumane and irresponsible, what we will focus on next is how these so-called advances are deteriorating the quality of the foods available. A far cry from the family-run farms of the past, the modern factory farm is home to our next EMD—unnatural feed and environment.

Unnatural Feed and Environment

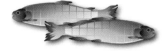

Wild Versus Factory-Farmed Fish

We have all heard that we should consume more fish because it is a great source of the essential fatty acids omega-3 and omega-6. However, is all fish created equal? Eighty percent of salmon on the global market today is factory-farmed. In the United States, it is estimated to be even higher—perhaps as high as 90 percent. Factory-farmed salmon has fewer omega-3s per ounce than wild salmon. According to the USDA Nutrient Database, wild fish can have up to 380 percent more omega-3 than factory-farmed fish. Additionally, the omega-3 to omega-6 ratio is far less health-promoting in factory-farmed fish. For instance, while the ratio of omega-3 to omega-6 in wild Coho salmon is 15.3 to 1 (optimal), the farm-raised Coho salmon has been shown to have a far less optimal 3 to 1 ratio.

Remember, as we outlined in Nutrition 101, the higher the ratio of omega-3 to omega-6, the greater the overall health benefits. And, much like the reduction of toxins from eating organic foods, eating wild fish reduces toxic exposure. Tests have shown that farmed salmon contains sixteen times more of the cancer-linked toxin PCB than wild salmon. Artificial colors are often induced in farmed salmon to make them a more appetizing "salmon" pink color, and one of the most commonly used coloring agents, canthaxanthin, has been linked to human eye defects and retinal damage.

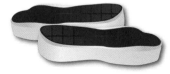

Grass-Fed Versus Grain-Fed Beef

A 2009 joint study between the USDA and researchers at Clemson University compared grain-fed beef with grass-fed beef and concluded that a traditional grass-fed diet was far superior to a grain-fed diet for many reasons.

- Grass-fed beef is loaded with more than 400 percent more vitamin A and vitamin E.
- It supplies higher levels of the B vitamins, thiamine and riboflavin.
- It has greater amounts of calcium, magnesium, and potassium.
- Grass-fed beef is two to four times richer in heart-healthy omega-3 fatty acids.
- Like wild salmon, grass-fed beef that consumes a diet natural to its species has a healthier ratio of omega-3 to omega-6 fatty acids.
- Grass-fed beef is higher in conjugated linoleic acid (CLA), which is a potential cancer fighter and fat metabolizer. Cattle that graze on grass have 300 to 400 percent more CLA than animals fattened on grain in a feedlot.

Factory-farmed cattle are often fed stale candy to reduce feed costs. According to Randy Shaver, Ph.D., of the University of Wisconsin, commercial cows are often fed stale chocolate and candy due to their low cost and high fat content. His review stated, "Upper feeding limits for candy or candy blends and chocolate are five and two pounds per cow per day, respectively." While this practice reduces feed costs, it also produces beef that is artificially high in fat and low in vitamin E, beta-carotene, omega-3 fatty acids, and CLA. HOLY COW!

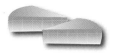

Cheese From Grass-Fed Versus Grain-Fed Cows

Have you ever wondered how the French stay so thin while gobbling up their creamy, world-famous cheese? One reason might be that they still take pride in the craft, using only the best dairy products from cattle that have been grazing on grass. This dairy has higher levels of the fat-metabolizing CLA than the typical American dairy produced by cows raised on grain-fed diets. How much more? Proceedings from the 2000 Inter-mountain Nutrition Conference—whose mission is to provide current information on nutrition and nutrition-related management issues pertinent to the dairy and beef industries—states that cheese from grass-fed cows is 400 percent richer in CLA. That gives the French cheese a large advantage in fat metabolization and cancer fighting. Ooh la la!

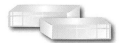

Butter From Grass-Fed Cows Versus Factory-Farmed Cows

Fresh grass is naturally rich in the essential vitamins E, A, and beta-carotene. Therefore, the butter made from cows that eat grass also contains high micronutrient values. The grass-fed dairy cows produce butter that has 50 percent more of the vitamins E and A, and nearly 400 percent more beta-carotene (which gives the grass-fed butter its deeper yellow color) than the butter produced from factory-farmed cows.

Just 3 ounces of grass-fed bison is a perfect "happy meal." According to the Carrington Research Extension Center at the University of South Dakota, grass-fed bison have as much as four times more selenium, an essential trace mineral with cancer-protective qualities, than grain-fed bison. Eating a mere 3 ounces of grass-fed bison can give you more than 100 mcg of selenium, a level that has been proven to have a mood-elevating effect after only two weeks.

Eggs From Pastured Hens Versus Commercial Eggs

When chickens are housed indoors and deprived of open fields and sunlight, they are deprived of their natural environment. In turn, their meat and eggs are depriving us of our essential micronutrients. Pastured hens, which are moved daily so they can hunt and peck for a new crop of grass and insects, produce eggs that contain as much as ten times more omega-3s than eggs from factory hens. Eggs from hens raised outdoors have from three to six times more vitamin D than eggs from hens raised in confinement.

Tests conducted by *Mother Earth News* magazine compared eggs from fourteen pastured flocks with commercial eggs, as listed in the USDA nutrient database. The test found that pastured eggs contained two times more omega-3 fatty acids, four to six times more vitamin D, two-thirds more vitamin A, three times more vitamin E, and seven times more beta-carotene. Another study in the *British Journal of Nutrition* found that pastured hen eggs had 170 percent more B_{12} and 150 percent more folate than their confined commercial counterparts.

For more information on locating these micronutrient-rich foods, visit the Rich Food Resource Center at www.caltonnutrition.com/rich-food

Pasteurization Through Heat and Radiation

The second EMD occurring during modern factory farming is *pasteurization*. While we may all be familiar with the term *pasteurization* regarding dairy products, you may not be aware of the practice of pasteurizing produce and proteins with radiation through a process called irradiation. Next, we will examine these two equally detrimental micronutrient-depleting processes.

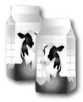

Unpasteurized Versus Pasteurized Milk

All of the milk we buy today in our supermarkets is pasteurized or ultra-pasteurized, but it wasn't so long ago that everyone drank fresh, natural, unpasteurized (raw) milk. However, due to some unsanitary urban farms back in the 1800s, a temporary solution called pasteurization was implemented. Pasteurization is a heat treatment that kills bacteria. However, as it turns out, pasteurization was a lot more cost effective than the maintenance of clean farms. When the large dairies saw the potential for mass production and increased profits using the new "cleaning" technique, they never looked back.

While drinking raw or pasteurized milk remained a personal choice through the 1800s and most of the 1900s, on August 10, 1987, the FDA published a final regulation that made unpasteurized milk difficult to procure. It became federal law that raw milk for human consumption cannot be sold across state lines. Additionally, it gave the individual states the rights to govern raw milk sales and place strict standards on its production. Not only does pasteurization kill the friendly bacteria (yes, there are some bacteria that are good for us, like probiotics), it greatly diminishes milk's natural micronutrient content. Ultrapasterurization heats milk to an even higher temperature, further extending its shelf life. Unfortunately, much of the organic milk on store shelves is often ultrapasteurized for fear it may not sell quickly. Make sure to check your labels when purchasing organic milk and steer clear of this micronutrient ultra-depleter.

Milk, in its unpasteurized, natural state, is full of essential micronutrients, including vitamins A, D, B_6, B_{12}, calcium, and CLA. Drinking raw milk can offer some incredible micronutrient benefits:

- Up to 60 percent more thiamine (vitamin B_1) and B_6 than pasteurized milk
- Up to 100 percent more B_{12}
- Up to 30 percent more folate (vitamin B_9)
- Increased amounts of calcium and phosphorus

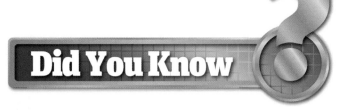

Radiation is measured in something called a kilogray. One kilogray contains the radiation output of 33 million chest X-rays. Most foods are irradiated using up to 1 kilogray, but fresh meat and poultry are irradiated using up to 4.5 kilograys, which equals the radiation output of approximately 150 million chest X-rays. If you see this radura symbol on your package, you can be assured that your food has experienced micronutrient depletion!

Cold Pasteurization—Irradiation

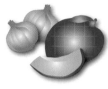

Food irradiation, which is often referred to as "cold pasteurization," has been practiced in the United States for almost fifty years. Irradiation is the process of exposing food to radiation to destroy microorganisms, bacteria, viruses, or insects that might be present in the food and extends its shelf life, making foods past their natural "due date" appear fresh and vibrant.

Today more than thirty-five countries have approved irradiation of some forty different food products, including potatoes, onions, bananas, apples, strawberries, mangoes, meat, poultry, fish, grains, seasonings, and spices. The volume of irradiated food is estimated to exceed 500,000 metric tons annually worldwide. But don't let the sheer volume of global food irradiation lull you into a false sense of security! Just because everyone is doing it doesn't mean it's safe.

While irradiation works to kill bacteria, it also disrupts the structure of everything it passes through. Specifically, irradiation breaks up a food's DNA, vitamins, minerals, and proteins and creates "free radicals" (atoms, molecules, or ions that contain unpaired electrons and crash into each other, multiplying exponentially) that contribute to many degenerative diseases, including heart disease, dementia, cancer, and cataracts.

In fact, in February 2003, the European Parliament revoked its earlier approval of irradiation and voted to allow spices, dried herbs, and seasonings as the "only approved foods for irradiation until adequate scientific evidence proving its safety is conducted." Irradiation also intensely depletes micronutrients. According to *New York Times* bestselling author, Dr. Joseph Mercola, "Irradiation destroys vitamins, nutrients, and essential fatty acids, including up to 95 percent of vitamin A in chicken and 86 percent of vitamin B in oats."

There is yet another problem with food irradiation, which we mentioned earlier: irradiation extends the shelf life of our fruits and vegetables—and as you already learned earlier in this chapter, storage time equals micronutrient loss. This means irradiated food can sit in a crate for a longer period of time without rotting, but this fresh-looking food continues to lose micronutrients long after non-irradiated food would have spoiled and been discarded. Consumers of irradiated food might be treated to a visual delight but in reality are eating nothing but naked calories.

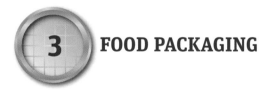

Did You Know

Food irradiation can leave food full of ick! Many factory farms, processing plants, and slaughterhouses produce meat contaminated by feces, urine, pus, and vomit—substances you would definitely not want to eat. Although the process of irradiation kills both *E. Coli* and *Salmonella* bacteria and allows the meat to pass through the inspection process, irradiation does not remove the offensive "icky" contaminants themselves. A better solution would be to clean up the factory farms and create sanitary environments. This would not only remove the "ick," it would also eliminate the bacteria that make you sick.

The following quote from *The Food Commission,* Britain's leading independent watchdog on food issues, says it best: "Food irradiation can result in loss of nutrients . . . This is compounded by the longer storage times of irradiated foods . . . which can result in the food finally eaten by the consumer to contain little more than 'empty calories.' This is potentially damaging to the long- and short-term health of consumers."

3   FOOD PACKAGING

Do you lead a busy life? Do you find that saving even a couple of minutes a day can make your life easier? Is stretching the dollar important to you? In this day and age, with the importance of convenience and managing money, many of us have turned to frozen or canned food. How do you think our next two EMDs, freezing and canning, fare when considering micronutrient loss?

Freezing and Canning

Store-bought packaged foods, like frozen or canned vegetables, often start out ahead of their conventional, fresh counterparts because they are often picked at their peak of ripeness, when they are at their most micronutrient dense. In contrast, fresh produce is often picked prior to peak ripeness to allow it to ripen during transport without becoming spoiled before arriving at the supermarket.

However, that is where the advantage ends. During the blanching process—the soaking of the vegetables in hot water, which takes place prior to the freezing process—the micronutrient content of many of the water-soluble vitamins are reduced by an average of 20 to 60 percent. Loss of antioxidants (which are needed to fight the free radicals we mentioned earlier) also occurs in the blanching and freezing process of most vegetables. While some of the micronutrients are lost in this process, the good news is the rest are locked into the frozen vegetables for up to twelve months.

Similarly in canned foods, micronutrients including the B vitamins (thiamine, B_6, and riboflavin), which are sensitive to heat and light, can be lost through the cooking process prior to canning. However, once the can is sealed, the micronutrients that remain are stable for approximately two years.

Researchers at the University of California, Davis, put it this way: "While the initial thermal treatment of canned products can result in loss, nutrients are relatively stable during subsequent storage due to the lack of oxygen. Frozen products lose fewer nutrients initially because of the short heating time in blanching, but they lose more nutrients during storage due to oxidation."

The losses incurred due to canning and freezing are similar to the data on micronutrient loss in vegetables during the first few weeks after being picked, when they would most likely be transported to the grocery-store produce section. According to the UK-based Institute of Food Research, freshly picked green beans lost 45 percent of their total micronutrients, broccoli and cauliflower 25 percent, carrots 10 percent, and peas up to 15 percent after just fifteen days.

So, if you buy from local farmers and eat your vegetables right away, you're better off eating them fresh. This will really add to your body's micronutrient bank account. However, if you see in the supermarket produce section that these "fresh" vegetables come from some place far away, then there is a good chance that the vegetables in your grocer's canned or frozen vegetable aisles may be just as micronutrient dense.

Remember:
Be aware and compare!
Make sure when choosing frozen and canned foods to investigate the ingredients closely. Many packaged foods contain high levels of sugar and sodium.

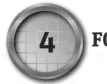

4 FOOD PREPARATION

We have discussed how the global distribution of food as well as factory farming and packaging methods can greatly diminish micronutrient content, thus diminishing our chances of micronutrient sufficiency. But how does the way we prepare food influence micronutrient content? You will find our next EMDs in the many aspects of food preparation, from peeling to pressure-cooking.

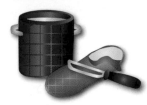

Peeling and Cooking

The first thing one might do to prepare a fresh vegetable for dinner is to peel it. While you may have been raised to peel your vegetables, this EMD greatly increases the loss of vitamin C, folate, and other vitamins in the vitamin B group. Even though it may look or taste better peeled, you may have just unknowingly thrown many of the micronutrients right into the trash.

Now, let's cook the vegetable. This EMD might also greatly affect the micronutrient content that finally makes it to your plate. A study done in Spain measured the level of flavonoids (a type of health-producing antioxidant) that remained in broccoli after it was cooked by four popular cooking methods—steaming, pressure-cooking, boiling, and microwaving. The authors found that the results proved "large differences among the four treatments in their influence on flavonoid content in broccoli."

When compared with raw, fresh broccoli, conventional boiling led to a 66 percent loss of flavonoids and high pressure-cooking led to a considerable 47 percent. Microwaving the broccoli proved catastrophic with an almost complete elimination at 97 percent. However, the Spanish scientists concluded that "steaming had minimal effects, in terms of loss" of the antioxidants. Why might this be true? If we think back to Chapter 3, we learned that some vitamins are water-soluble. It would seem logical then that placing them in hot water might compromise the micronutrients. Therefore, steaming broccoli with little water causes less micronutrient leaching. In fact, the water you pour down the sink after boiling your vegetables might actually be the healthiest part of your meal.

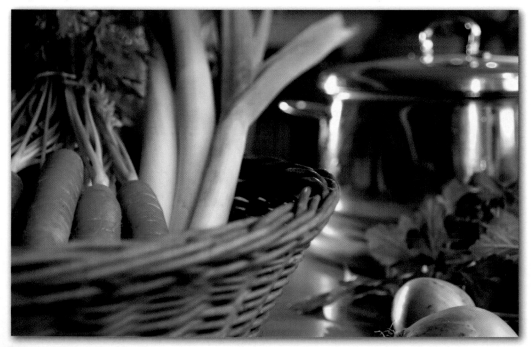

If you eat soup or any other food that has been kept on a stove for more than two hours, perhaps in a restaurant or at a buffet, you should know that it has lost up to 10 percent of its folate, vitamin C, and vitamin B_6, due to prolonged exposure to heat. Maybe you went out for a great dinner and could only eat a portion of the incredible entrée that you ordered. Did you realize that cooling, storing, and reheating leftovers leach away more than 30 percent of the folate and vitamin C?

Do you see how peeling and cooking can quickly strip your food of micronutrients? Do you remember how many micronutrients were lost in the transport of your food? Now, take that same vegetable, already micronutrient poor, and peel it, boil it, let it cool, and reheat it for lunch tomorrow. Or how about picking up a blanched, then frozen bag of broccoli and putting it in the microwave for your family's dinner? Consider the fact that the micronutrients lost due to cooking is greater in irradiated foods. That's right; irradiation can actually intensify the micronutrient loss caused by cooking. The picture gets grim quickly, doesn't it?

TABLE 5.1. VARIOUS COOKING METHODS AND THEIR IMPACTS ON MICRONUTRIENT LOSS IN SPECIFIC FOODS

FOOD	MICRONUTRIENT	METHOD	% OF MICRONUTRIENT LOST
Broccoli	Vitamin C	Blanching	47%
Carrots	Folate	Boiling	79%
Cauliflower	Beta-carotene	Canning	27%
Milk	Vitamin B_{12}	Boiling	30%
Mixed Vegetables	Vitamin C	Boiling (2–5 minutes)	55%
Navy Beans	Calcium	Cooking	49%
Navy Beans	Iron	Cooking	51%
Spinach	Magnesium	Blanching	36%

Source: Worlds Healthiest Foods Online

But all is not lost! We can influence or protect the amount of micronutrients in our food. After all, in most cities there is fresh, local produce. It may be harder to find and you may have to travel farther to get it, but it is available.

However, not everyone can find the time to enjoy a home-cooked meal these days, and even fewer people have time to spend hunting for the best locally grown produce to make it. A raw diet would certainly decrease the amount of micronutrients lost in food preparation, but that isn't something that everyone is interested in either, and we certainly understand the importance of saving money by eating leftovers. Our objective here is not to discourage or depress, but to make sure that we are aware of the severity of the micronutrient loss that can occur *before* we eat our food due to EMDs and to make this information the basis for **Naked Fact #5.**

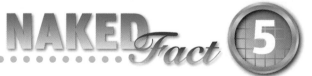

Global distribution, factory farming, food packaging, and preparation methods can cause large percentages of micronutrients to be depleted from your food before it reaches your plate.

5 Tips to Maximize Micronutrient Values

TIP 1: Try using the water from the boiling of vegetables for soup stock or for boiling rice. In this way, you put the lost micronutrients back on the plate.

TIP 2: Cut or juice your vitamin C–rich fruit right before eating to minimize micronutrient loss due to exposure to air (oxidation).

TIP 3: Riboflavin (vitamin B_2), found in milk and dried pasta, is sensitive to light (UV) exposure. Choose these foods in opaque, light-blocking containers to prevent this depletion. If you can see the food, then the light can deplete the micronutrients.

TIP 4: Cover the pot to preserve micronutrient loss on the stove. This reduces the loss of light-sensitive micronutrients, like vitamin B_2, while trapping water-soluble vitamins, so they won't escape through the steam.

TIP 5: While overcooking vegetables can cause micronutrient depletion, lightly cooking your vegetables in a healthy fat not only helps break down a plant's cellular structure to release its micronutrients, but the healthy fat will allow the fat-soluble vitamins (A, D, E, and K) to be absorbed.

5 PROCESSED FOODS

We've examined the impact of global distribution, factory farming, and food packaging and preparation on the micronutrient levels of fresh meats, fruits, and vegetables. However, up to this point we have been looking at EMDs as something that can steal micronutrients from your food—now we are going to look at foods that are EMDs.

Have you walked down the cereal aisle of your local grocery store lately? Do you fill your child's cereal bowl up with a hearty serving of Fruit Loops to kick-start their day? Maybe you prefer to start your morning with a nice cup of yogurt. Have you tried a YoCrunch yogurt with real Oreo-cookie toppings yet? Is your schedule so tight that you only have the time in the morning to pop a quick Toaster Strudel or a couple of slices of white toast in the toaster? These quick, convenient, processed foods make up a large part of the average diet. In fact, due to a startling increase in the consumption of these types of foods, scientists have coined a new term to describe them—EDNP foods.

The acronym EDNP stands for Energy-Dense, Nutrient-Poor. Energy refers to calories.

The acronym EDNP stands for Energy-Dense, Nutrient-Poor. *Energy* refers to calories. *Energy-Dense* refers to a high ratio of calories per gram. In other words, there are a lot of calories packed into a small amount of food. *Nutrient* refers to food's micronutrients, such as vitamins and minerals. *Nutrient-Poor* refers to the fact that a food has a low ratio of micronutrients per gram. This means that a piece of food has relatively few micronutrients for its size. When you put these two facts together, you get a recipe for disaster. EDNP foods include soft drinks, margarine, candy, pastries, ice cream, potato chips, sweetened coffee drinks, and many other commonly consumed edibles.

While EDNP foods are only supposed to occupy the very "tip" of the retired Food Pyramid and have been completely omitted from the USDA's updated My Plate recommendations, a recent study by Ashima K. Kant, Ph.D., published in the *American Journal of Clinical Nutrition,* found that Americans now get more than 27 percent of their daily calories from EDNP foods. If this statistic isn't shocking enough, for one-third of the population, EDNP foods make up an incredible 45 percent of their total daily calories. These foods are highly processed and are filled with excessive calories, unhealthy oils, and sugars. Dr. Kant compared her results to a similar study done in the 1970s and discovered that even with prior warnings on this subject, the American public had not improved in this arena. Public education efforts had not decreased the intake of these naked calories, and in fact, intakes have skyrocketed.

To understand how EDNP foods deplete you of your essential micronutrients, think of your body as a car. The car can only pick up as many people as can fit into it. Once the car is full, the car is full. Your body works the same way. You can only fit, or take in, a certain amount of food. If you stuff yourself with heavily processed EDNP foods, they literally crowd out the possibility of consuming more micronutrient-dense, natural foods. There just isn't enough room left for you to eat the micronutrient-rich foods that you need. In this way, EDNP foods work as Everyday Micronutrient Depleters (EMDs) that rob you of your essential micronutrients.

EDNP Foods

Many EDNP foods also contain one or more of three ingredients that we recommend cutting out of your diet; refined white flour, refined white sugar, and high fructose corn syrup. The refining of grain, which converts whole grain into white flour for pasta, bread, cereals, and baked goods, is one of the most detrimental practices in food science today.

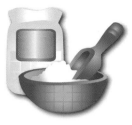

Refined Flour

Refined grains, or processed grains, have had both the bran and the germ removed from the grain kernel. Protein and fiber are found in the bran, which is the outer protective layer of the kernel. The germ contains the vitamins, essential fats, and the antioxidants. Once these micronutrient-rich pieces are removed, a fluffy white inner core called endosperm remains; it is with this core that processed white flour is made.

According to John Neustadt, N.D., coauthor of *A Revolution in Health Through Nutritional Biochemistry,* "Simply refining wheat into white flour wipes out 50 to 80 percent of the various B vitamins, 86 percent of the vitamin E, 85 percent of the magnesium, and 60 percent of the calcium."

You may notice that many food labels often read, "enriched white flour." It's true that many enriched or fortified foods may have had a few micronutrients added back into them; however, they did not replace the dozens of valuable micronutrients originally stripped. When you choose a product made from refined white flour, you are eating naked calories.

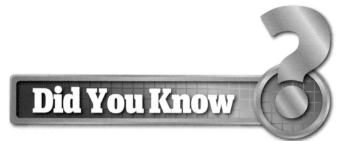

The refining of grains was studied by the Romans 2,000 years ago. History shows us that they understood the superiority of the whole grain over the refined grain as they insisted their athletes and warriors eat *only* unrefined grains.

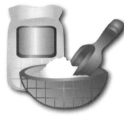

Refined Sugar

Just as micronutrient deficient as refined white flour, and probably just as common, is refined crystalline white sugar, commonly referred to as sucrose, or table sugar. White sugar is refined from cane or beet juice by stripping away all of its vitamins, minerals, protein, fiber, and water. In the next chapter we will explore the detrimental effects of sugar as an Everyday Micronutrient Depleter (EMD), but for now, we will focus on it as an undesirable ingredient in EDNP foods that are filling your body with naked calories.

If we take soft drinks as an example, research clearly shows that adults and children are drinking more of this EDNP food than ever before. Over the last forty years the consumption of soft drinks has doubled for adults and nearly tripled for children and teens. In fact, among children and teens aged two to eighteen, 29 percent of all beverages consumed are sweetened sodas—this makes soft drinks the most commonly consumed beverage.

Well, if more children are drinking soft drinks than ever before, then what did they stop drinking? Studies show that kids have cut their consumption of milk by 40 percent. As we all know, the calcium and vitamin D in milk helps grow strong bones. According to the National Institute of Child Health and Human Development, as much as 90 percent of adult bone mass is established during adolescence. Diminished intake of these micronutrients in childhood has been shown to result in the early onset of osteoporosis. To make matters worse, some of the milk now being offered in many schools today is almost just as sugar laden as the sugary soda itself. In Jamie Oliver's *Food Revolution,* the British chef brings to light the controversial practice of luring American kids to drink milk by giving them artificially colored, sugar-sweetened milk for school lunch. While these flavored milks have the benefit of micronutrients, they can also contain 4 teaspoons of sugar in every child-sized portion.

High Fructose Corn Syrup

The third common EDNP ingredient is high fructose corn syrup (HFCS.) This ingredient is known as glucose/fructose in Canada, and glucose /fructose syrup in the United Kingdom. Found commonly in fruit juices, cereal, bread, yogurt, ketchup, mayonnaise, candies, pastries, soft drinks, and sports drinks, HFCS is made by refining cornstarch. Its popularity rose in the 1970s when, due to manufacturing advances, it became cheaper to produce than sugar. In the U.S. today more HFCS is consumed than sugar.

According to Michael Pollan, author of *The Omnivore's Dilemma,* "Nearly 10 percent of the calories Americans consume now come from corn sweeteners; the figure is 20 percent for many children."

The CDC reports that Americans consume an average of 60 pounds of this sweetener per person every year. In the beginning of 2009, researchers from *Environmental Health,* a peer-reviewed environmental health journal, discovered high amounts of mercury (an element that causes damage to the brain, lungs, and kidneys), in nearly 50 percent of commercial HFCS samples. A second study, conducted by the Institute for Agriculture and Trade Policy (IATP), a non-profit watchdog group, found that of the fifty-five brand-name foods containing HFCS tested, one-third also contained mercury. "Mercury is toxic in all its forms," states the study's author, David Wallinga, M.D.

Another concern regarding HFCS is that, unlike sugar, it does not trigger the secretion of leptin, a hormone that tells your brain when you are full. Because of this, eating HFCS can lead to increased caloric intake and obesity. HFCS consumption can also lead to an increased risk of heart disease because it elevates triglyceride levels. As an ingredient goes, it is difficult to find one with worse press. It fills food with an intensely sweet flavor, but no nutritional value.

While many foods containing HFCS are EDNP foods that rob us of more micronutrient-dense food choices, the production of HFCS additionally acts as an EMD by contributing to soil erosion. HFCS is made from corn, and the farming of corn leaves a huge carbon footprint. Corn is cultivated in a monoculture system, meaning that the land it is grown on is used for corn cropping alone. This type of farming destroys the soil and depletes it of available micronutrients.

By depleting our soil, which depletes our minerals, HFCS is an Everyday Micronutrient Depleter (EMD). By filling our foods with naked calories and preventing the body's ability to trigger leptin secretion, we consider HFCS one of the most dangerous ingredients in Energy-Dense, Nutrient-Poor foods today.

So, how much of these EDNP foods are Americans actually consuming? According to the 2010 Report of the Dietary Guidelines Advisory Committee on the Dietary Guidelines for Americans, four out of the top five most-consumed foods are EDNP foods. Coming in at number one are flour-based desserts (including cakes, cookies, doughnuts, pies, crisps, and cobblers). These sweet treats (that almost always contain refined white flour, sugar, and/or high fructose corn syrup) provide, on average, 139 naked calories to each person, each day. Next, supplying an additional 129 naked calories per person per day are breads, which typically contain at least one of these EDNP ingredients. Sodas that are loaded with sugar and high fructose corn syrup, plus energy and sports drinks, are in fourth place, adding another 114 naked calories per day. Pizza with its processed flour crust takes the fifth spot and adds 98 naked calories per day to our bottom line. If we add up the calories from the foods in only these four categories, we can see that these EDNP foods contribute 480 naked calories to the caloric intake of each person in America, each

How many of these Energy-Dense, Nutrient-Poor (EDNP) foods do you consume?
Soft drinks, cookies, pastries, doughnuts, chips, pies, candy, sweetened coffee drinks, ice cream, syrup, buttered popcorn, chocolates, muffins, cake, tortilla chips, pudding, salad dressing, gravy

day. For a person eating a 2,000 calorie diet, that is nearly 25 percent of their daily caloric intake. This does not include the calories added by other commonly eaten foods such as chips, pretzels, buttered popcorn, candy, and ice cream. The calories these foods contribute raise the already startling percentage above and beyond. While the diet of the average American adult leaves much to be desired, the USDA report shows that the diet of U.S. kids is often worse: "Nearly 40 percent of total calories consumed (798 kcal/ day of 2027 kcal) by 2- to 18-year-olds in the U.S. are in the form of empty [naked] calories." Can you see how EDNP foods and the naked calories they contain can take up large percentages of your calories and act as Everyday Micronutrient Depleters (EMDs) in your life and the lives of your children?

• • • • • • • • • • • • • • • • • •

The Rich Food, Poor Food Philosophy

HOW MANY TIMES HAVE YOU SEEN a celebrity chef or health expert give advice on how we should eat in order to lose a few pounds or cut a few inches? It's like food swapping; first they show you meal "A," which is usually a mouth-watering plate of something sinfully yummy; then the camera pans to meal "B," a plate half full of something along the lines of meal "A," but with fewer calories, less sodium, or lower fat.

One well-known food-swapping guide, *Eat This, Not That*, suggested that readers substitute a regular-size chicken sandwich and fries from a well-known fast-food restaurant with a smaller honey-barbecue-coated chicken sandwich with a side of macaroni and cheese. Can you see the glaring problems with this? Did someone forget to tell them that refined white-flour rolls and pasta have little to no micronutrient value, or that the honey-barbecue sauce was a sugary mess? Did anyone other than us notice that there was nothing green, or fresh, on the plate? While there is no doubt that *Eat This, Not That's* suggestions lead to lower fat and sodium intake and thousands of saved calories, they accomplish nothing if your goal is micronutrient sufficiency. In our opinion, selecting a meal based on its fat, sodium, and calorie content misses the nutritional mark. In fact, so does choosing foods solely based on their carbohydrate count or because they fall into a 40/30/30 zone or because it is dictated by your blood type. None of these methods focus on what science has shown to be the most important factor of all in overall health—micronutrient sufficiency. Regardless of which diet profile you decide to follow, you should strive to consume as many micronutrient-rich foods as possible.

We define "healthy" foods based on their micronutrient content instead of their fat, sodium, calorie, carbohydrate, or protein contents. Therefore, we introduce to you our Rich Food, Poor Food philosophy.

Rich foods are natural, unprocessed, or minimally processed, high in micronutrient content, and help you increase your micronutrient-sufficiency level. *Poor foods* are often highly processed and are low or void of micronutrients. Like EDNP foods, *poor foods* often contain refined white flour, sugar, and high fructose corn syrup. The longer the ingredient list or the more the food is processed, the more likely it is to be a poor food, filled with naked calories. The Rich Food, Poor Food philosophy advocates eating an abundance of *rich foods* and avoiding *poor foods* and allows you to achieve optimal health through micronutrient sufficiency. Think of it as a new-and-improved method of food swapping, replacing micronutrient-poor foods with micronutrient-rich foods. To find hundreds of Rich Food swaps in every aisle of the grocery store to help you on your road to a more micronutrient-rich diet, grab a copy of our book, *Rich Food, Poor Food: The Ultimate Grocery Purchasing System (GPS)* and navigate your way to a healthier you today.

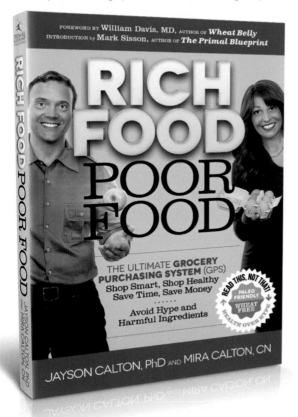

Can you see in Figure 5.2 how simply choosing the *rich food* option of fresh pineapple over the *poor food* option of canned pineapple could increase your chances of micronutrient sufficiency? The rich food option would deposit 531 percent more vitamin C alone into your body's bank account. Imagine how choosing *rich foods* over *poor foods* could increase your intake of all the micronutrients in an entire meal. How about the micronutrient advantage you might gain after a day or even a week? Would you be excited to learn that there may also be an added weight-loss benefit to following our Rich Food, Poor Food philosophy?

RICH FOOD vs. POOR FOOD

Compare our micronutrient bank account when we choose an equal amount of fresh pineapple instead of canned pineapple.

Fresh Pineapple

Canned Pineapple
(juice packed then drained)

YOUR MICRONUTRIENT DEPOSIT

50 kcal	Calories		50 kcal
10 g	Sugar	+20%	12 g
48 mg	+531%	Vitamin C	7.6 mg
18 mcg	+329%	Folate (vitamin B$_9$)	4.2 mcg
.11 mg	+57%	Vitamin B$_6$	.07 mg
35 mcg	+40%	Beta-carotene	.25 mcg

Did You Know?

In studies, vitamin C has been shown to increase fat loss, and beta-carotene is an antioxidant that helps boost immunity.

Did You Know?

Added sugar can spike insulin and increase fat storage.

The fresh pineapple option deposits many more vitamins into your micronutrient bank account.

The canned fruit option increases sugar content while robbing your bank account of essential micro-nutrients that keep you healthy.

Figure 5.2. Rich Food Versus Poor Food

A 2010 study out of Pomona College in California determined that individuals eating unprocessed or minimally processed foods (Rich Foods) burned more calories than those eating highly processed foods (Poor Foods). The researchers fed individuals two meals with the exact same number of calories. The only difference between them was the extent of processing. Half of the participants were given minimally processed cheese sandwiches made from multigrain bread and real cheddar cheese. The other half was fed highly processed foods, which, as we mentioned earlier, is a clear indicator that they would be considered poor food options. These participants ate cheese sandwiches with a processed cheese product on white bread made from refined white flour.

The scientists found that those individuals who ate the minimally processed cheese sandwiches burned nearly twice the number of calories afterward than those who ate the highly processed option. This is because highly processed food requires less effort to digest, which results in fewer calories expended. Therefore, when you choose rich foods over poor foods, avoiding highly processed foods, you enjoy a tastier meal filled with greater amounts of essential micronutrients and burn almost twice as many calories.

● ● ● ● ● ● ● ● ● ● ● ● ● ● ● ● ● ●

Becoming a Nutrivore

Take your first step

The Rich Food, Poor Food philosophy works no matter what type of diet you choose to follow. Our goal is to spread the message that heavily processed, micronutrient-poor foods containing naked calories are detrimental for vegans, vegetarians, low-fat, Primal/paleo, Mediterranean, and low-carbohydrate dieters alike. By encouraging individual choice and viewing nutrition as a science rather than an emotional doctrine, we can together demand that food retailers and restaurants focus on micronutrient-rich healthy food choices over micronutrient-poor processed options for all dietary philosophies.

To identify and unify this powerful new group of health-conscious visionaries, we have coined the term *nutrivore*. Nutrivores seek out rich foods over poor foods and recognize that micronutrient sufficiency is the basis of optimal health, regardless of their preferred diet philosophy. The quality of food is not measured by whether it is plant or animal or low-carbohydrate or low-fat; instead, foods are graded on their ability to supply all of the essential micronutrients. Whether eating an apple or an egg, a nutrivore attempts to obtain the freshest choice with the highest micronutrient content. A nutrivore strives to avoid nutritionally impaired poor foods, such as foods that have traveled long distances or that are highly processed and have little to no nutritional value.

Additionally, nutrivores are environmentally conscious and tolerant of the nutritional preferences of others. Based on their individual diet choices, nutrivores strive to eat as many wild-caught, grass-fed, non-genetically modified, raw, pastured, fresh, organic, and local foods that are rich in essential micronutrients as allowed by their chosen dietary philosophy. Following our Rich Food, Poor Food philosophy is the first step of our three-step plan toward becoming a nutrivore and achieving micronutrient sufficiency in order to maximize weight loss, prevent disease, and enhance your life. It is the same first step that Mira took to reverse her advanced osteoporosis. It worked for her, and it can work for you too. By embracing the Rich Food, Poor Food philosophy, you are taking your first step down the road toward optimal health. Later, you will uncover two additional steps of the nutrivore lifestyle. This brings us to **Naked Fact #6.**

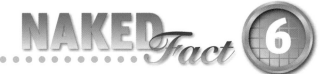

Avoiding heavily processed, Energy-Dense, Nutrient-Poor (EDNP) foods, and utilizing the Rich Food, Poor Food philosophy increases the likelihood of micronutrient sufficiency.

Thus far we have examined micronutrient loss from its beginnings in the soil, through its journey, to your table. Take a few minutes now to review all of the Naked Facts we have uncovered in this chapter. As you read through the Naked Facts, remember how dramatic some of these losses can be. Loss in your food's micronutrients means you're at a greater risk of micronutrient deficiency. Too many micronutrients lost may cause your body's bank account to eventually go bust.

Did you identify any Everyday Micronutrient Depleters (EMDs) in this chapter that are part of your lifestyle? Are there some you may be able to change? Could you increase your micronutrient-sufficiency level by implementing the Rich Food, Poor Food philosophy and take your first critical step in our three-step plan? Like Mira, might you consider eating a fresh, raw salad periodically, making frequent trips to the local farmers' market, or steaming your vegetables? When it comes to micronutrient sufficiency, our experience has taught us that it is not one big change that makes the most difference, but the many little changes you decide to make that add up.

In the next chapter, we're going to revisit Rob, our deflated employee who had just received his first paycheck, to witness what happens when he tries to spend the money he thinks is safely deposited in the bank.

Go online now to download your free nutrivore badge. Together we can make a difference. www.caltonnutrition.com/ nutrivore

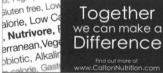

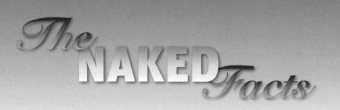

The **NAKED** Facts

- Global distribution, factory farming, food packaging, and preparation methods can cause large percentages of micronutrients to be depleted from your food before it reaches your plate.
- Avoiding heavily processed, Energy-Dense, Nutrient-Poor (EDNP) foods, and utilizing the Rich Food, Poor Food philosophy increases the likelihood of micronutrient sufficiency.

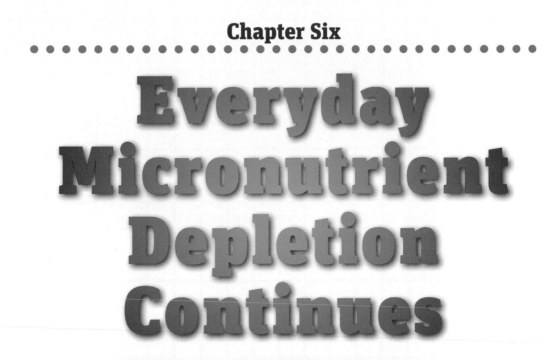

Chapter Six

Everyday Micronutrient Depletion Continues

Don't Count Your Chickens Before They Hatch

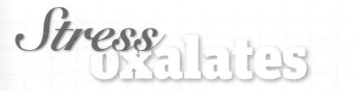

Stress

oxalates

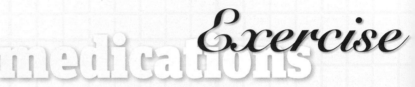

medications Exercise

> **"**Nothing is so good as it seems beforehand.**"**
> —George Eliot

Have you ever heard the proverb "Don't count your chickens before they hatch?" What does it mean? What are the proverbial eggs in your life that you are expecting to hatch into beneficial chickens? Is it a stock investment you are counting on to pay huge dividends? Or is it the money you spend on your daughter's piano lessons so that one day she might perform at Carnegie Hall? No matter what your unhatched eggs represent, the proverb works as a simple warning: While one can hope for certain things, no one can know for sure that they will happen—until they actually do happen.

As we learned in Chapter 5, Everyday Micronutrient Depleters (EMDs) can reduce the amount of micronutrients in your foods before you eat them—from farm to fork. They make it so you can't count on the micronutrients being *banked.* Does your new understanding of global distribution; factory farming; and food packaging, preparation, and processing practices assure you that your chickens will hatch? By avoiding these EMDs, are you guaranteed your micronutrients will be safe and securely deposited in your sufficiency bank account? Will your "health egg" be realized? Or is it possible that we have only uncovered half of the story?

Do you remember Rob, the young man in the previous chapter with the unexpectedly low paycheck? Let's rejoin him and see how he is coming along. Did the awareness of the deductions from his paycheck give Rob the true amount he would have available *after* his check was deposited? After accepting that his check had dwindled, Rob went to his local bank branch and deposited all of the funds. He knew that there wasn't enough money to purchase the television he had hoped for and he would have to use the week's pay to cover his expenses until his next paycheck arrived. Saturday night rolled around and Rob took his girlfriend out to an adorable little bistro that she wanted to try. On Sunday afternoon he went grocery shopping for a few bits. He figured that he would eat lunch out during the workweek with the extra funds he wasn't putting toward the television. Monday, Tuesday, and Wednesday all passed with no surprises. On Thursday afternoon Rob went to lunch with a few coworkers. When the bill came to the table, Rob handed over his debit card. The waitress returned just a few minutes later and quietly explained to Rob that his card had been declined. Embarrassed by the interaction, he quickly handed over his emergency credit card. *What could have gone wrong now?* he thought to himself.

So, where did Rob's money go? How did it vanish after Rob deposited it into his account? Have you ever been surprised when you checked your bank statement and there was less money in the account than you expected? In Rob's case, monthly bank fees caused his account to become overdrawn. Rob's bank removed some of his deposit before he could spend it.

Just like Rob, at some point in your life you may find less money in an account than you expected. Metaphorically these debits, or reductions in already deposited funds, represent the second group of Everyday Micronutrient Depleters (EMDs), which are caused by things that happen *after* your food is swallowed—when you think the micronutrients are "in the bank." These next five sneaky EMDs hide in categories that are common parts of our everyday lives: foods, drinks, medications, daily life, and dietary choices.

You already know the story of micronutrient depletion from the soil to the plate, but what happens *after* the food is swallowed—when we think the micronutrients are "in the bank"? The sad fact is that ingesting micronutrients does not necessarily mean your body will have a chance to use them. In this chapter you will learn the wide variety of EMDs that may be affecting your micronutrient-sufficiency level *after* you eat your food. Every EMD somehow blocks or depletes one or more of the essential micronutrients you need an adequate supply of, each day, to maintain basic health. While each Everyday Micronutrient Depleter (EMD) is important, it is less important which essential micronutrient it blocks. An easy way to think about EMDs is to imagine that they are like shovels full of earth. A few EMDs in your life and you have dug a small hole. Too many EMDs in your life and you have dug a hole so deep you might have a hard time climbing out of it.

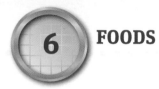

6   FOODS

We have all heard about the ability of the fiber in the foods we eat to lower cholesterol, but how many of us know how or why? This is the way it works: the soluble fiber, a component in some foods, binds (or chelates) to cholesterol-like compounds in the digestive tract, blocking their absorption into the bloodstream. This can ultimately produce a cholesterol-lowering effect in the blood. There are two other components in foods called phytates (phytic acid) and oxalates (oxalic acid) that act in a similar manner as fiber. However, rather than binding to cholesterol, they bind and block the absorption of micronutrients. Basically, that means that phytates and oxalates bind to specific vitamins and minerals and take them out of the body with them.

For this reason they are considered naturally occurring Everyday Micronutrient Depleters (EMDs), and they are found in more foods than you may think. This is how the foods you actually ingest can potentially lower your personal micronutrient-sufficiency level. That's right—some of your food choices may actually be causing additional micronutrient depletion to occur.

Phytates (Phytic Acid)

Whole-grain breads, corn, beans, seeds (including flaxseeds), nuts, grains (cereals), and soy isolates all contain our first EMD, phytates (phytic acid), which can block the absorption of calcium, magnesium, copper, manganese, chromium, iron, zinc, and niacin. In fact, it is phytic acid's blocking of niacin (vitamin B_3) that causes pellagra, a well-known micronutrient-deficiency disease. Additionally, Edward Mellanby, M.D., the discoverer of vitamin D, found that phytates accelerate the metabolism of vitamin D, causing the bone-softening vitamin D–deficiency disease called rickets.

According to a 2010 article in *Wise Traditions,* the quarterly journal of the Weston A. Price Foundation dedicated to exploring the scientific validation of dietary, agricultural, and medical traditions throughout the world, "Research suggests that we will absorb approximately 20 percent more zinc and 60 percent more magnesium from our food when phytate is absent." Additionally, according to a study in the *American Journal of Clinical Nutrition,* when phytates are removed from wheat, iron absorption is increased by 1,160 percent.

Did You Know

A study on Pakistani immigrants in the UK revealed that eating chapati (a Mediterranean-style bread) caused rickets and osteoporosis due to the high levels of phytates in the bread. We can protect ourselves from phytic acid's micronutrient-depleting effects by choosing to eat breads that have been made with sprouted grains. The sprouting of grains, or soaking them in water to transform them from seeds to seedlings, greatly reduces the phytic acid content.

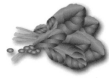

Oxalates (Oxalic Acid)

Spinach, collard greens, sweet potatoes, berries, rhubarb, and beans, including soy, are all foods that are good for you. But these very same foods are also sources of our second EMD, oxalic acid. Oxalates in your food bind to the calcium, magnesium, and iron in that same food (or in foods eaten with it), and block their absorption. In the case of spinach, this results in leaving a mere 2 to 10 percent of the seemingly plentiful supply of iron and calcium, respectively, and 65 percent of the magnesium available for absorption.

Imagine that throughout a day you have eaten one 10-ounce bag of spinach and calculated that you have ingested 281 mg of calcium, 160 mg of magnesium, and 7.7 mg of iron toward your overall sufficiency levels. However, because of the oxalic acid in the spinach, only about 28 mg of calcium, 104 mg of magnesium, and approximately 0.25 mg of iron can actually be absorbed, thereby significantly decreasing the amount of calcium, magnesium, and iron we thought we had working toward our daily sufficiency level.

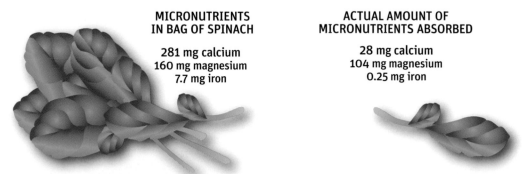

**MICRONUTRIENTS
IN BAG OF SPINACH**

281 mg calcium
160 mg magnesium
7.7 mg iron

**ACTUAL AMOUNT OF
MICRONUTRIENTS ABSORBED**

28 mg calcium
104 mg magnesium
0.25 mg iron

Vegetarians and vegans must be especially aware of oxalates. These two groups often eat large amounts of soy protein and spinach. Too many oxalates in a diet can not only lead to severe micronutrient depletion, but can also lead to kidney stones.

Now, if we've just mentioned some of your favorite foods, don't worry. After all, when eaten in moderation, both of the aforementioned EMDs may also prove to have several beneficial aspects.

We already mentioned one of fiber's most famous benefits—its cholesterol-lowering effect. Phytic acid (phytates) may also be beneficial in two ways. It has antioxidant properties, and it may be beneficial for diabetics by lowering blood glucose response. Phytic acid also releases inositol, a micronutrient that may reduce depression. Additionally, both phytates and oxalates have been suggested to have anticancer components. In animal studies, phytic acid showed a protective action in carcinogenesis.

You do not have to boycott different foods or change how you make your favorite salad. The mysteries of nature are far from being revealed and the benefits of these EMDs may someday far outweigh their micronutrient-depleting effects. What we want you to be aware of is this: **Many of the micronutrients that you think you are making available to your body may actually be negated by EMDs found in the very foods you are eating.**

As with the proverbial chickens, we can't assume that being micronutrient sufficient is as simplistic as calculating all of the micronutrients you eat and calling it a day. As we are learning, many factors must be evaluated before an accurate, personal micronutrient-sufficiency level can be assessed.

TABLE 6.1. EVERYDAY MICRONUTRIENT DEPLETERS IN FOOD

EMDS IN FOOD	WHERE IT IS FOUND	WEAKNESS? CONCERNS?	BENEFITS
Phytates (Phytic Acid)	Whole-grain breads, corn, beans, seeds of (including flaxseeds) nuts, grains (cereals), and soy isolates	Can block the absorption vitamin B$_3$ (niacin), calcium, magnesium, chromium, copper, iron, manganese, and zinc, and accelerates the metabolism of vitamin D	Antioxidant, anticancer components, lowers blood glucose response, releases inositol
Oxalates (Oxalic Acid)	Spinach, collard greens, sweet potatoes, quinoa, rhubarb, nuts, celery, green beans, rutabagas, wheat bran, wheat germ, soy products, and beans	Binds to calcium, magnesium, and iron, which blocks their absorption	Anticancer components

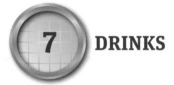 **7** **DRINKS**

Like foods, there are many EMDs hiding in our drinks. Many Americans enjoy alcoholic beverages, soft drinks, sport drinks, energy drinks, tea, and coffee. However, enjoying these daily pleasures contributes to micronutrient depletion.

There are six common EMDs hiding in our beverages: alcohol, phosphoric acid, caffeine, tannins, and our old friends, refined white sugar and high fructose corn syrup (HFCS). They all leach, deplete, or inhibit previously ingested micronutrients from nourishing your body. Some beverages contain only one of these EMDs, while others can potentially contain all six. Let's begin by examining alcohol, the first EMD on our list.

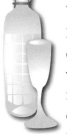

Alcohol

Does the pop of a champagne cork put a smile on your face? Does watching the Sunday football game usually include a couple of beers? Drinking alcohol in moderation, which includes all types of beers, wines, and spirits, is widely accepted and enjoyed in our society. But what is alcohol doing to our overall ability to achieve micronutrient sufficiency? Much has been said lately in the newspapers and on television about the potentially positive health benefits of low to moderate drinking. However, along with those benefits you will receive some unpublicized micronutrient-depleting consequences.

After our food is eaten it goes through a digestive process in order to release the essential micronutrients that are trapped inside. To achieve this, the pancreas secretes digestive enzymes to break down the food into usable micronutrients, which makes them available for absorption and utilization. Alcohol inhibits this breakdown of micronutrients by decreasing digestive enzyme secretion. But that's not all. This EMD also impairs absorption of the micronutrients that were made available for absorption by the digestive enzymes, such as thiamine (vitamin B_1) and folic acid (vitamin B_9). It does this by damaging the cells that line the stomach and intestines, and disabling transport of some micronutrients into the blood.

Now we don't want you to think we expect you to change how you celebrate, socialize, or unwind in your spare time. Our goal is to point out the necessity to replenish micronutrients that may become depleted if one partakes in the consumption of alcohol.

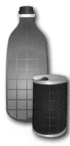

Phosphoric Acid

The second EMD that may be contained in drinks is phosphoric acid. Phosphoric acid is mainly found in carbonated soft drinks, carbonated energy drinks, and some flavored waters. This ingredient is a chemical additive often used to help keep the carbonated bubbles from going flat and/or to cut the sweetness of the 7 to 10 teaspoons of sugar found in most non-diet or sugar-sweetened formulas.

Research shows phosphoric acid can negatively affect calcium in two ways: it increases its excretion and impairs its absorption. Our bodies are always trying to maintain a one-to-one balance between phosphorus and calcium. When phosphoric acid is introduced into our system, calcium from our bones and teeth is released into our bloodstream to balance it. When the phosphoric acid is released through urination, the calcium goes with it. This is how the seemingly harmless habit of drinking anything that contains phosphoric acid may lead to essential micronutrient loss by means of excretion.

In the stomach, hydrochloric acid is needed to help digest our food and absorb micronutrients, especially calcium. Phosphoric acid is known to neutralize hydrochloric acid in our stomachs and bind with calcium and magnesium to form salts, thus prohibiting our body's absorption of both. Although these processes have been studied, the extent and effect of these micronutrient losses have yet to be determined.

Caffeine

Caffeine can be found in caffeinated soft drinks, coffee drinks, tea, cocoa beverages, and energy drinks and is the third EMD found in our drinks category. While it is accepted that caffeine can cause calcium depletion through urination, many scientists believe that adequate calcium consumption can offset this potentially negative effect. You may want to consider supplementation of calcium if the third EMD, caffeine, is present in your daily routine. Remember, only 30 percent of the individuals in the USDA study were sufficient in calcium before drinking caffeinated beverages. These statistics did not take into consideration the amount leached through the intake of caffeine or any of the EMDs we have discussed thus far. While caffeine has also been shown to have some medicinal benefits, when evaluating your chances for micronutrient sufficiency for calcium, do not forget the need for extra calcium if you consume this EMD.

CAFFEINE EYE-OPENER

- More than 50 percent of Americans over age eighteen drink coffee every day.

- Seventy percent of the U.S. population is deficient in calcium.

- Only 43 percent of Americans report taking a supplement that contains calcium.

- Most multivitamins contain barely any calcium.

- Your Grande Vanilla Frappuccino has a whopping 60 grams of sugar —three times the daily intake recommended by the American Heart Association.

Tannins

When you are savoring your morning coffee or tea, you are not only consuming the third EMD caffeine, but you are also drinking in the fourth EMD found in this category—tannins. While enjoying a glass of red wine you may not only be sipping in the EMD, alcohol, but that dry, mouth-puckering sensation is letting you know that tannins are also present. Like oxalates and phytates (from our foods category), tannins are naturally occurring molecules that bind with micronutrients in the intestine and decrease their absorption.

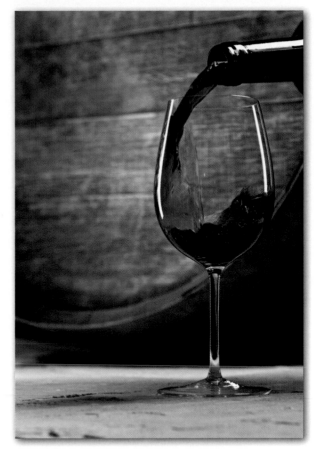

As is the case with many of the EMDs we are examining, tannins can be found in both drinks and foods. In addition to coffee, tea, and red wine, these menacing molecules are found in more places than you might think—fruits, berries, beans, fruit juices, spices, and nuts all contain varying levels of this EMD. Tannins negatively influence iron and calcium absorption, and some studies indicate that magnesium and zinc may also be affected. It is recommended that individuals who are susceptible to iron deficiency avoid tannins at mealtimes, to allow for proper absorption of this essential micronutrient.

Refined White Sugar

The fifth EMD potentially found in your drinks is refined white sugar. We have already identified refined white sugar as a common micronutrient-stripping ingredient in many Energy-Dense, Nutrient-Poor (EDNP) foods. In this section we will examine it as an EMD.

Refined white sugar is used in some soft drinks, juice drinks, coffee drinks, cocoa drinks, sport drinks, energy drinks, flavored teas, and many other beverages. It is also abundant in the food you eat. It can be found in obvious places such as baked goods, ice cream, and candy. Did you know that it can also be found in your mayonnaise, ketchup, salad dressing, and seasoning mixes?

Did You Know

A recent study out of the University of Bordeaux, France, concluded scientifically that refined sugar, including both fructose and sucrose, is far more addictive than cocaine. Food manufacturers have over twenty names they use to hide sugar on your food labels. Don't be fooled. Take a closer look for these sinister aliases.

Agave nectar	Glucose
Brown sugar	High fructose corn syrup
Cane crystals	Honey
Cane sugar	Invert sugar
Caramel	Lactose
Corn sweetener	Maltose
Corn syrup	Malt syrup
Crystalline fructose	Molasses
Dextrose	Raw sugar
Evaporated cane juice	Sucrose
Fructose	Syrup
Fruit juice concentrates	

If you thought the increase in the rate of soft drink consumption in Chapter 5 was startling, sit down, because that was nothing. In the last twenty years, we have increased sugar consumption in the U.S. from 26 pounds to 135 pounds of sugar per person per year! That is more than one-third of a pound of sugar per person per day. Sugar is commonly referred to as the white devil or the anti-nutrient because, unlike many of the other EMDs, there is no evidence of any health or nutritional benefit of refined white sugar. It has both micronutrient-depleting effects as well as micronutrient-blocking effects.

Sugar upsets the mineral relationships in your body. It can cause chromium and copper deficiencies and blocks the absorption of calcium and magnesium. For decades, sugar has been responsible for weakening the human immune system. In order to have a healthy immune system your body requires vitamin C. This vitamin C is needed in high doses for your white blood cells to gobble up a bad bacteria or virus.

Vitamin C and glucose—a type of sugar—have similar chemical structures. Much like in our earlier discussion about the competition between micronutrients, vitamin C and glucose also compete for entry into your cells. In fact, even slightly elevated blood sugar levels can weaken your immune system. It is due to these micronutrient-depleting factors and hundreds of other negative consequences that the American Heart Association reduced the recommended daily intake of sugar in August 2009 to a maximum of 6 teaspoons of refined white sugar per day. Each can of sugar-sweetened regular soft drinks contains approximately 8 teaspoons. This means that the American Heart Association recommendation would not allow an individual to drink even one regular soft drink per day.

TRY THIS!

Spoon out 8 level teaspoons of sugar to show your children how much sugar is in a 12-ounce can of regular soda. Spoon out an incredible 11 level teaspoons for a 20-ounce bottle. Can you imagine how much sugar you're giving your child (or yourself) when you order the 44-ounce soda to enjoy at your favorite movie theater?

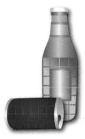

High Fructose Corn Syrup (HFCS)

We have already identified high fructose corn syrup (HFCS) as a common ingredient in many EDNP foods and labeled it an EMD for the role it plays in soil erosion. We are now going to examine HFCS for a third reason. High fructose corn syrup is the final EMD that depletes our essential micronutrients in the drinks category.

As we discussed earlier, HFCS is found in a variety of beverages, including soda, energy drinks, juices, and alcoholic mixers. It acts as an EMD, because in order to use the fructose in high fructose corn syrup, your body must contribute a number of minerals such as chromium, magnesium, zinc, and copper. The more HFCS you consume, the more your body becomes depleted of these essential minerals.

Recent studies on HFCS in soft drinks shed light on the seriousness of this EMD. While federal law mandates that HFCS not exceed 55 percent fructose (the ingredient depleting our micronutrients), a recent study in the journal *Obesity* tested the HFCS levels of twenty-three sweetened beverages and found levels exceeding 55 percent. The researchers found that many soft drinks contain HFCS with fructose levels as high as 65 percent. Remember, the greater the amount of fructose, the greater risk for micronutrient depletion.

HARD TIMES FOR SOFT DRINKS

 In the United States the consumption of carbonated soft drinks has exploded over the past forty years and has more than doubled since 1971.

 Soft drinks account for more than one out of every four beverages consumed in America.

 As the single most consumed beverage in America, soft drinks provide more than 7 percent of all calories, according to the National Health and Nutrition Examination.

 Soft drinks provide the average twelve- to nineteen-year-old boy with about 15 teaspoons of refined sugar a day and the average girl with about 10 teaspoons a day.

 The manufacturers of soft drinks are the largest single user of refined sugar in the country.

According to the Childhood Obesity Research Center at the University of Southern California, high fructose intake can cause an increased risk for high blood pressure, kidney stones, fatty liver, and fat gain.

It isn't just the coffee or the soft drinks that are loaded with refined white sugar and high fructose corn syrup; many of the "healthy" drinks are just as guilty. A single bottle of Energy Citrus Vitamin Water contains 33 grams of sugar, while a bottle of SoBe Green Tea contains a whopping 61 grams. Parents often try to steer their children away from the soft drinks, and for this we applaud them. However, what about that juice box? Even 100-percent real fruit juice contains a lot of natural sugar and tannins. Although natural sugars are not the same as refined white sugar, they still raise insulin levels. Insulin is a fat-storage hormone, and high levels of insulin can contribute to type 2 diabetes.

The medical community substantiates that it is far more beneficial to eat your fruit than to drink it—children and adults alike. Fruit does more to fill you up and has far fewer calories than juice. Many bottled juices that are advertised to children are far worse than their natural juice counterparts. They may contain "some fruit juice," but when you see that phrase on a label, you should really be reading it as, *contains large quantities of refined white sugar and/or high fructose corn syrup*. Here are a few examples of the sugar and HFCS content of beverages available in the "juice" aisle of grocery stores.

Minute Maid Cran-Grape Juice: An 8-ounce serving contains almost 10 teaspoons of sugar. High fructose corn syrup and refined white sugar have been added.

Tropicana Grape Juice Beverage: An 8-ounce serving contains almost 10 teaspoons of sugar. High fructose corn syrup has been added. An individual bottle is 15.2 ounces. This creates a bottle with almost 20 teaspoons of sugar packed inside!

Did You Know

According to research at the Hospital for Sick Children in Canada, penicillin, in solution form, is 80 percent sugar. Three of the other top ten children's medications came in above 60 percent sugar. This gives a whole new meaning to Mary Poppins's magic spoonful.

HOW MUCH LIQUID CANDY ARE YOU DRINKING?

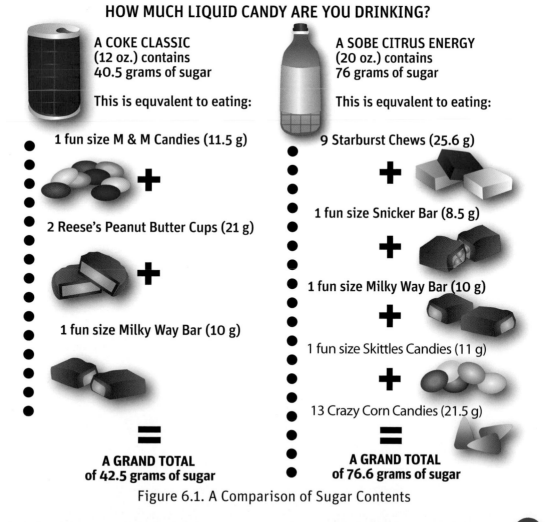

A COKE CLASSIC (12 oz.) contains 40.5 grams of sugar

This is equvalent to eating:

1 fun size M & M Candies (11.5 g)

+

2 Reese's Peanut Butter Cups (21 g)

+

1 fun size Milky Way Bar (10 g)

=

A GRAND TOTAL of 42.5 grams of sugar

A SOBE CITRUS ENERGY (20 oz.) contains 76 grams of sugar

This is equvalent to eating:

9 Starburst Chews (25.6 g)

+

1 fun size Snicker Bar (8.5 g)

+

1 fun size Milky Way Bar (10 g)

+

1 fun size Skittles Candies (11 g)

+

13 Crazy Corn Candies (21.5 g)

=

A GRAND TOTAL of 76.6 grams of sugar

Figure 6.1. A Comparison of Sugar Contents

Finally, this discussion would be incomplete without mentioning sports and energy drinks, which are the fastest-growing beverages in the United States and can contain large amounts of both refined white sugar and HFCS. The millions of athletes who choose to replenish their electrolytes with such drinks may also be filling their fit bodies with nearly 60 grams of sugar per 32-ounce bottle.

Consumers spent 4.8 billion dollars on energy drinks in 2008, an increase of more than 400 percent from 2003!

According to the latest research from Mintel International Group, a market research firm, consumers spent 4.8 billion dollars on energy drinks in 2008, an increase of more than 400 percent from 2003! While millions of people around the world use these drinks to combat fatigue, the levels of phosphoric acid, caffeine, sugar, and HFCS in these drinks can do more to your body than give you a temporary jolt.

While a cup of coffee may serve up 100 mg of caffeine, many of the energy drinks zap you with almost double that amount. That same energy drink can contain up to 60 grams or 14 teaspoons of sugar. It may contain HFCS and phosphoric acid as well. Do you see how these EMD factors are adding up? At universities around the country, college students consume these drinks to stay up and study at night. However, they are also enjoying these beverages at bars mixing them with alcohol. When this happens, bartenders are serving up five of the drink category's EMDs in a single collegiate concoction!

Have you ever ordered a dessert coffee, perhaps an Irish coffee? An Irish coffee has alcohol, caffeine, tannins, and sugar. How about a cosmopolitan martini? A classic cosmo calls for vodka, Rose's Lime Juice (a sugary lime-flavored syrup made by Dr. Pepper), and cranberry juice (most likely filled with tannins, HFCS, and sugar).

Sometimes the EMDs may be less obvious. You may go to dinner and have a cocktail at the bar while waiting for your table to be ready. At dinner you enjoy wine, and after the meal you have a cup of coffee. As you can see, you may be enjoying more of these drinks-related EMDs than you previously thought. This brings us to **Naked Fact #7.**

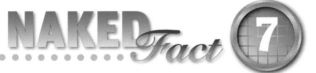

Many of the foods and drinks one may choose
every day can block or deplete micronutrients,
thereby reducing micronutrient sufficiency.

8   MEDICATIONS

> **"**What's remarkable is how most conventional doctors have it completely backward when it comes to vitamins and minerals . . . Doctors tend to only use vitamins if medications don't work. They should be prescribing the vitamins in the first place . . . Imagine a drug that could cure within days or weeks a fatal disease using a very small dose, without toxicity and with a 100% success rate. Such a drug does not exist and will never exist. But that is the power and potential of nutrients.**"**
> —Mark Hyman, M.D.

While the EMDs in the categories of foods and drinks are, for the most part, everyday items that we can all choose, the EMDs in the medications group can be a bit more complicated. Many of us are told by physicians that prescription medications are necessary to treat some medical conditions. Others choose to treat themselves by turning to over-the-counter options. Either way, our micronutrient sufficiency is being directly attacked by the medications we take.

Prescription Medications

According to a 2010 report by the CDC's National Center for Health Statistics, one-half of Americans take at least one prescription medication. One out of every five children and nine out of every ten adults age sixty and over take at least one prescription drug. In fact, almost 40 percent of older Americans take five or more prescription drugs per month.

With such a large percentage of the population taking prescription medications, it is extremely important that we discuss what effect they might have on one's personal micronutrient sufficiency.

According to Hyla Cass, M.D., author of *Supplement Your Prescription: What Your Doctor Doesn't Know About Nutrition,* "Drug-induced nutrient depletion is far more common than we thought." Yet, it seems that most of the individuals who take these medications are unaware of this serious side effect. While the prescriptions in America may come with "may cause drowsiness" warnings, they do not come with "causes micronutrient depletion" warnings.

However, according to Dr. Cass, this is not the case throughout the world. She explains, "Health Canada, which is the federal department responsible for helping Canadians maintain and improve their health, requires that manufacturers of statin drugs include warnings about related CoQ_{10} deficiencies."

There have been numerous studies on long-term drug use and micronutrient deficiencies, and there is conclusive evidence that states that prescription drugs deplete vital micronutrients in three distinct ways. First, as is the case with Ritalin and Adderall, which are prescribed for attention deficit disorder, some prescribed medications reduce appetite. If you aren't particularly hungry, you may decide to eat only once or twice a day, which decreases the likelihood of receiving enough of the essential micronutrients required for good health. In contrast, other drugs, including antipsychotics, antidepressants, and steroids, cause blood sugar swings, which in turn cause cravings for simple carbohydrates like white bread, pasta, and sugary snacks—processed EDNP foods that contain little to no micronutrient value.

Finally, we have medications that *directly* deplete the micronutrients from your body. Let's examine three micronutrients, the prescription drugs that directly deplete them, and some of the effects of their depletion.

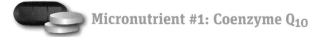 ## Micronutrient #1: Coenzyme Q_{10}

As our first example in illustrating the direct micronutrient-depleting effect of prescription medication, we will use the micronutrient coenzyme Q_{10} (CoQ_{10}). This accessory micronutrient plays a critical role in the synthesis of ATP (an energy molecule that fuels all cells) and is crucial in the protection against free radicals. Remember, in Chapter 5 we stated that free radicals are pretty much just like their name implies—free moving, unattached electrons that crash into other molecules, causing other electrons to detach and become free radicals. The more free radicals there are, the more cellular damage is done.

Initially, a deficiency of this crucial compound can make someone lethargic. Coenzyme Q_{10} can be depleted by a variety of different drugs that include antidepressants, cholesterol-lowering statin drugs, beta-blockers, antidiabetic drugs, and antihypertensive drugs. (Lipitor, which is in the top 10 percent of all drugs sold in the United States, would be included here.) According to a report from the National Center for Health Statistics, nearly 45 percent of people over the age of sixty now take cholesterol-lowering prescription medicines—a statistic that has more than doubled since 1999.

Most cardiologists recommend their patients take CoQ_{10} because the heart requires a great deal of it for energy production; some studies suggest that congestive heart failure is primarily a CoQ_{10} deficiency disease. Would it shock you to discover that drugs prescribed to heart patients result in lowered levels of CoQ_{10}? While treating a patient with a poor heart, physicians are prescribing prescription medications that deplete CoQ_{10}, a micronutrient known to be essential to that same organ.

Another benefit of CoQ_{10} is its ability to boost the effectiveness of other antioxidants and destroy free radicals. It is so powerful that it can actually stop the harmful effects of some toxic medications. In fact, it can stop the toxic effects of beta-blockers. Wait a second. Did you catch that? It can stop beta-blockers' toxic side effects. This would be a good thing, of course, if we didn't already know that beta-blockers deplete CoQ_{10}.

While we would never tell an individual to stop taking a medication without first discussing it with their physician, we want you to be aware of the array of medications that act as micronutrient depleters. A small deficiency in CoQ_{10} can turn into an even greater deficiency when medications are prescribed. Do not let this happen to you. Examine in Table 6.2 (on page 117) which of the micronutrients are being depleted by your medications and replenish those vital micronutrients

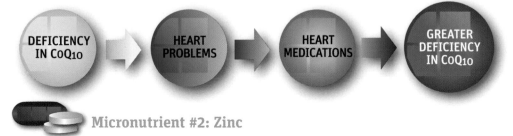

Micronutrient #2: Zinc

Micronutrient deficiency of zinc is widespread. Deficiency rates increase with age, due to poor absorption of micronutrients in older adults and diets high in phytate-containing processed grains. Zinc deficiency can commonly be seen in conditions such as diabetes, liver and kidney diseases, macular degeneration, and melanomas. A zinc deficiency can be detrimental because zinc is needed for the cell activity of more than 300 enzymes. It detoxifies alcohol, aids in protein digestion, regulates gene expression, aids in regulating insulin receptors, and facilitates your thyroid hormones. It can protect your DNA from damage, and it greatly enhances immunity. Many medications that you may be taking inhibit the absorption of zinc. These can include oral contraceptives, ACE inhibitors, diuretics, antiulcer medications, as well as cholesterol-lowering drugs.

Micronutrient #3: Folic Acid (Vitamin B9)

Let's change our focus to folic acid (vitamin B9), which is one of the most common deficiencies in America. While many women learn during pregnancy that supplementation of folic acid is important to decrease the risk of spina bifida, they are unaware of the consequences of stopping this crucial supplementation. According to the U.S. Centers for Disease Control and Prevention, approximately 80 percent of U.S. women use oral contraceptives at some point between the ages of fifteen and forty-four. These medications leach folic acid.

The same can be said of the many hormone-replacement therapy drugs containing estrogen. Folic acid deficiencies have been linked to hysterectomies and cervical dysplasia in the United States.

Folic acid, by means of lowering homocysteine, may also aid in the prevention of osteoporosis. A depleted level of folic acid, due to birth control pills, may result in osteoporosis, which ironically, is also commonly treated by the same physicians who prescribed the birth control in the first place. Confusing, right? Let's pause here to review. In order to avoid pregnancy, one might take birth control pills. These birth control pills may cause lowered folic acid levels. Lowered folic acid levels may cause osteoporosis.

Folic acid has also been proven to aid in the prevention of heart disease. It shouldn't surprise us that recent studies have linked folic acid–depleting oral contraceptives to plaque buildup in the arteries. According to a 2008 study conducted by researchers at the University of Ghent, Belgium, and presented at a conference of the American Heart Association, every ten years of oral contraceptive use correlated with a 20 to 30 percent increase in plaque buildup. You may also find it ironic that while folic acid has been shown to alleviate the pain of arthritis, many arthritic medications, which are primarily anti-inflammatory drugs, actually deplete levels of folic acid. This means that the same drug used to reduce the pain you feel from arthritis actually depletes folic acid, which causes the arthritis to feel worse.

Is all of this soaking in? We do not believe that, in most cases, the medications themselves are the causes of the original conditions or diseases. Physicians, upon diagnosis, prescribe medications in an attempt to control existing conditions or diseases. As we have learned from some of the most brilliant minds in nutritional medicine, most, if not all, modern conditions and diseases can be traced to micronutrient deficiency. The medicines we take simply act to further deplete us of micronutrients. In some cases, they deplete us of the very same micronutrient whose depletion most likely caused the condition or disease in the first place. In this way the medications them-

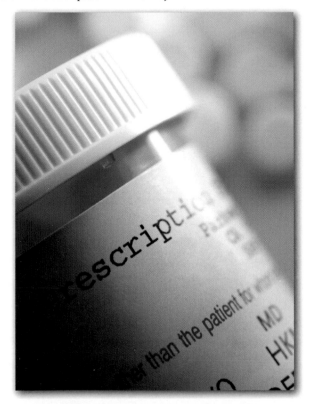

selves now become Everyday Micronutrient Depleters (EMDs), potentially causing an exacerbation of the original condition, or initiate an entirely new one.

It is interesting to think about how many millions of prescriptions might not have been needed if specific micronutrients had never become deficient or were properly replenished. Mehmet Oz, M.D., stresses, "In evaluating patients' symptoms, we doctors must assess whether symptoms are due to the illness, to side effects of the drugs, or to drug-induced nutrient depletion. Considering the inadequate nutritional status of most people, consider that the illness itself may even be due, at least in part, to nutrient deficiency."

TABLE 6.2. PRESCRIPTION DRUGS AND MICRONUTRIENT DEPLETIONS

DRUG	INDICATION FOR USE	MICRONUTRIENTS DEPLETED
Opiates Hydrocodone, Acetaminophen *(Tylenol)*	Pain relief	Folic acid, vitamin C, iron, potassium
Statin Drugs Atorvastatin *(Lipitor),* Fluvastatin *(Lescol),* Lovastatin *(Mevacor),* Pravastatin *(Pravachol),* Rosuvastatin *(Crestor),* Simvastatin *(Zocor)*	Lower cholesterol	Coenzyme Q_{10}
ACE Inhibitors Lisinopril *(Prinivil, Zestril),* Ramipril *(Altace),* Quinapril *(Accupril),* Enalapril *(Vasotec)*	High blood pressure	Zinc
Thiazide Diuretics Hydrochlorothiazide *(Esidrix, Hydrodiuril, Oretic)*	High blood pressure	Vitamin D, calcium, magnesium, phosphorus, potassium, zinc, coenzyme Q_{10}
Beta-Blocking Drugs Atenolol *(Tenormin, Senorman),* Nadalol *(Corgard),* Metoprolol *(Lopressor, Toprol XL)*	High blood pressure	Coenzyme Q_{10}, chromium, melatonin
Loop Diuretics Bumetanide *(Bumex, Burinex),* Ethacrynic acid *(Edecrin),* Furosemide *(Lasix),* Torsemide *(Demadex)*	High blood pressure, heart failure	B_1, B_6, vitamin C, calcium, folic acid, magnesium, phosphorus, potassium, zinc, iron, chromium
Proton Pump Inhibitors Lansoprazole *(Prevacid),* Omeprazole *(Losec, Prilosec),* Rabeprazole *(Aciphex),* Pantoprazole *(Pantoloc, Protonix)*	GERD; severe gastric ulceration	Beta-carotene, vitamin C, B_1, B_{12}, folic acid, calcium, zinc
Biguanide Metformin *(Glucophage)*	Diabetes, prediabetes	Folic acid, B_{12}, B_1
Bisphosphonates Alendronate *(Fosamax),* Risendronate *(Actonel),* Ibandronate *(Boniva),* Tiludronate *(Skelid)*	Osteoporosis	Calcium, magnesium, phosphorus
Fluoroquinolone Antibiotics Ciprofloxacin *(Cipro),* Enoxacin *(Penetrex),* Gatifloxacin *(Tequin),* Levofloxacin *(Levaquin),* Lomefloxacin *(Maxaquin),* Moxifloxacin *(Avelox),* Norfloxacin *(Noroxin),* Ofloxacin *(Floxin),* Sparfloxacin *(Zagam),* Trovafloxacin *(Trovan)*	Bacterial infection	Biotin, B_1, B_2, B_3, B_6, B_{12}, healthy intestinal bacteria, calcium, iron, magnesium, zinc

DRUG	INDICATION FOR USE	MICRONUTRIENTS DEPLETED
Potassium Sparing Diuretics Amiloride *(Midamor)*, Spironolactone (Aldactone), Triamterene *(Maxzide, Dyazide, Dyrenium)*	Heart failure, high blood pressure	Calcium, magnesium, phosphorus
Conjugated Estrogen *Alora, Cenestin, Climara, Estinyl, Estrace, Estraderm, Estratab, FemPatch, Menest, Ogen, Premarin, Premphase, Prempro, Vivelle;* Estrogen-containing Oral Contraceptives	Hormone replacement therapy (HRT)	B_6, vitamin D, calcium, magnesium, zinc, folic acid, B_{12}
Beta-2 Adrenergic Receptor Agonists Albuterol *(salbutamol, Proventil, Ventolin)*, Bitolterol *(Tornalate)*, Isoetharine, Levalbuterol *(Xopenex)*, Metaproterenol *(Alupent)*, Pirbuterol *(Maxair)*, Salmeterol *(Serevent)*, Terbutaline *(Brethine)*	Asthma, COPD	Potassium, and possibly calcium, magnesium, phosphorus
Corticosteroids Cortisone *(Cortone)*, Hydrocortisone [*Cortisol*] *(Cortef, Hydrocortone)*, Prednisone *(Deltasone, Meticorten, Orasone, Panasol-S)*, Prednisolone *(Delta-Cortef, Prelone, Pediapred)*, Triamcinolone *(Aristocort, Atolone, Kenacort)*, Methylprednisolone *(Medrol)*, Fluticasone *(Flonase, Veramyst)*, Beclomethasone *(Beconase, Qvar, Vancenase, Vanceril)*	Severe inflammation, autoimmune disease, immune system suppression, asthma, allergic rhinitis	Beta-carotene, B_6, folic acid, vitamin C, vitamin D, calcium, magnesium, potassium, selenium, zinc, melatonin
Calcium Channel Blocking Drugs Amlodipine *(Norvasc)*, Felodipine *(Plendil)*, Nifedipine *(Procardia, Adalat)*, Nimodipine *(Nimotop)*, Nisoldipine *(Sular)*	High blood pressure	Vitamin D
Sulfonylureas Glyburide *(Diabeta, Glynase, Micronase)*, Glipizide *(Glucotrol)*, Glimepiride *(Amaryl)*	Diabetes	Coenzyme Q_{10}
Cardiac Glycoside Digoxin *(Lanoxicaps, Lanoxin)*	Heart failure, arrhythmias	Calcium, magnesium, phosphorus, potassium, B_1

DRUG	INDICATION FOR USE	MICRONUTRIENTS DEPLETED
Antibiotics Amoxicillin *(Amoxil, Trimox),* Erythromycin *(Robimycin),* Azithromycin, *(Zithromax),* Clarithromycin *(Biaxin)*	Infection	Healthy intestinal bacteria, B_1, B_2, B_3, B_6, B_{12}, vitamin K, folic acid, biotin, inositol
Psychoactive Drugs Benzodiazepines *(Valium, Xanax, Ativan, Klonopin),* and SSRIs *(Prozac, Paxil)*	Antianxiety	Vitamin C, B_{12}, coenzyme Q_{10}
Tricyclic Antidepressants Amitriptyline, Doxepin, Desipramine *(Norpramin)* Imipramine *(Tofranil, Tofranil-PM),* Asendin, Elavil, Protriptyline *(Vivactil)*	Depression	Coenzyme Q_{10}, B_2, sodium

Source: InviteHealth.com, Natural Medicines Comprehensive Database University of Maryland

What does Jeffrey Blumberg, Ph.D., director of the Jean Mayer USDA Human Nutrition Research Center on Aging at Tufts University (HNRCA), have to say about drug-induced micronutrient depletion?

> One other thing that I would stress is that older people as a group take more medications more frequently and for longer periods of time than any other age group. And yet we know there are many drug-induced nutritional deficiencies. This is a problem that is significantly underappreciated and that often goes unrecognized despite the simple solution available to prevent it. It is rarely diagnosed, in part because many of the sub-clinical nutrient deficiencies induced by pharmacotherapies lead to signs like lethargy and bone pain, which are simply attributed to aging. But these signs and symptoms are not caused by aging but by the use of multiple drugs prescribed for long periods, often the patient's lifetime. There is an extensive database of drug actions that impair nutrient bioavailability and alter nutrient metabolism and excretion. For example, cimetidine lowers the absorption of folic acid, statins inhibit the synthesis of coenzyme Q_{10}, and isoniazid reduces the hydroxylation of vitamin D.

Over-the-Counter (OTC) Medications

Have you ever wondered how an antacid works in your body? Do you take aspirin at the first sign of a headache? Do you rub hydrocortisone cream on your inflamed skin to treat your minor rash? How many times a week do you use an over-the-counter medication? While the number of people taking prescription medications is high, millions more use their non-prescription OTC counterparts. Over-the-counter medications are our second EMD in the medication group and include common remedies such as aspirin, acetaminophen, nonsteroidal anti-inflammatory drugs (NSAIDs), antacids, laxatives, and H2 blockers (found in heartburn medication). Although they may seem harmless because you can buy them without a prescription, these popular medications can deplete a wide variety of micronutrients and can be some of the most overlooked Everyday Micronutrient Depleters (EMDs).

According to Dr. Jeffrey Blumberg of Tufts University, vitamin B_{12}, folic acid, and calcium require an acidic environment to be absorbed. If pH levels are elevated, as they are by antacids, which are used by half of the American adult population, absorption of these micronutrients can decrease by more than half. He recommends taking a supplement containing B_{12}, folic acid, and calcium if one takes antacids.

Another class of over-the-counter medication used for heartburn is H2 blockers. This class of medication includes brand names such as Axid, Pepcid, Tagamet, Zantac, and others. These over-the-counter medications can deplete calcium, folic acid, iron, B_{12}, vitamin D, and zinc. Below is a list compiled by the University of Maryland Medical Center of micronutrients depleted by means of antacids, along with the related side effect of such depletion.

Calcium: Bone loss leading to possible osteoporosis, bone pain, muscle cramps, irregular heartbeat

Copper: Anemia, changes in structure of hair, heart damage, growth retardation, impaired bones, lung disease

Iron: Anemia, weakened immunity, dizziness, fatigue, irregular heartbeat

Magnesium: Muscle cramps, heart irregularities, insomnia, high blood pressure, diabetes, osteoporosis

Phosphorus: Bone pain, mental confusion, anorexia, anemia, low immunity, respiratory difficulties, seizures

Potassium: Loss of appetite, nausea, drowsiness, excessive thirst, irrational behavior, fatigue, muscle pain, weakness especially in lower legs, irregular heartbeat

Zinc: Loss of appetite or taste, impaired immunity, growth retardation, skin changes, increased susceptibility to infection

Did you notice how serious some of these deficiencies could be? Knowing this, why would anyone consider taking an antacid, or any over-the-counter medication, without properly replenishing his or her depleted micronutrients through diet and/or supplementation? It may interest you to know that many prescription medications can cause heartburn, and if heartburn is chronic, it is usually a symptom of something more serious. By taking a micronutrient-depleting antacid you may be masking the symptom of something far worse, while creating a gap in your micronutrient sufficiency where more illness can grow.

How many times have you heard that it could be good for your heart to take an aspirin every day? While this may help your heart, it is also depleting folic acid, vitamin C, iron, and potassium.

Are you taking any of the over-the-counter medications listed in Table 6.3? Which micronutrients could they be depleting from your body? Could avoiding these depletions increase your personal micronutrient sufficiency and bring you closer to achieving optimal health? Just like their prescription drug counterparts, the OTC medications you take deplete micronutrients.

TABLE 6.3. OVER-THE-COUNTER MEDICATIONS AND POSSIBLE MICRONUTRIENT DEPLETIONS

MEDICATION	INDICATION FOR USAGE	MICRONUTRIENTS DEPLETED
NSAIDs Ibuprofen *(Advil, Motrin)*, Naproxen *(Aleve, Midol)*	Inflammation, pain	Folic acid, iron, melatonin, zinc
Aspirin *Bufferin, St. Joseph,* Bayer	Pain, inflammation, fever (adults)	Folic acid, vitamin C, iron, potassium, zinc
Acetaminophen *Tylenol*	Pain, fever	Coenzyme Q_{10}, glutathione
Antacids *Gaviscon, Gelusil, Maalox, Mylanta*	Gastritis, GERD	Beta-carotene, folic acid, vitamin D, calcium, chromium, iron, zinc, magnesium, phosphorus, copper
Laxatives with Bisacodyl *Carter's Little Pills, Correctol, Dulcolax, Feen-a-Mint*	Constipation	Calcium, potassium
H2 Inhibitors *Pepcid, Mylanta, Tagamet, Zantac*	Ulcer, GERD	Folic acid, B_1, B_{12}, vitamin D, calcium, iron, zinc

Source: InviteHealth.co, University of Maryland

The next time you decide to take a prescription or over-the-counter medication, remind yourself that they are Everyday Micronutrient Depleters (EMDs), and then replenish your micronutrient levels. This brings us to **Naked Fact #8.**

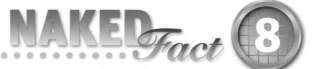

Prescription and over-the-counter medications deplete essential micronutrients, which can either exacerbate the same condition or initiate a new deficiency condition or disease.

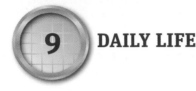

9 DAILY LIFE

This next category of Everyday Micronutrient Depleters is daily life. Here you will find common daily realities such as stress, smoking, pollution, hurried lifestyle, and exercise.

Stress

Stress is something that most, if not all, of us have in our lives more often than we would like. For the majority of people stress comes mostly from the workplace or from home. However, stress hides everywhere. Stress can be hiding even in the most pleasurable situations. On vacation, stress may be lurking at ticket counters, security checkpoints, and at the destination itself (poor weather or lost luggage). Stress has been shown to contribute to many common diseases such as ulcers, hypertension, arthritis, and heart disease. However, you may never have thought of stress in terms of its being an EMD.

According to Rudolf Ballentine, M.D., author of *Radical Healing,* when a person becomes stressed or frightened, certain metabolic events cause the body to use up more of certain micronutrients. Vitamin C levels decrease as one responds to stress, explains Dr. Ballentine, and supplementation of vitamin C is helpful in stress-related disorders. Humphrey Osmond, M.D., of the University of Alabama, and Abram Hoffer, M.D., a psychiatrist from British Columbia, contend that weight for weight, vitamin C is "as active as Haldol," a drug prescribed to help people deal with stress.

As it turns out, stress also depletes the body's resources of certain B vitamins. "The B vitamins came to be known as anti-stress nutrients because they are often the first deficiencies to develop during times of stress," said Michael Rosenbaum, M.D., author of *Super Supplements.* "Water-soluble nutrients such as the B vitamins, vitamin C, and all of the minerals are generally excreted at a faster rate during periods of stress. Because [they] are not stored to any great extent, deficiencies can develop rather quickly."

A study published in the *Archives of Internal Medicine,* conducted by the Mayo Clinic in Rochester, Minnesota, revealed that if a subject was only given half the daily requirement of thiamine (vitamin B_1), the subject became "irritable, depressed, quarrelsome, uncooperative, and fearful that some misfortune awaited them." Riboflavin (vitamin B_2) helps the body produce antistress hormones. Therefore, as you become stressed you deplete the very micronutrient that helps you fight stress. Does this pattern sound similar to the prescription medication scenario we described earlier, in which the drug prescribed for the condition depletes the same micronutrient that contributed to the deficiency in the first place? We are all bound to get stressed. While the stress itself may be unavoidable, the micronutrient depletion from it can be remedied. Micronutrient supplementation and/or replenishment through food may not only reverse the depletion, it may actually alleviate the stress you feel.

Smoking and Pollution

Smoking is another daily-life EMD that depletes the body of micronutrients. Although we could create lists of how bad cigarettes are for your overall health, show graphic examples of the destruction it does to your lungs, and supply you with an abundance of studies on associated health risks, we are only providing the data on smoking as it pertains to micronutrient depletion.

- A study at University of California at Berkeley concluded that a wide variety of fat-soluble vitamins, including A and E, were degraded with cigarette smoke.

- The National Health and Nutrition Examination Survey (NHANESII) showed that smokers of twenty or more cigarettes per day had 28 percent less vitamin C intake and a significant reduction in serum levels compared to nonsmokers.

- A study at Kansas State University exposed rats to cigarette smoke. This exposure induced vitamin A depletion, as well as emphysema, in the rats.

- Research conducted at Johns Hopkins revealed that exposure to passive smoking (second-hand smoke) may result in decreased concentration of selected micronutrients. That's right. Smoking also robs those around you of their micronutrients!

It is important to add that studies suggest if you are exposed to ozone pollution, as is the case in many large cities, you should consider supplementation, as the effects may be similar to that of smoking. Living with air pollution can cause increased cases of asthma, and studies indicate that supplementing with antioxidants, including vitamin C, beta-carotene, lycopene, and selenium, may reduce the symptoms of asthma. And, if your environment causes asthma, most likely you will be prescribed an inhaler and other medications that in and of themselves can be further robbing you of micronutrients!

• • • • • • • • • • • • • • •

Toxic Chemicals

YOUR BODY COMES INTO CONTACT with numerous toxic chemicals every day. Some you ingest, some you clean your home with, and others you slather on to beautify and protect your skin. However, you may never have thought of these toxic chemicals as EMDs that affect your micronutrient levels. Could your choice of rice, seafood, and poultry, or your preferred shampoo, dish soap, and toothpaste be causing your body to utilize the micronutrients you ingest for detoxification, leaving you at risk for other conditions caused by their deficiencies? And perhaps more important, could becoming sufficient in your essential vitamins and minerals protect you from the toxicity of these environmental factors?

Toxic Chemicals in Food

Living in this modern, industrialized world means that many things in our lives have been made simpler and more productive. On the other hand, recent research shows that this "simpler" existence may have some fairly unwanted consequences. First, it has caused a contamination of the water supply due to industrialized *runoff*. Additionally, the desire to grow animals for human consumption at an unnatural pace has found use of toxic chemicals as a means to increase poultry size and potential profits. For these and many other reasons, we find our modern foods contaminated with lead, arsenic, and mercury.

However, did you know that nutritional science has shown micronutrients to be your body's best defense from these dangerous toxic chemicals? That's right. As it turns out, micronutrients work as the body's natural detoxifiers, affecting both the absorption and excretion of these toxic contaminants. They have also been shown to be highly effective at reducing the effects of toxicity, such as oxidative stress.

Take some time to read the table below. Where is your highest exposure to these toxic chemicals coming from? Do you think you could reduce your exposure by limiting your intake of their sources? Remember, you don't have to be an *extremist,* and frankly we would not want you to stop eating fish because of possible mercury contamination. Just remember that being sufficient in your essential micronutrients is your best defense against the inevitable reality of toxic exposure.

TABLE 6.4. TOXIC CHEMICALS FOUND IN FOODS AS EVERYDAY MICRONUTRIENT DEPLETERS

TOXIC CHEMICALS	WHERE IT IS FOUND	CONCERNS	MICRONUTRIENTS TO PREVENT TOXICITY
Lead	Rice, juice, and foods containing synthetic nitrates	Fatigue, headaches, irritability, uneasy stomach, reduced IQ and attention span, impaired growth, reading and learning disabilities, hearing loss, mental retardation, coma, convulsion, and death	Calcium, iron, phosphorous, selenium, zinc, vitamins B_1, B_6, C, and E, as well as alphalipoic acid and quercetin have the ability to scavenge free radicals and chelate lead ions. While vitamin D usually increases the absorption of calcium, magnesium, and zinc, if those minerals are deficient, then vitamin D may work to increase intestinal absorption of lead instead.

TOXIC CHEMICALS	WHERE IT IS FOUND	CONCERNS	MICRONUTRIENTS TO PREVENT TOXICITY
Arsenic	Rice, juice, and foods containing synthetic nitrates and poultry from conventional farms	Nerve damage, scaling skin, Skin pigment changes, increase of lung, bladder, kidney, skin and liver cancer, circulatory problems	Phosphorous, Selenium, Vitamins A and E
Mercury	Fish, usually the largest predatory fish, like swordfish and shark, who have eaten the greatest majority of toxin-containing smaller fish for the longest period of time	Sensory impairment (vision, hearing, speech), disturbed sensation, lack of coordination, profuse sweating, faster-than-normal heartbeat, increased salivation, and high blood pressure	Selenium and Vitamins C and E

Toxic Chemicals in Household Products

Today many household and personal care products are loaded with unpronounceable ingredients that have been show to have deleterious side effects. Have you ever considered how many of these potentially dangerous items you come into contact with every day?

For example, both the triclosan, commonly found in antibacterial soaps, as well as the sodium lauryl sulfate (SLS), found in many toothpastes, laundry detergents, hair coloring, shampoos, and other foaming products, have been shown to cause the formation of dioxins. According to the Environmental Working Group's *Skin Deep: Cosmetic Safety Reviews* research, studies on SLS have shown it to potentially cause irritation of the skin and eyes, organ toxicity, developmental and reproductive toxicity, neurotoxicity, endocrine disruption, ecotoxicology, and biochemical or cellular changes, as well as possible DNA mutations and cancer. They explain that the danger is based on the level of exposure, but considering many of these products are used at least once a day, researchers believe that the buildup over a few years could be quite high. In order to fight off the effects from only these two ingredients, your body would need to use a host of vitamins and minerals. These include, but are not limited to, vitamins C and E to prevent damage due to oxidative stress, selenium to retard DNA damage and inhibit the production of carcinogens, folic acid and B_{12} to minimize chromosome damage, and vitamin D to prevent cancer.

If we look at this sample of micronutrients needed to protect you from these two toxic chemicals, we must consider the ramification of their potentially becoming depleted. What functions and responsibilities might they be falling short in achieving?

TABLE 6.5. MICRONUTRIENTS UTILIZED DUE TO DIOXINS AND ASSOCIATED CONDITIONS IF DEFICIENT

MICRONUTRIENT UTILIZED	ASSOCIATED CONDITIONS OF POTENTIAL DEFICIENCY
Vitamin C	Coronary heart disease, delayed blood clotting, cancer
Vitamin E	Cataracts, Alzheimer's disease, cardiovascular disease, cancer
Selenium	Impaired immunity, cancer, cardiovascular disease, thyroid disease
Folic Acid	Megaloblastic anemia, neural tube defects, cardiovascular disease
Vitamin B$_{12}$	Gastritis, peptic ulcer, anemia, dementia, tingling in limbs, constipation

As you can see, there are vast ramifications of the introduction of only these two toxic chemicals. Would it surprise you to know that according to the United Nations Environmental Programme (UNEP) approximately 70,000 chemicals are commonly used across the world, with 1,000 new chemicals being introduced every year? Imagine the micronutrients your body must utilize in order to protect you from all of them. You can see how this ever-expanding list of toxic chemicals works as an EMD, utilizing the micronutrients you think are in the bank, reserved for other key health-promoting activities.

• • • • • • • • • • • • • • •

Hurried Lifestyle

HAVE YOU EVER FELT LIKE there isn't enough time to accomplish everything you need to get done? Your harried day may not only cause stress, but it may also cause you to make some not-so-smart food choices or skip meals entirely. It takes time to plan and prepare a healthy meal, and a hurried lifestyle can be an impediment, even if we desire to be mindful about nutrition. The alternative is to grab EDNP foods in an attempt to curtail our hunger while on the run. It's common to see people every day at convenient stores and coffee shops choosing EDNP foods that are crowding out the micronutrient-rich foods they need.

In addition, when we eat and run we tend not to chew our foods well. Your mouth is the beginning of your digestive tract, and swallowing things whole or partially chewed causes the digestive process to begin poorly. Your teeth begin the digestive process by breaking your mouthful of food into smaller particles with more surface area so that the enzymes, the chemical food processors in your saliva, can do their job. When you swallow your food prematurely, your body isn't allowed the time to sufficiently coat the foods with these enzymes; therefore, insufficient breakdown of the foods ingested takes place.

In a study in the *American Journal of Clinical Nutrition,* researchers discovered that when almonds were chewed at least twenty-five times, they released greater amounts of vitamin E than almonds chewed only ten times.

Exercise

"There are 1,440 minutes in every day. Schedule thirty of them for physical activity!" This is the recommendation of the Centers for Disease Control and Prevention.

Although we agree that cardiovascular exercise and weight training are essential components to overall health, many micronutrients are depleted through these beneficial activities. Often when people get excited about losing weight, the first thing they do is run off to the gym to work off the pounds. We support your efforts, but caution that you may be unknowingly jeopardizing your micronutrient-sufficiency level when you exercise without effectively replenishing micronutrients lost as a result of your well-intended physical exertion.

Believe it or not, exercise can be an Everyday Micronutrient Depleter (EMD) too, and the amount of micronutrients lost through exercise correlates with the intensity and the duration

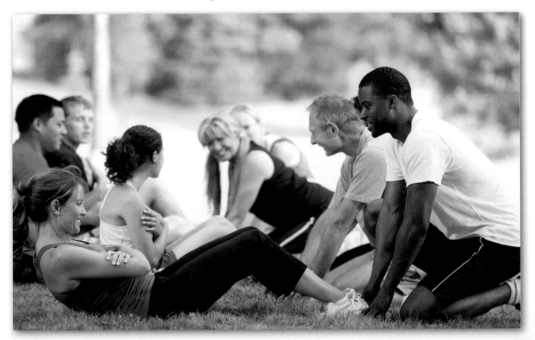

of the activity. For those exercising fewer than four hours a week, iron deficiency is no more of a concern than it would be for a sedentary person. However, individuals who train for more than six hours a week often have iron-deficiency anemia. This is because intense training stimulates an increase in red blood cell and blood vessel production, which increases the demand for iron. The harder the workout, the faster the iron is depleted, and the greater the need for replenishment.

A study in the *American Journal of Clinical Nutrition* found that athletes, both male and female, were deficient in magnesium and only consumed an average of 70 percent of the Dietary Reference Intake (DRI) for magnesium in the first place. This already diminished supply of magnesium is further lost through sweat and urine. In this study, men who road stationary bicycles in the heat for eight hours compounded these deficiencies by losing another 4 to 5 percent of their total magnesium intake.

In a German study, potassium loss for athletes who ran in 70 degrees Fahrenheit for forty minutes was 435 mg/hr. Potassium is found in intracellular fluid and is essential for regulating total body water and muscle contractions. In addition, it was found that supplementing with potassium during training increased markers of recovery.

While exercise wear and tear causes cellular damage in your body, a French study proved that selenium could help to repair this damage. By supplementing some men with selenium, researchers were able to determine that the men receiving selenium supplements had less cellular damage after exercise than the men receiving a placebo.

Another micronutrient shown to be beneficial for athletes is zinc, which aids in post-workout tissue repair. Spanish scientists compared volleyball players during a stressful two-month training period to a control group and discovered increased zinc excretion and altered zinc metabolism in the players who didn't receive any days off. The study concluded that these lowered levels of zinc actually increased fatigue and decreased endurance, which made for poorer overall performance.

Do you know what an antioxidant is? Do you know how antioxidants affect your health? Do you get enough of them? Antioxidants are extremely important for athletes who perform aerobic activity. This is because these individuals undergo more oxidative cell damage, causing the formation of free radicals. Antioxidants like vitamin A, C, E, CoQ_{10}, quercetin, and alpha lipoic acid are fantastic free radical scavengers and can help to reduce this cellular damage.

Antioxidants are extremely important for athletes who perform aerobic activity.

These are just a few examples of the many micronutrients that are depleted through exercise and how certain micronutrients have been shown to enhance physical performance. Being proponents of exercise, we know that its benefits are far reaching. However, the very same workouts that are keeping our muscles strong and our waistlines trim are also depleting us of the vital micronutrients that we have ingested through our foods.

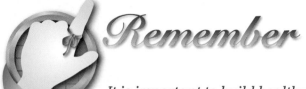

Remember

It is important to build healthy habits early in a child's life. Sports are great for both physical and psychological development—however, children's bodies are also depleted of essential micronutrients through exercise.

10 DIETARY CHOICES

This final EMD category includes diets as a means to achieve weight loss (including accompanying weight-loss surgeries and supplements), as well as diets chosen as a lifestyle, due to medical, health, or for personal preference issues.

Diets for Weight Loss

To complicate matters further, our last EMD exercise often occurs simultaneously with our next EMD—diet. Here we will examine the many aspects of diet that contribute to micronutrient deficiency. Let's face it: Most people who head to the gym are doing so in an effort to lose weight, and most people who are trying to lose weight end up changing their eating patterns in one way or another. The problem is that many diet plans restrict calories. Lowering the amount of food you take in will obviously lower the amount of micronutrients you take in as well. Choosing a low-carbohydrate diet, such as an Atkins-style plan, causes decreased intakes of fruits, vegetables, and grains. On this plan, nutritionists often recommend supplementation to ensure proper micronutrient levels.

You might choose a low-fat diet. Low-fat diets, as the name implies, would decrease your overall fat intake as well as your essential fatty acids. In addition, when fat is removed from the diet there are only two

Let's face it: Most people who head to the gym are doing so in an effort to lose weight, and most people who are trying to lose weight end up changing their eating patterns in one way or another.

other options to replace it—proteins and carbohydrates. While your choice may be protein, more often than not, most people will choose carbohydrates. The problem with this is that many of the carbohydrates chosen today, as you have learned in Chapter 5, are EDNP foods (often containing refined white sugar, processed white flour, and HFCS) and are low in micronutrients.

Also, some high-glycemic carbohydrate-based foods can dramatically increase insulin levels, which stimulate the body to store fat, which can eventually lead to diabetes. When dieting, many people eat pre-packaged or frozen diet meals. If we remember the discussion in Chapter 5, eating both frozen food as well as microwaving our foods is not always in our best interest. Many dieters opt to pre-make meals, carefully measuring them out according to diet recipes and take them to work to ensure success. This helps greatly with convenience and portion control, but storage time and reheating of meals are also EMDs.

Some dieters may decide to skip meals altogether. According to Carrie Ruxton, Ph.D., R.D., in her study published in the British Nutrition Foundation's publication, *Nutrition Bulletin,* "A survey of U.S. female college students found that 32 percent skipped breakfast in order to control weight, while a UK survey of 1,000 regular dieters found that 21 percent admitted to skipping meals." Obviously, this is not a pathway to micronutrient sufficiency. To make matters worse, many dieters tend to choose the same foods over and over again. The point is, the more often you choose the same foods and the lower your calorie level, the less likely you will be to receive all of your required micronutrients.

 Dieters Beware!

We want to take a moment to address a potentially dangerous aspect of diet that is becoming extremely popular: weight-loss aids. We evaluate them here only based on how they can affect your micronutrient-sufficiency levels. Weight-loss aids can either be administered by prescription, over the counter in the form of supplements, or through actual medical procedures. A market research survey conducted by Mintel International Group found 24 percent of the 1,000 current or former dieters surveyed had used weight-loss pills at some stage. One such over-the-counter diet aid is Alli. Previously known

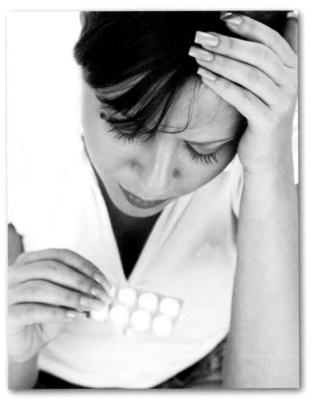

as the prescription medications Xenical and Orlistat, Alli works by blocking the absorption of fat after it has been ingested. The problem with this is that if we block fat, we lose our ability to absorb important essential fatty acids and fat-soluble vitamins (A, D, E, and K).

For example, Alli can reduce the absorption of the essential micronutrient vitamin E by 60 percent. Why would we want to reduce the amount of something that has the word "essential" in its name? Here is another little fact that the makers of Alli don't share with you: German studies have shown that this "diet aid" may actually raise appetite sensations and increase food consumption.

Another weight-loss medication is the prescription drug Meridia, which works by suppressing appetite. When we don't feel hungry, we don't eat, and if we don't eat we are basically starving ourselves and eliminating many essential micronutrients. Hoodia, a natural supplement, also claims to work through appetite suppression. A more recent addition to diet aids, Sensa, promotes sprinkling scented food flakes on your food. These sprinkles send signals to your brain to indicate your body is full or satisfied, causing you to reduce food intake, thus micronutrient intake. In addition, many eager dieters try to hurry up the weight-loss process by taking caffeine-filled over-the-counter fat burners. These stimulant-based, diuretic, over-the-counter medications also deplete vital micronutrients.

The most dangerous type of diet aids, when considering micronutrient sufficiency, may be surgical procedures such as laparoscopic banding (lap band) and gastric bypass surgery. These medical procedures cut out or "band off" a portion of patients' stomachs so they cannot eat large portions, which in turn ensures they will not be able to fully absorb their micronutrients. For patients undergoing either of these procedures, supplementation is imperative.

> *The most dangerous type of diet aids, when considering micronutrient sufficiency, may be surgical procedures such as laparoscopic banding (lap band) and gastric bypass surgery.*

For gastric bypass surgery patients, specific vitamins and minerals must be taken for the rest of the patient's life, usually in liquid or chewable tablet form. This is due to decreased stomach size, decreased absorption of vitamins and minerals in the small intestine, and a lack of gastric juices in the "new stomach" that would normally help break down micronutrients.

Food as Lifestyle Choice

While losing weight is one of the most popular reasons to diet, for many people dieting has become less about losing weight and more about lifestyle. For instance, leading a vegetarian or vegan lifestyle is more widespread than ever; nevertheless, it has its own set of micronutrient-related challenges. Vegetarians and vegans tend to be low in iron, due to the absence of meat in their diets. Their diets also tend to be high in legumes, spinach, soy, and grains. As we learned earlier in this chapter, these foods contain phytates and oxalates—EMDs that can further leach iron. Remember, this same increase in phytic acid and oxalic acid consumption can also cause calcium, magnesium, copper, chromium, manganese, zinc, and niacin to be depleted.

Milk is the primary source of vitamin D in the United States, and all vegans as well as vegetarians who exclude dairy products should consider supplementation of vitamin D. Calcium should also be supplemented by vegetarians and vegans, because of elevated levels of oxalates and decreased levels of calcium found in their diet profiles.

In a study published in 1999 in the *American Journal of Clinical Nutrition,* 245 lactovo-vegetarians and vegans who were not taking vitamin B_{12} supplements were evaluated. It was found that 73 percent of those tested had low serum vitamin B_{12} concentrations. Vegans and vegetarians must pay close attention to B_{12} levels and should consider supplementation because this vitamin cannot be found naturally in any plant-based sources and is only found in animal products. Additionally, two important amino acids should be considered: carnosine, which facilitates longevity, and carnitine, which helps with fat metabolization. Both are only found in animal products. Finally, the omega-3 fatty acids EPA and DHA are also only found naturally in animal-based foods; therefore, vegans and vegetarians should be aware of the considerable risk of EPA and DHA deficiency.

Another lifestyle diet is eating gluten-free—the only medically accepted treatment of celiac disease. A gluten-free diet can be beneficial in eliminating many adverse food reactions and allergies. However, the elimination of foods containing gluten, a protein found in certain foods like wheat or barley, also eliminates many of the natural sources of micronutrients in those foods. Gluten-free foods are often low in calcium, vitamin D, iron, zinc, magnesium, and the B vitamins.

A gluten-free diet can be beneficial in eliminating many adverse food reactions and allergies.

In fact, when individuals following a gluten-fee diet were studied, more than half were found to be deficient in both vitamin B_6 and folic acid (vitamin B_9). Celiac patients, as well as others following this eating profile, should discuss with their physicians whether they should be taking B vitamins or a properly formulated multivitamin supplement.

Proponents of a raw food diet believe that the health benefits include increased energy, improved skin appearance, better digestion, weight loss, and reduced risk of heart disease. A study published in the *Journal of Nutrition* found that consumption of a raw food diet successfully lowered cholesterol and triglycerides.

Critics of the raw food diet are quick to point out that statistically, these diets are micronutrient deficient in calcium, iron, and B_{12}. In fact, a *Journal of Nutrition* study found that strict raw food diets often cause vitamin B_{12} deficiencies that can lead to increased levels of homocysteine—an amino acid released as the body digests protein. Increased levels of this amino acid have been linked to cardiovascular disease.

After reviewing all of the Everyday Micronutrient Depleters in the Daily Life and Dietary Choices categories, there should be no doubt in your mind as to the validity of our **Naked Fact #9**.

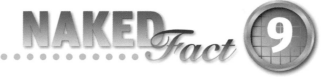

Stress, smoking, pollution, toxic chemicals, hurried lifestyle, exercise, weight loss, and lifestyle diets are all possible Everyday Micronutrient Depleters (EMDs).

Phew! There are certainly an abundance of Everyday Micronutrient Depleters lurking in our lives. But don't fret—you are getting close to the light at the end of this tunnel. You are well on your way to completing the second step of our three-step plan and becoming a nutrivore. Remember that the first step was to choose *rich foods* over *poor foods* whenever possible to increase the micronutrient value of the foods you eat. The second step is to become aware of the number of EMDs that occur in your life. When Mira took this second step, she realized that by eating her daily spinach salad filled with calcium and magnesium-depleting oxalic acid; her sugar-laden, calcium and magnesium-depleting fat-free muffin; and her numerous cups of calcium-leaching black coffee, she had actively been participating in the deterioration of her bones. Add to that the hours of dance classes, daily stress, and prescription birth control medication, and she had a recipe for early onset osteoporosis. Reducing and eliminating these EMDs was an important second step in reversing her condition and building back her bones. Attempting to reduce as many of these stealth micronutrient thieves as you can will get you one step closer to achieving optimal health.

We have just shared with you the abundance of EMDs that rob you of essential micronutrients *before* and *after* you eat. You may still be debating if a healthy diet can supply you with an adequate amount of micronutrients. It's time now to answer the fundamental question first posed in Chapter 4. *Can I get all the essential micronutrients I need from a balanced diet, or do I need to take a multivitamin?* Does this diet exist? Is it possible to find a balanced diet that meets minimum RDI micronutrient sufficiency? In Chapter 7, we tackle the biggest face-off in nutritional history as we explore the "balanced diet" to determine if it is indeed fact or fiction.

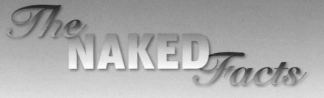

The **NAKED** *Facts*

- Many of the foods and drinks one may choose every day can block or deplete micronutrients, thereby reducing micronutrient sufficiency.

- Prescription and over-the-counter medications deplete essential micronutrients, which can either exacerbate the same condition or initiate a new deficiency condition or disease.

- Stress, smoking, pollution, toxic chemicals, hurried lifestyle, exercise, weight loss, and lifestyle diets are all possible Everyday Micronutrient Depleters (EMDs).

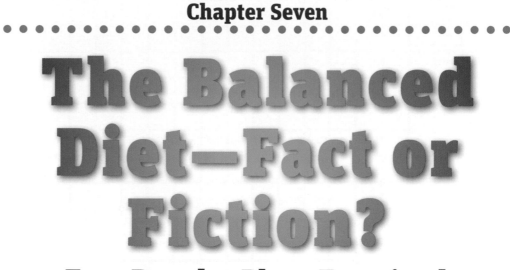

Chapter Seven

The Balanced Diet—Fact or Fiction?

Four Popular Plans Examined

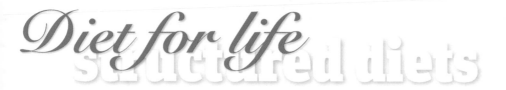

Diet for life   structured diets

Diet industry

menu plans

Popular diets   reduce the risks

❝It may be that chronic micronutrient insufficiency from food alone is more fact than fantasy.**❞**

—William Misner, Ph.D.

D o you remember David, the rocket scientist you read about way back in Chapter 4? When we last left the story, we were sitting at a table with David and several others, at a dinner party, when he sat back in his chair, wiped his mouth, and asked, "So tell me this: Can I get all the essential micronutrients I need from a balanced diet, or do I need to take a multivitamin?" Upon hearing the question the table became quiet, and everyone leaned in to hear the answer once and for all. We discussed with them the mineral depletion in the soil; pertinent statistics on the global micronutrient-deficiency pandemic; and the numerous EMDs that one encounters *before*, as well as *after,* consuming food.

At this point in the conversation, the waiters brought the first course. Everyone at the table received magnificent salads full of a variety of garden vegetables—everyone, that is, except David. David was brought a beautifully prepared beef carpaccio topped with arugula, Parmesan shavings, and drizzled olive oil. When someone at the table asked about his special request, he told us that at the suggestion of his physician, in order to lower his cholesterol and lose a few pounds, he was following the Atkins for Life diet.

A petite blonde woman across the table interjected, "Well if that is what you eat, then you probably can't get all of your micronutrients. There simply aren't enough vegetables in that program. I follow The Best Life Diet, and eat a ton of salads and whole grains. I saw it on *Oprah,* and I am sure that Bob Green wouldn't steer her wrong."

David, always the scientist, answered the woman defensively, "My diet was written by a medical doctor, it was recommended to me by my physician, who is also a medical doctor, and I am following the meal plans perfectly. I think that the reason the USDA study found so many Americans micronutrient deficient was because they weren't evaluating people who ate specific menu plans, just people who were eating randomly."

The petite woman sat up taller in her chair, and the debate continued. "Just because you are on a structured diet does not mean that you are getting all of the vitamins and minerals you need. That type of a menu just can't offer as many micronutrients as my diet does." We shared a quick knowing glance across the table and decided that it was time to stop the "great diet debate" before it escalated further. We agreed with David first. He was right; the USDA had simply evaluated people following a random eating pattern. Although some of them were more than likely following a diet of some kind, they were not instructed on what to eat.

With a nod to the blonde woman, we added that we also agreed with her. Just because someone is following a popular diet doesn't mean they are going to be micronutrient sufficient, and that a restrictive diet, like the Atkins for Life diet, would seem to be less likely to fulfill one's micronutrient needs. We then told the table that a few years back we had decided to seek out the answer to the very question that our dinner companions were now debating. *Do popular, structured diets, like the mainstream weight-loss plans that become bestsellers each year, provide micronutrient sufficiency?*

To find out, we researched published studies that looked at the possibility of obtaining micronutrient sufficiency while following a diet—any diet. First, we came across a study by William Misner, Ph.D., published in the *Journal of the International Society of Sports Nutrition (JISSN)*. Dr. Misner used a statement made by the American Dietetic Association (ADA) as the foundation for his study. It stated, "The best nutritional strategy for promoting optimal health and reducing the risk of chronic disease is to wisely choose a wide variety of foods." Dr. Misner's objective was to see if a diet that was not supplemented, consisting of a wide variety of foods, could provide 100 percent of the daily essential micronutrient requirement.

To do this, seventy diets from the menus of both athletes and sedentary subjects were reviewed. Twenty subjects (ten men and ten women ages twenty-five to fifty) with the highest variety of foods in their menus (matching most closely the ADA's statement on choosing the widest variety of foods) were evaluated. This group included:

- two professional cyclists (athletes)
- three amateur triathletes (athletes)
- one amateur runner (athlete)
- three amateur cyclists (athletes)
- five eco-challenge amateur (athletes)
- six sedentary subjects (non-athletes)

Their menus were then computer-analyzed for their ability to deliver 100 percent of the RDA for ten essential vitamins and seven essential minerals (vitamins A, D, E, K, B_1, B_2, B_3, B_6, B_9, B_{12}, iodine, potassium, calcium, magnesium, phosphorus, zinc, and selenium).

The results might surprise you:

- *All* of the dietary analyses fell short of providing 100 percent of the RDA from food alone.
- Males averaged deficiencies in 40 percent of the vitamins and 54.2 percent of the minerals.
- Women averaged deficiencies in 29 percent of the vitamins and 44.2 percent of the minerals.
- One of the subjects was deficient in fifteen out of the seventeen essential micro-nutrients (88 percent deficient).
- A whopping sixteen out of the twenty subjects were 99 to 100 percent deficient in at least one of the seventeen essential micronutrients.

Even with the American Dietetic Association's "best nutritional strategy" in place, these diets were found to have gaping nutritional holes. The study concluded, "Food alone in all twenty subjects did not meet the minimal Recommended Daily Allowances (RDA) micronutrient requirements for preventing nutrient-deficiency diseases." The study goes on to say, "It may be that chronic micronutrient insufficiency from food alone is more fact than fantasy."

This first study demonstrates that it is not just the USDA that has deemed our diets deficient in essential micronutrients. However, so far we have only looked at studies that have examined the adequacy rates of random diets. These diet menus have been designed by individuals who may not have any idea how they are supposed to eat in order to achieve RDA or RDI sufficiency. The researchers, in both the previous study and the USDA studies, gave no direction or suggestions to the subjects as to which foods they should eat in order to increase their overall chances of reaching sufficiency. Surely, if a qualified "professional" sat down with paper and pen they could easily put together a variety of delicious, daily menus that would show us all just how easy it is to meet sufficiency while eating a balanced diet, right? Let's see.

Next, we found a study published in the *Journal of the American Dietetic Association* titled, "Problems Encountered in Meeting the Recommended Dietary Allowances for Menus Designed According to the Dietary Guidelines for Americans." As part of the study, a group of dietitians designed menus based on the Dietary Guidelines for Americans—a program published by the U.S. Department of Health and Human Services (HHS) and the USDA that serves as the basis for federal food and nutrition education programs—that meet the RDAs while providing 2,200 to 2,400 *palatable* calories. Using software designed specifically for creating a healthy diet, these trained dietitians were unable to accomplish the study's objective. According to the researchers, "Only 11 percent of the menus met the RDA for zinc. Half of the menus did not meet the RDA for vitamin B$_6$ and one-third did not meet the RDA for iron." If a group of trained health professionals cannot produce menus that consistently reach the RDAs and dietary guidelines within an average amount of calories that promote leanness while being universally palatable, how is the general public expected to do so? Is it even possible?

It should be no surprise to most of you that the diet industry is a big business. In fact, dieting could be considered one of America's most popular pastimes. Research indicates that approximately 70 million people at any given time are on a diet of some kind. While each diet is unique and seems to attract its own group of followers, all diets share one common element: They were all written by someone, or a team of someones, with a higher-than-average degree of knowledge of nutrition. The creators of these plans have many times dedicated their lives to the study of their particular style of diet. They are often considered "experts" in their fields and can commonly be seen on TV or at seminars explaining exactly how and why their plan works so well.

So I, Jayson, half of the brain behind this writing team, decided to conduct a study that became the basis for my dissertation and was ultimately published in the *Journal of the International Society of Sports Nutrition (JISSN)*. It examined the sufficiency level of twenty-seven essential micronutrients as recommended by the RDI, in four popular diet plans. I wanted to see if the very act of dieting itself could be creating a micronutrient-deficient state in the typical American dieter.

First, I wanted to make sure the diets I chose to study were popular; i.e., ones that the average person can find in a bookstore. Next, I wanted all three major types of diets represented: low-carbohydrate diet (Atkins for Life), Mediterranean-style diet (The South Beach Diet), and low-fat diet (The Best Life Diet). Then, I added a medically based diet created and tested by some of the best minds in the business, the DASH diet. DASH stands for Dietary Approaches to Stop Hypertension, and as its name implies, it was not originally designed to be a weight-loss diet. There are now subsequent books, however, that boast the DASH diet's weight-loss benefit, including *The DASH Diet for Hypertension* by Thomas Moore, M.D.

It turns out that Thomas Moore, M.D., and well over 100 other qualified medical and nutritional professionals, were members of a special team that created and tested the DASH diet. The team was called the DASH Collaborative Research Group. These researchers were from such esteemed institutions as Brigham and Women's Hospital, Harvard Medical School, Duke University Medical Center, Johns Hopkins University, Kaiser Permanente Center for Health Research, National Heart, Lung and Blood Institute, and the Pennington Biomedical Research Center at Louisiana State University. When I dug deeper, I discovered that the DASH diet is recommended by virtually all medical professionals and has millions of people using it to naturally

> *All three major types of diets represented: low-carbohydrate diet (Atkins for Life), Mediterranean-style diet (The South Beach Diet), and low-fat diet (The Best Life Diet).*

lower blood pressure and reduce their risk of heart disease, stroke, cancer, kidney disease, and osteoporosis.

The website www.dashdiet.org states that, in addition to being recommended by your physician, DASH is recommended by:

- The National Heart, Lung, and Blood Institute (one of the National Institutes of Health, of the U.S. Department of Health and Human Services)
- The American Heart Association
- The 2010 Dietary Guidelines for Americans
- U.S. guidelines for treatment of high blood pressure

The website also informs that the DASH diet formed the basis for the USDA MyPyramid.

In addition, I discovered that in 2011, *US News & World Report* rated DASH the #1 American diet, and that the prestigious Mayo Clinic endorsed and recommended the DASH diet to its patients. I ultimately used the Mayo Clinic's suggested daily menus to conduct my study. I was sure that within my compiled group of four popular diet programs, one of the authors, or in the case of the DASH diet, group of "authors," who were all acutely aware of the RDI guidelines for essential micronutrients, would have created suggested menus that met these minimum requirements.

After all, Robert Atkins, M.D., of *Atkins for Life;* Arthur Agatston, M.D., of *The South Beach Diet;* and Bob Greene, O.P.R.A.H., (no M.D. or Ph.D. necessary) of *The Best Life Diet* are all #1 *New York Times* bestselling authors. Also, the DASH diet is recommended by numerous organizations and leading medical authorities. Millions upon millions of people around the world had studied these plans and followed their suggested daily menus in an attempt to achieve their specific health goals. *Could these diets be causing micronutrient deficiencies in millions of people? And if they were, what were the potential ramifications of this effect? Does the very act of dieting create a micronutrient deficient state in the typical dieter?*

I started the study by selecting three complete daily menus from each of the four selected diets. The resulting twelve menus were then evaluated exactly as they were suggested in their respective texts, official companions, or websites. Each ingredient of each meal and snack for all twelve daily menus were evaluated for calorie content, as well as for its content of twenty-seven essential micronutrients, based on RDI guidelines. The twenty-seven essential micronutrients measured in this study were vitamin A, thiamine (vitamin B_1), riboflavin (vitamin B_2), niacin (vitamin B_3), pantothenic acid (vitamin B_5), vitamin B_6, biotin (vitamin B_7), folic acid (vitamin B_9), vitamin B_{12}, vitamin C, vitamin D, vitamin E, vitamin K, choline, calcium, chromium, copper, iron, iodine, potassium, magnesium, manganese, molybdenum, sodium, phosphorus, selenium, and zinc.

The same database used in the USDA adequacy rate research—the USDA National Nutrient Database for Standard Reference—was used to calculate micronutrient levels. The daily menus examined in this study were intricately designed and suggested to millions of people as competent, healthy, balanced diets that would help them achieve not only their weight-loss goals, but perhaps more important, the ultimate goal of better health—which is why the outcome of this research was extremely disturbing, and was one of the main reasons we decided to write this book and educate people on the importance of micronutrient sufficiency.

Ironically, the entire concept of the DASH diet is that one can lower blood pressure naturally by achieving micronutrient sufficiency in potassium, magnesium, and calcium. This is the same micronutrient-sufficiency concept that we are talking about in this book. The difference is that the diet's authors stopped at high blood pressure. Our goal is to expand that concept to include almost all disease and create a clear pathway to optimal health via sufficiency in *all* of the essential micronutrients. We should state that the overall accomplishments and theories of these diet plans, including the DASH diet, are not in question. They have all been proven to work and help millions of people to achieve weight loss and/or improved health, but at what cost? Let's examine the results of the study and then discuss further their possible long-term ramifications.

When following each diet plan's suggested daily menus/meal plans (using food alone), the study determined that *NONE* of the four popular diet plans provided minimum RDI sufficiency for the twenty-seven essential micronutrients necessary for optimal health. Here is what did happen.

TABLE 7.1. INDEPENDENT DISSERTATION RESEARCH ON FOUR POPULAR DIET PROGRAMS

NAME OF DIET	TYPE OF DIET	% RDI SUFFICIENT	# OF MICRONUTRIENTS THAT MET RDI	# OF CALORIES AVERAGE DAILY INTAKE
Atkins for Life	Low carbohydrate	44%	12	1,786
Best Life	Low fat	56%	15	1,793
DASH	Medical	52%	14	2,217
South Beach	Mediterranean	22%	6	1,197
Average		44%	11.75	1,748

As it turns out, the blonde woman at our table was right. According to this study, the Best Life Diet did provide more micronutrients at about the same calorie level as Atkins for Life. However, as you can see in the table above, even the Best Life Diet did not provide 100 percent sufficiency. In fact, it was found that a typical dieter using one of these four popular diet plans would be, on average, *only 44 percent sufficient* in obtaining the minimum RDI requirements and would meet sufficiency in *less than twelve out of the twenty-seven* essential micronutrients required every day to prevent micronutrient-deficiency diseases. Again, if we look at this data from another angle, we can see that individuals following any of these diets' menus would be on average 56 percent *deficient* in micronutrients and would be deficient in *more than fifteen out of the twenty-seven* essential micronutrients required every day to prevent micronutrient-deficiency diseases.

> *Individuals following any of these diets' menus would be on average 56 percent deficient in micronutrients . . .*

Are you surprised? Probably not after seeing the other studies earlier in the book. However, some of you must have been surprised that even when the diet is being designed by some of the greatest minds in the field of medicine and nutrition, not one was able to achieve the very basis of our overall well-being—minimum micronutrient sufficiency. While these are disturbing results, to quote a popular phrase, "You ain't seen nothing yet." The first part of this research sadly shows that on average, popular diets are deficient in more than half of the micronutrients we all need every day to protect us from common health conditions and diseases, even when a professional has suggested exactly what we should eat *down to the last gram.*

However, as you might have noticed, one of the suggested menus only averaged 1,197 calories, while another averaged 2,217. Based on the results in Table 7.1, wouldn't it stand to reason that if the South Beach Diet's suggested 1,197 calories were practically doubled to match the DASH diet's 2,217 calories, the South Beach Diet would provide a much higher level of sufficiency? While the answer may be yes, we also have to remember that unlike the DASH diet, the main goal of the South Beach Diet is weight loss, and if the calories go up, the weight-loss effect may go down. Be this as it may, I decided to examine exactly how many calories it would take to reach 100 percent RDI sufficiency for each diet plan, putting aside any weight-loss benefit.

Since a diet's success and beneficial results are due to the specific food choices it recommends, changing food choices would alter each diet from its original science. I decided instead to simply raise the amount of each ingredient in each meal proportionally, until RDI sufficiency for all twenty-seven essential micronutrients was met. Thereby, I simply created larger meals of exactly the same suggested daily menu plan. In doing this, it was guaranteed that no macronutrient (carbohydrates, fats, and proteins) ratios or food selections would change, and minimum calories needed to achieve RDI sufficiency could be determined for each unique diet plan.

Here are the results. The Atkins for Life diet required the most calories, at an average of 37,500 calories per day to become 100 percent sufficient in the minimum RDI level for all twenty-seven micronutrients. The DASH diet required an average of 33,500 calories to do the same. The Best Life Diet required an average of 20,500 calories, and the South Beach Diet ended up requiring the least, at an average of 18,800 calories. Overall, the four diets required an average of 27,575 calories per day to become 100 percent sufficient in all twenty-seven essential micronutrients—well over any calorie level in which weight loss and/or health benefits could be achieved. That is the calorie equivalent of *54 McDonald's Big Macs or 120 six-inch Veggie Delite Subway sandwiches* per day.

TABLE 7.2. NUMBER OF CALORIES NEEDED IN FOUR POPULAR DIETS TO ACHIEVE 100% RDI SUFFICIENCY

NAME OF DIET	CALORIES REQUIRED TO REACH 100% RDI SUFFICIENCY FOR ALL 27 MICRONUTRIENTS
Atkins for Life	37,500
Best Life	20,500
DASH	33,500
South Beach	18,800
Average	27,575

This study empirically determines that an individual following one of these popular diet plans would have to eat on average *27,575 CALORIES A DAY, EVERY DAY,* to achieve minimum RDI sufficiency in all twenty-seven essential micronutrients. If not, micronutrient deficiency in at least one of the twenty-seven micronutrients is inevitable. Are you shocked? Did you think it would be easier to achieve micronutrient sufficiency? Did you assume that the professionals would have led you on a more micronutrient-sufficient path?

Now, to be fair, some of the authors of these diets do recommend that followers of their diet take a daily multivitamin, but not all of them. How many of you out there have started a diet program and jumped in, so eager to see the weight loss that you skipped ahead to the "how-to" portion of the program and disregarded any possible recommendations that may have been mentioned in

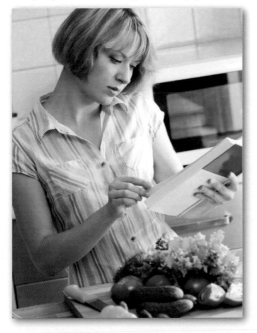

the rest of the text? Have you ever followed a diet that suggested taking a multivitamin and decided not to? The truth is many dieters simply don't think they need micronutrient supplementation when they are following a popular diet program. They think that the foods make up a balanced diet, and that a balanced diet is all they need to be micronutrient sufficient. However, you can see from all of the studies we have examined together, that *every one* of the diets, whether random or popular, are deficient in providing minimum RDI sufficiency in multiple essential micronutrients.

Some of you may be wondering what the daily menus included. How many meals were the dieters eating? Did the menus offer variety? We present them here for your review.

South Beach Diet

SAMPLE MENU

The South Beach Diet, 2-Week Quick Start Plan, page 29

Breakfast: juice and omelet

6 oz vegetable juice

2 large eggs

80 grams light sour cream

1.75 grams salt

.03 tsp pepper

½ tsp margarine

18.5 grams red bell pepper

6.25 grams scallion

.79 oz turkey bacon

Snack 1

80 grams celery

1 tbsp spreadable cream cheese

Lunch: three-bean salad

2 oz green beans

2 oz yellow beans

¼ lb ground turkey breast

.75 grams salt

.03 tsp pepper

½ tbsp pine nuts

½ tsp soy sauce

.25 gram basil leaves

1 oz mozzarella cheese

½ clove garlic

4 large leaves Boston lettuce

¼ small cucumber

¼ tbsp fresh ginger

18.5 grams mint leaves

¼ tbsp Asian fish sauce

Snack 2

1 cup hummus

1 carrot

Dinner: fish and coleslaw

6 oz halibut

¾ tbsp olive oil

½ tbsp fresh dill

1 cup vegetable coleslaw

.935 grams mustard

Dessert snack

½ cup part-skim ricotta

½ tsp unsweetened cocoa

½ tsp vanilla extract

SAMPLE MENU

Atkins for Life, page 161, Meal Plan 1: 60 gm net carbohydrate option

Breakfast: cereal and fruit

½ cup Fiber One cereal

½ cup whole milk

½ cup blueberries

Lunch: burger and peas

100 grams 90% lean ground beef

104 grams cabbage

¼ carrot

1 tbsp sour cream

.75 grams salt

⅓ cup green peas

½ tbsp mayonnaise

Meal 3

6 oz Atlantic-farmed salmon

1 cup broccoli

¾ cup edamame

½ cup raspberries

Snack

2 oz Swiss cheese

1 oz macadamia nuts

SAMPLE MENU

The Best Life Diet, page 180

Breakfast: cereal and berries

1 cup nonfat milk

1 cup strawberries

2 tbsp unsalted almonds

¼ cup All Bran (cereal)

⅔ cup Weetabix (cereal)

½ cup Cheerios (cereal)

Snack 1

1 cup light chocolate or vanilla soy milk

3 squares cinnamon or honey graham crackers (preferably whole wheat)

Dinner: snapper with couscous salad

½ Ruby Red grapefruit

½ tbsp olive oil

¼ tsp of sea salt

¼ avocado, peeled, cored, and diced

1 slice red onion (⅛ of a small red onion)

1½ cups of fresh arugula

4 oz snapper or white fish

1 cup whole wheat couscous

1 tbsp lemon juice

1 tbsp parsley

Lunch: sandwich, salad, apple

2 slices of whole wheat bread

2 oz reduced-fat cheddar cheese

1 tomato

4 basil leaves

1 cup spinach

½ cup button mushrooms

1 tbsp olive oil

1 tbsp balsamic vinegar

1 small apple

Snack 2

1 cup nonfat milk

1 cup raspberries

Anytime Snack

1 granola bar

The DASH Diet

SAMPLE MENU

Day 1, www.mayoclinic.com/health/dash-diet/HI00046

Breakfast: juice and bagel

1 whole wheat breakfast bagel

2 tbsp peanut butter

1 medium orange

1 cup nonfat milk

Lunch: milk and fancy salad

1 cup nonfat milk

1 pear

1/3 cup unsalted peanuts

12 reduced-sodium whole wheat crackers

4 cups spinach

1/2 cup mandarin orange sections

Dinner: cod with vegetables

90 grams cod fillet

1 sourdough roll

1 tsp margarine

1/2 cup green beans

20.34 grams honey

16.75 grams sage & onion stuffing mix

1 cup bulgur

1 cup blueberries

Anytime snack

4 vanilla wafers

1 cup light plain yogurt

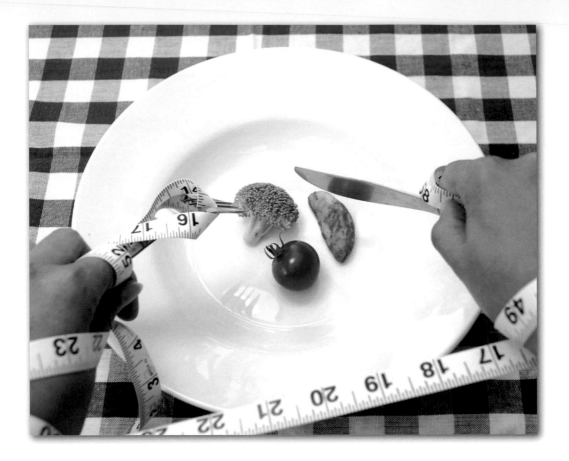

As you can see, the study did not use small, restrictive menus in order to manipulate a low overall micronutrient-sufficiency level. The micronutrient deficiencies quoted in the study were determined using the exact sample menus you just examined. Does your average daily menu look as varied or complete? The fact is, even when two of the diets had their followers eating six times a day, they were still deficient in numerous essential micronutrients.

Paleo and Primal Make Six

In the year following the initial publication of this book, we were often asked how a paleo or Primal diet would have fared in this study. Would these newly popular ancestral-based diets, focused largely on eating unprocessed, micronutrient-dense foods, fare any better? While our gut instinct was that they would, we decided to address these queries by examining these programs using the same method as with the other diets we had studied earlier. To do this, we chose three days' worth of menu suggestions from the "Squeaky Clean Paleo" meal plan section of *Practical Paleo,* as well as the Ken and Kelly Korg suggested eating plans from *The Primal Blueprint,* along with one day from author Mark Sisson's own typical weekday eating log.

Practical Paleo

SAMPLE MENU
Practical Paleo, page 219

Breakfast: pumpkin pancakes and breakfast sausage

2 eggs

¼ cup canned pumpkin

½ tsp pure vanilla extract

1 tbsp pure maple syrup

½ tsp pumpkin pie spice

½ tsp cinnamon

⅛ tsp baking soda

½ tbsp butter

2 sausage links

Dinner: lamb lettuce boats with avo-ziki sauce

½ lb lamb stew meat

1.5 grams sea salt

.06 tsp pepper

¼ tsp oregano

½ tbsp coconut oil

3 large romaine leaves

½ cup tomato

½ cup cucumber

1½ lemons juiced

½ avocado

½ clove garlic

1 tbsp olive oil

½ tsp dill

Lunch: beef stir-fry with mixed vegetables

½ lb skirt steak

1 tbsp coconut oil

½ cup red onion

½ cup broccoli

½ cup string beans

½ bell pepper

½ tbsp sesame seeds

1 tbsp green onion

⅛ cup water chestnuts

1 tbsp coconut aminos

1 clove garlic

½ tsp ginger

The Primal Blueprint

SAMPLE MENU
The Primal Blueprint, page 250

Breakfast: steak and fruit

4 oz flank steak

½ cup blueberries

½ peach

1 cup green tea

Lunch: chicken club lettuce wrap

3 large lettuce leaves

4 oz cooked chicken

½ red pepper

1 tomato

½ avocado

1 tsp mayonnaise

Dinner: beef stir-fry

4 oz beef steak

2 tbsp olive oil

1 zucchini

1 cup sliced mushrooms

1 cup spinach

½ cup sliced bamboo shoots

¼ oz sesame seeds

Snacks

1 large hardboiled egg

1 apple

1 tbsp almond butter

After analyzing their menus, we were not surprised to find that both the paleo- and Primal-style diets were at the head of the pack in reaching micronutrient sufficiency. Both the paleo and the Primal meal plans met sufficiency in fifteen of the twenty-seven essential micronutrients examined, at 2,160 and 1,911 calories respectively. However, while they tied the Best Life Diet for the most micronutrient sufficient of the programs analyzed, you can still see that neither the paleo nor Primal diet was really able to pull ahead and raise the bar in this area. When we examined exactly how many calories it would take to reach 100% RDI sufficiency for each diet plan, we found yet again that while these program were superior and needed fewer calories, the calories required would still be well outside the range of a medically wise dietary program.

TABLE 7.3. INDEPENDENT RESEARCH ON TWO ADDITIONAL POPULAR DIET PLANS

NAME OF DIET	% RDI SUFFICIENT	# OF MICRONUTRIENTS THAT MET RDI SUFFICIENCY	# OF CALORIES IN AVERAGE DAILY INTAKE	CALORIES REQUIRED TO REACH 100% RDI FOR ALL 27 MICRONUTRIENTS
Practical Paleo	56%	15	2,160	17,000
Primal Blueprint	56%	15	1,911	14,100

In support for these programs, however, we should add that both ancestral programs steer their followers to source local produce, grass-fed meat, wild-caught fish, and pastured eggs and poultry whenever possible. But because the USDA's database did not always contain these higher-quality products, we could not accurately reflect the full potential increase in micronutrient intake in the data.

However, after careful evaluation as to the possible increase in micronutrients the inclusion of these higher-quality products would deliver, it is our belief that it would not change the number of sufficient micronutrients in a statistically significant way—the specific micronutrients these diets were deficient in would not be greatly affected by the foods involved. For example, the sizable deficiencies in calcium, chromium, and biotin in both ancestral diets would not be removed even if we examined the potential micronutrient benefits of choosing pastured eggs over conventional. We should also add that while the two texts both encourage their readers to include organ meat (offal) and bone broth in their menus, these high-micronutrient foods were not included in the daily menus that were examined, nor were they contained in the majority of the menus suggested by either text.

Are you surprised that neither the paleo diet nor the Primal diet are able to reach micronutrient sufficiency or really do that much better than the other popular diets? We certainly were.

We do feel that the inclusion of high-quality, micronutrient-rich foods probably would increase the amount of micronutrients ingested for both the paleo and the Primal diets over what is reflected in our data. But to be fair, following Step One of this program, following our Rich Food, Poor Food philosophy, and including these high-quality foods would increase the sufficiency for all the popular diet plans examined.

The goal of this study was to determine the approximate micronutrient levels being delivered to the typical person who follows one of these dietary philosophies as outlined in the respective texts. These people could then be educated as to whether they are reaching micronutrient sufficiency from food alone.

The facts are that none of the diet plans, paleo and Primal included, deliver 100% sufficiency for the 27 essential micronutrients examined within a realistic and medically wise calorie range.

Similar studies have examined micronutrient inadequacies in other popular diet plans as well. A study conducted by the Children's Nutrition Research Centre of the Royal Children's Hospital in Australia found that following the Atkins Diet resulted in significant reductions in intake of vitamin B_2, folate, calcium, magnesium, potassium, and iron, while the Weight Watchers diet reduced intake of riboflavin, niacin, potassium, calcium, magnesium, iron, and zinc. Research published by the National Institute of Hygiene in Poland evaluated the effects of a low-calorie diet, such as those typically prescribed for obesity, on a group of ninty-six overweight patients. After following the prescribed 1,000-calorie a day diet for eighteen weeks, intakes of vitamins A, B_1, B_2, C, E, and niacin were all found to be insufficient. These studies add to our body of evidence that many popular and prescribed diet plans are deficient in essential micronutrients.

Based on the studies we have examined, which include random and structured popular diets, let's make the following statement our **Naked Fact #10.**

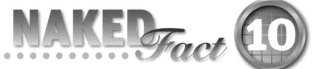

*According to published research, random,
low-carbohydrate, Mediterranean, low-fat, paleo,
Primal, and medically based diets from food alone
have all been shown to be deficient at delivering
minimum RDI levels of essential micronutrients
within medically wise calorie ranges.*

You can now answer David's question for yourself. *"Can I get all the essential micronutrients I need from a balanced diet, or do I need to take a multivitamin?"* You have seen the research that proves the balanced diet to be more fiction than fact. While it may be possible to use computer programs and databases to formulate a specific food combination that would supply your RDI requirements, the consumption and sustainability of such a diet would be up for serious debate. Ultimately, our response to David and the many others worldwide who have asked the first part of the above question is always the same: No, research has shown that you cannot get all of your essential micronutrients from a balanced diet. (We'll get to the multivitamin part of this question a little bit later in Chapter 9.)

All right, before we move on let's take a moment to play detective and apply some of the things we have discovered in past chapters. Take a look at the suggested menus again. Did you notice if any of the menus suggested spinach, whole-wheat breads, grains, nuts, berries, fruits, or cereals? Remember, these foods all contain Everyday Micronutrient Depleters (EMDs), such as oxalates, phytates, and tannins. We should also remember that in all of the studies, micronutrient content was evaluated before any of the Everyday Micronutrient Depleters (EMDs) were applied. But what if someone following one of these diets drank alcohol, took medication, or had a stressful job? What if they cooked everything in the microwave or exercised hours a day?

As we have learned, much of what has been calculated toward RDI sufficiency will be further reduced or, in some cases, negated by many the EMDs that can be found in our everyday life. Now that we have followed micronutrient loss from soil to your plate and have seen what happens to our food after it is eaten, would you recognize the EMDs in your own life? Let's examine a day in the life of a typical person living today. We'll call her Peggy. In the following section, underline each time that Peggy encounters an Everyday Micronutrient Depleter (EMD) throughout her day. (We'll give you the answers on page 155—don't peek!)

• • • • • • • • • • • • • •

A Portrait of Peggy

PEGGY STARTS HER DAY, like millions of us, with her morning coffee. This particular morning she chooses a low-fat muffin to go with her black coffee; other days she just has the coffee. On the way to the office, Peggy is on the phone managing a problem that has come up concerning an important, stressful project. Her morning continues with a short, but tense meeting, followed by another cup of coffee, some time at her desk, and more coffee.

Peggy is trying to lose a few pounds, so for lunch she heats up a popular processed, frozen, diet meal in the microwave. Peggy takes prescription medications for her high cholesterol and anxiety. She takes these medications every day after lunch with a Coke and then again before bed. By mid-afternoon Peggy's stomach announces, with gurgles and churns, that the 300-calorie muffin she had for breakfast and the 350-calorie lunch was just not enough. She grabs some chips (baked) and a cran-grape juice drink for a much-needed, mid-afternoon boost.

Tonight Peggy's children will be staying at their dad's house, so she will get to go to the gym. Like many people, she has decided to treat herself to a personal trainer twice a week, and tonight is one of those nights. Peggy loves working out with Ricardo, her trainer, because he really pushes her to do more than she would do on her own. Before Peggy gets to the gym, she drinks an energy drink, which she finds helps her get the most out of her workout.

Ricardo starts Peggy out with a twenty-minute warm-up on the Stairmaster before their typical one-hour weight-training routine. At the end of her session, Ricardo reminds Peggy that it is "weigh-in" night. Once a week Ricardo weighs her, to see how close she is to attaining her fifteen pounds of desired weight loss. Peggy has lost four pounds already. Tonight her weight is 156, the same as last week. Ricardo reminds Peggy that if she wants to lose the weight, she will have to eat less and work out more. He also suggests that she may want to try a popular fat burner, which has helped many of his other clients lose weight quickly. Stressed and slightly depressed about her weight, Peggy returns home to an empty house, microwaves a 400-calorie frozen pizza made from whole-wheat flour, and finally gets to enjoy a much-deserved glass of wine, or two, before taking her medications and going to bed.

How Does Your Day Compare?

How does Peggy's day compare to your day? How many times did you count EMDs in Peggy's story? According to our count, EMDs entered Peggy's life at least thirty-six times throughout her day, and with Ricardo's suggestion to increase her workout duration and decrease her calorie intake, Peggy's overall micronutrient-sufficiency level would only incur greater depletion. On top of this, taking fat burners would add an over-the-counter weight-loss aid to her already long list of EMDs.

Using your new understanding of the caloric intake that would be required to reach micronutrient sufficiency as well as the micronutrient-depleting effects of EMDs, how likely is it that Peggy is sufficient in all of her essential micronutrients? As this chapter has shown, based on the average amount of calories required to reach sufficiency from food alone, Peggy could never be completely sufficient. This is because she had a full, busy day; based on the RDI, in order to eat the amount of calories Peggy would need to be micronutrient sufficient, she would have to have done nothing except eat all day. However, if Peggy ate the average 27,575 calories it would take to become micronutrient sufficient, instead of losing fifteen pounds, she would quickly gain weight and eventually become obese.

Where Did Peggy Encounter All 36 EMDs?

1 & 2	Coffee containing caffeine and tannins (2 Drink EMDs)
3 & 4	Low-fat muffin containing white flour and white sugar (EDNP Food & EMD)
5	Stress on phone (Lifestyle EMD)
6 & 7	Coffee containing caffeine and tannins (2 Drink EMDs)
8	Stress from tense meeting (Lifestyle EMD)
9 & 10	Coffee containing caffeine and tannins (2 Drink EMDs)
11–13	Lunch: microwaving (Food Preparation EMD) Frozen prepackaged meal (Food Packaging EMD) Diet meal restricting calories (Lifestyle EMD)
14 & 15	Medication for cholesterol and anxiety (2 Medication EMDs)
16–19	Coke, containing phosphoric acid, caffeine, and high fructose corn syrup (EDNP food & 3 Drink EMDs)
20	Bag of chips (EDNP food)
21–23	Cran-grape juice drink containing tannins, high fructose corn syrup, and white sugar (3 Drink EMDs)
24–26	Energy drink containing sugar, caffeine, and phosphoric acid (3 Drink EMDs)
27	Gym workout (Exercise EMD)
28–32	Dinner: wheat crust contains phytic acid and sugar in tomato sauce (2 EMDs) Microwaving (Food Preparation EMD) Frozen prepackaged meal (Food Packaging EMD) Diet meal restricting calories (Lifestyle EMD)
33 & 34	Wine containing alcohol and tannins (2 Drink EMDs)
35 & 36	Medication for cholesterol and anxiety (2 Medication EMDs)

YOUR ASSIGNMENT

Write down all of your daily activities and examine the EMDs you encounter.

With the number of obese adults and children worldwide skyrocketing, we can no longer ignore this dangerous and debilitating pandemic. The frustrating thing about dieting is that most people go on a diet and think that if they follow the diet religiously for the required amount of time, they will live happily ever after at their new lower weight. But this just isn't true.

According to an article published in *Medicine & Science in Sports & Exercise,* the official journal of the American College of Sports Medicine, researchers from Wake Forest School of Medicine reported, "Nearly all overweight/obese people have difficulty maintaining weight loss. In most persons, one-third to two-thirds of their lost weight will be regained within the first year, and the rate of regain does not diminish as time elapses, with an estimated 66 percent of lost weight regained within two years and 95 percent regained within five years."

In the next chapter we explore the connection between the seemingly unstoppable obesity pandemic and the micronutrient-deficiency pandemic we have introduced in this book. We will explore research that supports this link and show you how micronutrient sufficiency could be the missing puzzle piece to controlling your weight forever.

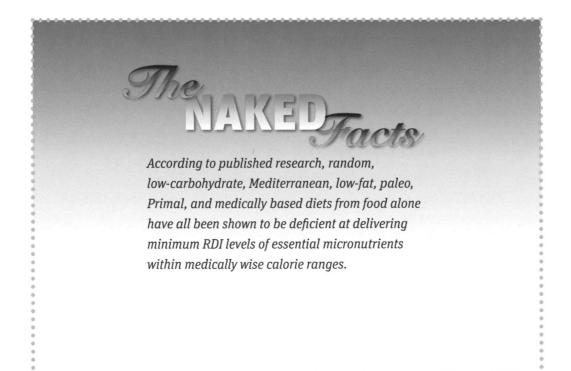

The NAKED *Facts*

According to published research, random, low-carbohydrate, Mediterranean, low-fat, paleo, Primal, and medically based diets from food alone have all been shown to be deficient at delivering minimum RDI levels of essential micronutrients within medically wise calorie ranges.

Chapter Eight

The Obesity Puzzle

Micronutrient Sufficiency—
The Missing Piece

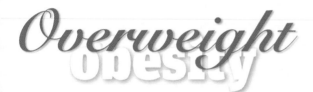

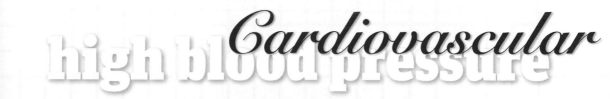

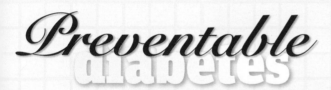

> ❝The insidious, creeping pandemic of obesity is now engulfing the entire world.❞
> —Professor Paul Zimmet, Chair of the 10th International Congress on Obesity

Returning to Delhi was a shock to our senses. The solitude of the Dera sand dunes in Rajasthan, India, was now behind us. Camel treks to visit remote communities nestled between peaceful fields of golden wheat, full of warm and friendly faces, were replaced by overcrowded city streets filled with bustling bodies, clattering sounds, and traffic jams. Cars, cows, and bicycle-drawn *tuk tuks* all tried to maneuver their way through the same narrow streets. A massive maze of exposed wires filled the sky above us, supplying power to the enormous population of this lively capital city.

The city was filled with many exotic and lingering smells—the good and the bad awaiting us around every corner. We were on our way to a visit with a local family to conduct research for the Calton Project, and we knew from the amount of traffic that we would not make it on time. Our driver, a soft-spoken Sikh named Seva Singh, noticed our impatience. "No worries," he assured us. He told us that he had all three things necessary to be a good driver in India: a good car to carry us in, a good horn to make the cows get out of our way, and most important, good luck. We had a brief chuckle and settled back into our comfortable SUV. Watching the bustling city around us was fascinating. The vibrant colors of the women's saris danced past the windows. The men, now mostly wearing suits, were a stark contrast from the loose-fitting punjabis we had been accustomed to seeing them wear in the rural areas. Then, at a stoplight, a startling discovery was

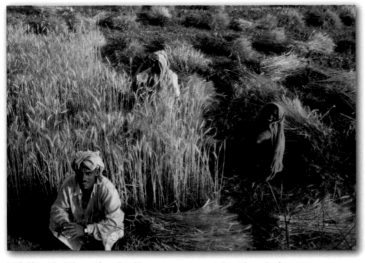

While visiting the Indian countryside, the Caltons were impressed by the lean men and women who worked long hours in the fields.

The Caltons witnessed women sitting on the streets of urban India with stalls of candy and packaged foods all around them.

made. We didn't have to get out of the car, search the back-streets, or ask a local scientist numerous questions to uncover it. There, stopped at the corner was a school bus. A stream of uniform-clad children, both boys and girls, were being deposited in front of the small brick building. No longer were the children thin and in shape, walking through fields to get to school as we had seen in the countryside. Here in Delhi, they arrived by school bus, looking rounded and fat, expending no energy of their own. We looked at each other in shock. The obesity pandemic had arrived.

According to Richard H. Carmona, M.D., the former Surgeon General of the United States, "Obesity is the terror within; unless we do something about it, the magnitude of the dilemma will dwarf 9/11 or any other terrorist attempt." Obesity rates have tripled over the past forty years for children and teens, increasing their risk of diabetes and other diseases. For the first time, children are being diagnosed with high blood pressure. "Where will our soldiers and sailors and airmen come from? . . . Where will our policemen and firemen come from if the youngsters today are on a trajectory that says they will be obese, laden with cardiovascular disease, increased cancers and a host of other diseases when they reach adulthood?"

These statements might put obesity in a whole new light for some of you. If you consider the fact that children are our future, it appears that our future may be in grave danger. In fact, according to a study in *Pediatrics,* the official journal of the American Academy of Pediatrics, "All indications are that the current generation of children will grow into the most obese generation of adults in U.S. history."

It is hard to imagine there is anyone who over the past ten years has not heard about the world's overweight and obesity pandemic. In America, obesity has affected just about everyone in some way; whether personally through family or friends, or in the rising costs of health care.

According to the World Health Organization (WHO), currently 74.1 percent of Americans over the age of fifteen are overweight or obese, and the predictions concerning the future of obesity are even more sobering.

According to Johns Hopkins researcher May Beydoun, Ph.D., MPH, staff scientist at the National Institute on Aging, "Obesity is likely to increase, and if nothing is done, it will soon become the leading preventable cause of death in the United States." Annually, the United States Government, which really means all of us, spends well over 100 billion dollars on obesity alone. More than 300,000 Americans die yearly from illnesses related to being overweight or obese. The excess weight America is putting on daily has lead to an increase in type 2 diabetes, high blood pressure, osteoarthritis, heart disease, stroke, gallbladder disease, sleep apnea, and cancer. With obesity such a hot topic in the media, most of us are more than familiar with its dangerous and debilitating effects. So instead of talking about the "weighty" consequences, we dedicate this chapter to exploring the connection between being overweight or obese and micronutrient deficiency.

The truth is that Americans have tried just about everything to lose weight. With the popular diet programs, gym memberships, hypnosis, acupuncture, endermologie, cellulite creams, body wraps, infomercial contraptions, diet pills, prescription drugs, liposuction, aerobic classes, health spas, electronic abdominal stimulators, personal diet coaches, gastric bypass surgery, lap bands, fat-free foods, low-carbohydrate foods, foods whose macronutrient ratios add up to 40/30/30, vibration machines, yoga, saunas, appetite suppressants, diet drinks, exotic herbs, fasting, body cleansing, and aerobic pole dancing, Americans should be the skinniest people on the planet. But we're not . . . why? Although one of the major government objectives for 2010 was to reduce the number of obese people in America to less than 15 percent, instead of declining, the number of obese people rose.

According to the Surgeon General, there are approximately 300,000 deaths each year in the United States that are a result of being overweight or obese. This is equivalent to three jetliners . . . filled to capacity . . . crashing every day.

A 2011 report by the Centers for Disease Control and Prevention (CDC) shows that since 1990, a dramatic increase of obesity has occurred in the United States. It cited that in 1990 no states were recorded as having a prevalence of obesity equal to, or greater than, 15 percent. In contrast, the latest data from 2010 shows no state having a prevalence of obesity less than 20 percent, thirty-six states had greater than 25 percent, and twelve states had obesity prevalence greater than 30 percent (Alabama, Arkansas, Kentucky, Louisiana, Michigan, Mississippi, Missouri, Oklahoma, South Carolina, Tennessee, Texas, and West Virginia).

Although most of this data may make it seem that America is alone in this *epidemic,* let us be clear in stating that obesity is a global *pandemic.* According to WHO, there are more than 1 billion overweight adults worldwide—at least 300 million of them obese. Since 1980, obesity rates have risen more than 300 percent in some areas of the United Kingdom, Eastern Europe, the Middle East, the Pacific Islands, Australasia, and China.

Crude projections suggest that by the year 2025, levels of obesity, not including individuals who are merely overweight, could be as high as 30 to 40 percent in Australia, England, and Mauritius and over 20 percent in Brazil. The obesity pandemic is not restricted to industrialized societies; often, obesity rates accelerate more rapidly in developing countries than in the developed world. It is imperative that we take action now.

Obesity—Not a Disease of Wealth

According to the World Health Organization (WHO), America ranks ninth on the list of the most overweight countries with 74.1 percent of people over the age of fifteen considered overweight.

The South Pacific island of Nauru tops the list with an alarming 94.5 percent of its adult population overweight and over 80 percent of its population obese.

The Federated States of Micronesia, Cook Island, Niue, and Tonga all have overweight populations of over 90 percent.

U.S. obesity rates are increasing at approximately 1 percent per year.

At this rate, 95 percent of the American population over the age of fifteen will be overweight or obese by 2030.

So, what can we do? How can we reduce obesity rates? It is obvious that we must be missing an important piece of the puzzle when it comes to stopping, reversing, and eventually eradicating obesity. Maybe we just aren't looking in the right place. To be honest, based on the list of potential weight-loss methods that we cited earlier, we haven't left very many stones unturned in our search for a thinner us.

The question we are posing to you and the nutritional and medical world at large is: **Could micronutrient deficiency be the missing puzzle piece in the fight against obesity?**

While obesity has been researched from almost every conceivable angle, in our quest to answer this question we needed to find a scientific study that identified a direct link between micronutrient deficiency and obesity. As it turns out we found such a study, and the statistics were more staggering than we could have ever imagined.

In this landmark study, published in December 2007 in the journal *Economics and Human Biology,* researchers revealed that micronutrient-deficient women had an 80.8 percent higher chance of being overweight or obese than non-deficient women. That's right—a direct link between being micronutrient deficient and being overweight or obese had been found.

Upon first examination of that study, you may not see the silver lining. However, it turns out that the link between being overweight or obese and micronutrient deficiency could be the best news *ever* in the fight against obesity. This is because if you take the study and turn it upside down and reexamine it, it indicates that being micronutrient sufficient could protect one from becoming overweight or obese by that same 80.8 percent! If being deficient showed an 80.8 percent increase in risk, then it would stand to reason that being sufficient would show the same 80.8 percent decrease in risk.

You may be thinking that all of this sounds a little too good to be true. We thought so too, until we dug a little deeper and found a few more studies to confirm our hypothesis. We started by searching for studies that included specific micronutrient level analysis with their data. We were hunting for studies that determined if micronutrient deficiency was common in subjects who were overweight and obese. The first such study we discovered was out of Sweden. The researchers studied 230 four-year-old children and found:

- Nearly 20 percent (one out of five) of the children were already overweight or obese by the age of four.
- Twenty-five percent of their total food intake came from "junk food" (another name for EDNP foods or poor foods that we have already learned cause micronutrient deficiencies).
- Almost all of the children were deficient in vitamin D, iron, and omega-3.

Did you notice that the Swedish children were found to be deficient in vitamin D, iron, and omega-3 fatty acids? Could deficiencies of these three micronutrients unlock the secrets of obesity? Let's take this step by step, and begin with the first micronutrient that was listed as deficient in the Swedish study, vitamin D.

Researchers from the Medical College of Georgia who were also curious about vitamin D deficiency set out to determine if vitamin D played a role in childhood obesity. The study, presented to the American Heart Association, found that when 650 children between the ages of fourteen and nineteen were tested, the students with the lowest vitamin D intake had the highest percentages of both body fat and abdominal fat. These results, which proved a correlation between childhood obesity and vitamin D deficiency, are particularly important because abdominal (visceral) fat has been linked to an increased risk of heart disease, stroke, high blood pressure, and diabetes. So, if vitamin D deficiency is linked to childhood obesity, and childhood obesity rates are steeply rising, then how many children in America have a vitamin D deficiency?

In a 2009 study by Albert Einstein College of Medicine, American children were found to be a whopping 70 percent insufficient in vitamin D. "We were astounded at how common it was," says study author Michal Melamed, M.D. "There is a lot of data that suggests adults with low vitamin D levels are at risk for diabetes, high blood pressure, cardiovascular disease, and a lot of cancers, and if kids start out with low levels and never increase them, they may be putting themselves at risk for developing all of these diseases at a much earlier age."

According to Michael F. Holick, Ph.D., Professor of Medicine, Physiology and Biophysics at Boston University School of Medicine and the author of *The Vitamin D Solution,* we should not be surprised at this high percentage. He explains, "[Parents should know] their child is likely to be vitamin D deficient if the child does not take a supplement of 400 IU (international units) vitamin D a day and receive some unprotected sun. It is next to impossible to get enough vitamin D from diet, and the sun-phobic attitude has made the problem much worse."

Therefore, we've determined that children with vitamin D deficiency are at a greater risk for obesity, and that the vast majority of children are vitamin D deficient. Do you think that similar results were found in studies on adults as well? Hold on to your hats because the next study is incredible.

A study from Children's Hospital in Los Angeles found that women who were deficient in vitamin D were, on average, 16.3 pounds heavier than women who were not vitamin D deficient. The researchers believe that vitamin D may slow the growth of fat cells; furthermore, vitamin D deficiency lowers blood levels of leptin, a hormone that tells your brain you are full. If you often find yourself eating more than you should, you may want to consider the possibility that due to a vitamin D deficiency, your brain simply doesn't get the message that you are full. Individuals deficient in vitamin D, which is now being touted as the "skinny" vitamin, are at a higher risk of obesity. This is great news because this means that being sufficient in vitamin D could then reduce this risk.

 Fast Facts on Vitamin D

Vitamin D is the only vitamin that can be derived from both food and sunshine; however, getting enough vitamin D may still be difficult. Here are four fast facts to enhance your vitamin D knowledge:

 If you live anywhere on the planet on a latitude north of Atlanta (approximately 33 degrees north), it's impossible to produce vitamin D from the sun during the winter months.

 People with fair skin need to be exposed for at least ten minutes every day to the midday sun wearing no sunscreen and at most shorts and a tank top, in order to get the RDI of vitamin D.

3 The levels of vitamin D in a mother's body while she is pregnant matters more than all the vitamin D in the milk her child will drink in the first nine years of life.

4 Dark-skinned individuals and the elderly don't produce vitamin D as efficiently as those younger and fairer.

Now that we have seen that vitamin D deficiency is linked to obesity, let's move on to iron, the next micronutrient found deficient in the Swedish four-year-olds. Perhaps an iron deficiency is also linked to obesity. In a study published in the *International Journal of Obesity*, overweight Israeli children and adolescents were examined to determine if a link existed between iron deficiency and weight. It was determined that when the children were divided into groups based on weight and body mass index (BMI), the children highest in both showed significantly higher levels of iron deficiency.

Is it possible that if we examined omega-3, the third micronutrient found to be deficient in the Swedish study, we would be three-for-three in finding a link between a micronutrient deficiency and obesity? The answer, as you may have guessed, is yes.

In a study presented at the North American Association for Study of Obesity (NAASO), twenty women with severe obesity who were already on a restricted low-calorie diet were observed. Researchers divided the women into two groups and gave one group omega-3 fatty acids. The women that were given the omega-3 fatty acids reduced their weight 20 percent more than the placebo group and reduced their BMI by up to 15 percent in only three weeks. This means that an increase in omega-3 brought an increase in weight loss *and* a decrease in BMI.

Science has also established that omega-3 increases oxidation of fat by activating genes that break down fat. In a study on animals that were overeating, much like obese humans, the introduction of omega-3 not only intensified fat breakdown, it also reduced the number of overall fat cells.

> *Stress actually increases body fat—particularly, belly fat.*

Do you remember back in Chapter 6 when we identified stress as an Everyday Micronutrient Depleter (EMD)? Well, stress actually increases body fat—particularly, belly fat. Science has pinpointed cortisol—a stress-induced steroid made by your body—to be the culprit behind belly fat.

As the body experiences stress it secretes cortisol into the bloodstream, which spikes appetite and increases fat deposits in the belly region. It also breaks down the lean muscle—the type of tissue that burns calories most efficiently. Supplementation with omega-3 can reduce the body's stress-induced production of cortisol by 22 percent. In fact, in a study at Gettysburg College in Pennsylvania, individuals supplementing with omega-3 had significantly lower cortisol levels. These same test subjects were able to shed three and a half times more body fat, while increasing lean muscle mass.

Do these studies confirm that we have the answer to obesity? Is it possible that these three micronutrient deficiencies are at the root of this global pandemic? The truth is that we didn't solve the mystery of obesity; rather, we found scientific clues as to what may be causing it. What we have discovered is that a deficiency in essential micronutrients, in these cases vitamin D, iron, and omega-3, has been linked in some way to being or remaining overweight or obese. Do you think there are other micronutrients that may also be pieces of the greater obesity puzzle? Let's look.

● ● ● ● ● ● ● ● ● ● ● ● ● ● ●

The Crave Cycle

HAVE YOU EVER FELT THAT YOU JUST COULDN'T STOP eating a bag of potato chips? Or perhaps you found yourself making a late-night run to the store because you craved something sweet? More likely than not, you have at some point felt a desire for a specific type of food, be it salty or sweet. What you might not have realized is, there is a good chance that the craving was your body's way of telling you that you were becoming deficient in a micronutrient. The problem was that you and your body weren't speaking the same language. While your body was screaming for calcium, all you heard was a cry for salty French fries.

According to Michael Tordoff, Ph.D., a researcher at Philadelphia's Monell Chemical Senses Center, craving salt is due to a calcium deficiency. Sodium temporarily increases calcium in the blood, which tricks your body into thinking the calcium deficiency is over. However, while this may temporarily satisfy your salt craving, the secreted bone calcium leads to an exacerbated calcium deficiency and further salt cravings. In animal studies, researchers found similar findings. It was observed that animals would devour table salt if calcium, potassium, or iron were deficient.

For all you *sweet tooths* out there, we have good news for you, too. Studies show that deficient mineral levels, such as magnesium, can induce sugar cravings. However, once these levels are increased, the cravings diminish. But what happens if you give in and grab something sugary sweet? Similar to salt cravings, giving in is actually making your cravings worse.

Can you think of anything we told you back in Chapter 6 about sugar that would make this true? Sugar is an EMD that blocks the absorption of essential minerals, including magnesium and calcium. So, you feel a craving for something sugary, you eat it, and the sugar in the food itself blocks the absorption of the minerals calcium and magnesium, causing further depletion.

Now, not only is your magnesium deficiency causing you to feel a desire for more sweets, the calcium depletion is causing you to crave something salty on top of it. According to Michael Steelman, M.D., past president of the American Society of Bariatric Physicians, "It becomes like a dog chasing its tail."

THE **CRAVE** CYCLE

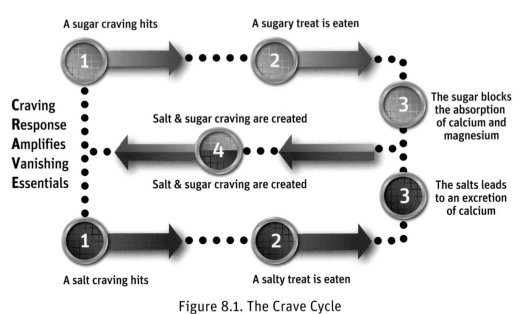

Figure 8.1. The Crave Cycle

Can you see how micronutrient deficiency may lead someone to overeat or cheat on a diet? A lack of discipline may not be the cause of overeating or failed diet attempts. Cravings are your body's deep cries for essential micronutrients.

Zinc has also been shown to have its own link to obesity. It turns out that zinc is one of the micronutrients responsible for taste-bud sensitivity. By the age of sixty, taste-bud sensitivity is greatly reduced. In studies done on rats, zinc deficiency caused the rats to ingest more of the foods they preferred. In other words, not being able to taste food made lab rats eat more of it.

Obesity affects many of us, and what we can learn from those suffering from this condition may help us all better understand what lies at the root of this global pandemic. A small number of nutritional theorists are thinking outside the box and connecting the dots between micronutrient deficiency and obesity in a whole new way. In a paper titled, "The Metabolic Tune-Up: Metabolic Harmony and Disease Prevention," Bruce N. Ames, Ph.D., writes about the connection between micronutrient deficiency and obesity. "We hypothesize that a micronutrient deficiency counteracts the normal feeling of satiety [feeling full] after sufficient calories are eaten. This may be a biological strategy for obtaining missing nutrients, which is important in fertility. Thus part of the reason for the obesity epidemic may be that energy-dense, micronutrient-poor diets leave the consumer deficient in key micronutrients, e.g., calcium, and constantly hungry."

If these contemporary theoretical perspectives were to be combined with current scientific research concerning the link between micronutrient deficiency and obesity, being overweight or obese would be viewed in an entirely different light. Instead of being wrongfully perceived as lazy, undisciplined overeaters, overweight and obese people would be seen for what they most likely are—individuals who are simply biochemically more in tune with their body's need for their required essential micronutrients and are trying to achieve micronutrient sufficiency the only way that their bodies know how—by eating more food.

• • • • • • • • • • • • • • • •

Antioxidants Aid in Battling Obesity

WHY IS IT THAT THE FRENCH CAN EAT GOURMET, high-fat cheeses and still stay thin? As we have seen, their traditional, artisan cheeses from grass-fed cows contain higher levels of many micronutrients. But could their love of wine also play a role? Although we learned in Chapter 6 that alcohol is an Everyday Micronutrient Depleter (EMD), like many other EMDs wine (or the polyphenols in wine) has been shown to have health benefits.

Polyphenols in grape seeds are loaded with antioxidants. As we discussed earlier, antioxidants work to protect our bodies from free radicals that damage cells. In fact, grape seed extract has sixty times more potent antioxidant activity per milligram than vitamin E.

In a 2009 study from France's University of Montpellier, a group of "lucky" hamsters was fed a daily diet high in fat and grape seed extract from chardonnay grapes. A second group of hamsters was fed only the high-fat diet, while a third group was fed a standard diet. After twelve weeks the hamsters on the high-fat diet alone had gained significant weight and had increased their blood sugar levels, insulin levels, triglycerides, and abdominal fat. In contrast, the researchers found that animals given grape seed did not have increased abdominal weight. Researchers concluded that this is "the first time that chronic consumption of grape phenolics is shown to reduce obesity development." In fact, the researchers concluded that the grape seed extract group showed limited oxidative stress, which led to an "antiobesity effect."

Could other antioxidants also help in our fight against obesity? A recent study from Oregon State University and the University of Washington discovered the connection between alpha lipoic acid, commonly referred to as the "universal antioxidant," and obesity. Alpha lipoic acid is a unique antioxidant. Unlike other antioxidants, alpha lipoic acid can work both in water, like vitamin C, and in fatty tissue, like vitamin E. This means that it can work throughout your entire body. Also, unlike other antioxidants, alpha lipoic acid may help to regenerate other antioxidants after they are depleted by free radicals. This makes alpha lipoic acid a very powerful antioxidant indeed.

The study examined two groups of mice, half of which had received alpha lipoic acid supplementation. Although the mice were fed identical diets, the alpha lipoic–supplemented mice gained 40 percent less weight than the mice that were not supplemented. Mice receiving alpha lipoic acid ate less than those without supplementation, even when offered an equal supply of food. The alpha lipoic acid seemed to have an appetite-suppressing effect on the rodents. The supplemented mice also exercised more than the non-supplemented mice, even when kept in the same environments. Does it sound to you as if alpha lipoic acid may help you to control your desire for food and increase your energy levels?

In another study focusing on antioxidants, researchers at the National Institute of Food and Nutrition in Warsaw, Poland, studied 102 overweight women. They determined that these women had higher deficiency levels of the "antioxidant" vitamins A, C, and E than average-weight women. Perhaps the vitamins A, C, and E, as well as their antioxidant "accessory nutrient" counterparts grape seed extract and alpha lipoic acid, can help protect us from obesity.

If you think back to earlier examined facts, you may be able to recognize why we should expect vitamin C to be deficient in overweight individuals. Do you remember that vitamin C has been shown to be extremely effective at reducing stress? According to Neil Nathan, M.D., author of *On Hope and Healing,* "Vitamin C is a critical player in stress reactions in the body . . . research shows that the demand for vitamin C increases by up to tenfold during periods of stress."

Do you remember what is secreted in times of stress? If you guessed cortisol, you're right, and you probably also remember that cortisol causes body fat to increase, especially around the midsection. According to the University of Maryland, even slight deficiencies of vitamin C can increase cortisol output. Perhaps vitamin C should be considered a supplement that not only stress-proofs the body, but fat-proofs it too.

Perhaps vitamin C should be considered a supplement that not only stress-proofs the body, but fat-proofs it too.

Another reason vitamin C may be linked to obesity is that it is an important component in the creation of carnitine, which helps your body turn fat into fuel. Researchers at Arizona State University proved that individuals with low levels of vitamin C burned 25 percent fewer calories during the same period of exercise than those who had adequate vitamin C levels. So, becoming sufficient in this single essential micronutrient can curb your cortisol to minimize your middle and create carnitine to augment your ability to burn calories.

Antioxidants' ability to create an "antiobesity effect" is most likely due to their ability to destroy free radicals. Back in Chapter 6, in our discussion of prescription medications, we introduced you to CoQ_{10}, a powerful coenzyme. It is also an antioxidant that has been studied and proven to be crucial in the protection against free radicals. It should not surprise you then that multiple studies have been conducted linking a deficiency of CoQ_{10} to obesity. In a Belgium study, Luc Van Gaal, M.D., Ph.D., Professor of the Department of Endocrinology, Metabolism & Clinical Nutrition-Faculty of Medicine from University Hospital Antwerp, Belgium, examined twenty-seven obese patients and discovered that over one-half of these patients were significantly deficient in CoQ_{10}. These significantly deficient obese patients were then given 100 mg of CoQ_{10} daily, and after nine weeks they had lost an incredible average of 30 pounds.

However, it is not just antioxidants that have been shown to help individuals with the "battle of the bulge." A study titled "VITAL" (VITamins And Lifestyle), sponsored by the National Cancer Institute, examined 75,000 men and women over a ten-year period to determine the effectiveness of supplementation for weight management. It was determined that the consistent consumption of micronutrients vitamin B_6, vitamin B_{12}, and chromium were all indicators of stabilized weight over that ten-year period.

So, how does this all add up? Let's examine our clues and see, if when combined, they create the missing puzzle piece we have been looking for.

Did You Know

The U.S. Government has set guidelines for the amount of free radical–fighting antioxidants one should take in daily. The USDA recommends that we consume 3,000 to 5,000 ORAC units daily. Eighty percent of the population is consuming less than 1,000 ORAC units.

So what is ORAC ? ORAC stands for Oxygen Radical Absorption Capabilities. It is how we measure the ability of an antioxidant to fight free radicals. The USDA recommended "5-a-day" fruit and vegetable servings will give you an ORAC score of about 1,750 units. Following these U.S. Government guidelines will leave you with a deficiency of approximately 1,250 to 3,250 ORAC units daily. This reveals that the USDA fruit and vegetable recommendations alone would not fulfill the USDA's recommendations for ORAC and supports the need for antioxidant supplementation. Grape seed extract can have an ORAC value of up to 50,000 units.

CLUE 1

Swedish children were deficient in vitamin D, iron, and omega-3 and were obese by the age of four.

CLUE 2

Vitamin D deficiency is common and probable in overweight and obese individuals.

CLUE 3

Iron deficiency was found to be prevalent in overweight and obese populations.

Omega-3 supplementation caused men and women to lose weight.

Food cravings have been scientifically proven to be our body's way of telling us we are deficient in micronutrients like calcium, magnesium, potassium, and iron.

Zinc deficiency can cause decreased taste-bud sensitivity, which can lead to overeating.

Antioxidants such as grape seed extract, alpha lipoic acid, and vitamins A, C, and E are linked (in a good way) to obesity. Supplementation caused an "antiobesity effect" from decreased appetite, increased activity levels, and decreased abdominal fat. Individuals with these deficiencies had increased likelihood of being overweight or obese.

CoQ_{10} was determined to be significantly deficient in obese and overweight subjects, and supplementation produced an average weight reduction of an astounding 30 pounds in nine weeks.

Vitamin B_6, vitamin B_{12}, and chromium supplementation prevented weight gain over a ten-year period when compared to individuals who did not supplement these micronutrients.

While these clues only constitute a section of the missing puzzle piece, we can start to make out the image before us. Is it possible that obesity is really a condition of being micronutrient deficient? Two of our previously accumulated Naked Facts state that a global micronutrient-deficiency pandemic exists, and that a deficiency of an essential micronutrient may ultimately cause health-related conditions or diseases. We now know that numerous essential micronutrients have been studied, and it has been concluded that micronutrient deficiency increases the chances of becoming overweight or obese. Therefore, according to all of these studies, being overweight or obese is a related condition of being micronutrient deficient. This solidifies **Naked Fact #11.**

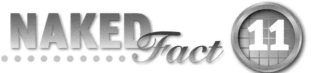

NAKED *Fact* 11

Obesity has been shown to be a
condition of micronutrient deficiency.

While we have established the link between obesity and micronutrient deficiency, it's only one of two vital factors that contribute to becoming overweight or obese. The other critical piece of this puzzle is calories. Yes, obesity is a condition of micronutrient deficiency, but in order for one to become obese one would have to take in a large amount of calories from food. What do you think micronutrient deficiency would look like with a deficiency of calories, or little to no food? It would look like a malnourished, underweight individual. However, when you look at impoverished, malnourished countries today you may be surprised by what you find. These days, the poor are becoming obese, and not because of an abundance of natural, micronutrient-*rich* food, but rather due to the detrimental increase of the processed poor foods now available to them.

In his book *In Defense of Food,* Michael Pollan states, "A diet based on quantity rather than quality has ushered a new creature onto the world stage; the human being who manages to be both overfed and undernourished, two characteristics seldom found in the same body in the long natural history of our species."

In the year 2000, the number of overweight adults surpassed the number of those who are underweight for the first time in history. According to an article by the Food and Agriculture Organization of the United Nations (FAO), "Obesity is deceptive. Although obese people may appear well fed, they are often deficient in essential nutrients, leading to poor health and disease. The underweight and overweight share high levels of sickness and disability, shortened life spans, and reduced productivity."

Mr. Neville Rigby, the former director of the International Obesity Taskforce, concurs, "It is not about being rich and well fed. Obesity is most often related to poverty, low economic status, and exclusion from the health system."

We can see that the two groups, the hungry underweight and the well-fed overweight, both suffer from many of the same health conditions. What may not be as apparent is that they also share malnutrition in the form of micronutrient deficiency. This is caused by a lack of essential vitamins and minerals due to micronutrient-*poor* food (naked calories). Mr. Daniel Epstein of WHO states, "Obesity has become a problem of poverty; poor people have an easier time of eating junk food. People fill up on things that have a high-caloric value but little nutritional value."

We want to be clear here—micronutrient deficiency is a form of malnutrition that in the absence of food (calories) appears as hunger, identified by a malnourished, underweight appearance. However, when energy-dense poor foods are ingested in large quantities, the face of micronutrient deficiency changes to that of obesity. Mervyn Deitel, M.D., founding editor of *Obesity Surgery*, puts it this way, "The commonest form of malnutrition in the western world is obesity." They are really just two sides of the same micronutrient-deficiency coin.

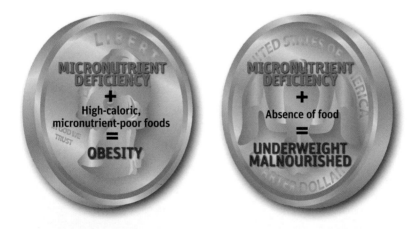

Figure 8.2. The Two-Sided Micronutrient-Deficiency Coin

Let's examine a study that further proves this point. In the *European Journal of Clinical Nutrition,* scientists evaluated individuals who were malnourished as well as those who were overweight and obese to determine whether micronutrient deficiencies existed. They tested for vitamins A, C, E, folic acid (B_9), and B_{12}. It was revealed that the micronutrient deficiencies were present equally in both the malnourished, as well as the overweight and obese patients. This brings us to our **Naked Fact #12.**

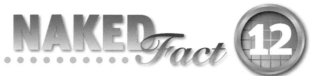

Malnourishment and obesity are both conditions of micronutrient deficiency. The only thing that differs is the caloric intake.

Multivitamins: The Next Big Weight-loss Supplement?

WITH THE KNOWLEDGE THAT MILLIONS of malnourished, underweight people are globally expanding to become billions of overweight and obese people, financially straining many of the world's global superpowers, the obesity pandemic is quickly becoming something we can no longer ignore. We have seen that specific micronutrients have proved beneficial for weight loss through a variety of pathways. With all the evidence pointing to obesity as a condition of micronutrient deficiency, it might seem reasonable to assume that supplementation of these essential micronutrients in the form of a multivitamin may eliminate, or at least shrink, the obesity pandemic.

Studies have been conducted on the effectiveness of multivitamin supplementation as a possible means to lose weight. A study in the *British Journal of Nutrition* recruited forty-five obese, non-consumers of multivitamins and minerals. These individuals were all put on the same calorie-restricted diet. One group was given multivitamins and minerals while the other group was given a placebo. At the end of the study, researchers observed two very interesting things:

 Those subjects who took the multivitamins and minerals reported a natural appetite-suppressing effect and felt more satisfied with the diet's smaller portions for longer periods of time.

 Both of the groups had lost the same amount of weight.

It shouldn't surprise any of us by now that the subjects taking the micronutrient supplements would receive some benefit. In this case, the benefit was that they were more satisfied than the placebo group. This coincides with our earlier findings on the appetite-suppressing effects of antioxidants as well as with Dr. Ames's hypothesis, and would certainly help a lot of people *stay* on a diet program. However, some of you may be surprised by the second piece of data from this study. It states that both groups lost the same amount of weight. How can this be? Doesn't this second piece of data seem counterindicative to our earlier studies?

In the studies previously presented, supplemented groups lost a significantly larger amount of weight than their non-supplemented counterparts. What changed? Did you notice that in the previous studies micronutrients were delivered in an isolated form? When all the micronutrients were piled into one vitamin and mineral supplement in the study in the *British Journal of Nutrition,* the increased weight-loss benefits of the micronutrients were negated. Why? What could be blocking the benefits of the micronutrients when delivered in the form of a multivitamin? To answer these questions, we turn to the ABCs of Optimal Supplementation.

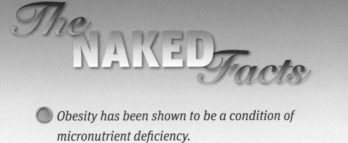

- *Obesity has been shown to be a condition of micronutrient deficiency.*
- *Malnourishment and obesity are both conditions of micronutrient deficiency. The only thing that differs is the caloric intake.*

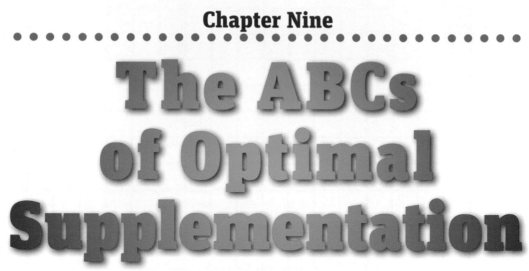

Chapter Nine

The ABCs of Optimal Supplementation

A Recipe for Success

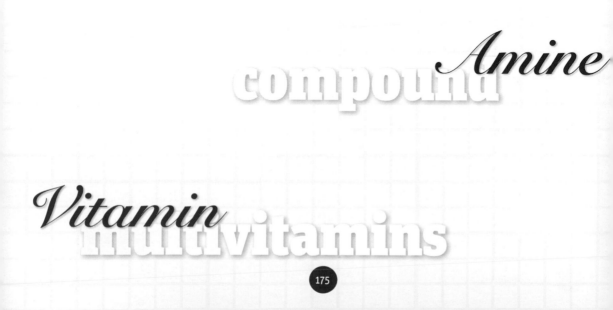

Vitalis vital

Amine

compound

Vitamin multivitamins

175

ara stood at her cooking station and awaited the instructions. Today her culinary teacher, Chef Marie, was going to teach the class how to make a lemon meringue pie. Their first task would be to separate the eggs. Sara felt confident she could do this without a problem because she made egg-white omelets for her family almost every Sunday morning. When instructed, she cracked the first egg, then dripped the clear egg white over the edge of the egg's shell and into the first glass bowl. She then discarded the yolk into a second glass bowl.

"No, Sara, not like that," scolded Chef Marie. Sara could feel the eyes of the other students on her, and her face immediately flushed. She couldn't imagine how she could have messed up something as simple as separating an egg. Chef Marie pointed out, "Look, there is a dash of yolk in your white. The fat in the egg yolk will collapse the delicate egg white foam. How can you expect to make perfect meringue with sad, collapsed foam?"

As Chef Marie began writing on the blackboard she said, "Separating eggs and whisking the whites into meringue foam is not as simple as all of you may have thought. There are many ways to ruin your egg whites. Note them so that we don't make these mistakes again."

Sara took out her notepad and wrote down the list from the blackboard.

Don't whisk in plastic bowls.

Never whisk eggs on humid days.

Any fat in the white, either from the yolk or from oil on your hand, will deflate the whites.

Eggs should be cold and at least four days old.

Make sure the whisk itself is very dry.

Did you have any idea that there were so many rules to consider when whisking an egg? After all, an egg only has two components that we can see, the white and the yolk. In this chapter, we discuss the multivitamin. Like the egg, it is also far more complicated than it appears. In the next two

Although it was 1753 when Lind published his *Treatise on the Scurvy*, a document of his research on the effective treatment of scurvy with citrus, it took the British Admiralty until 1795 to mandate lemon juice for all sailors.

This caused over 100,000 more British sailors to die needlessly of scurvy in that forty-two-year period. Even back then it took a long time for scientific research to affect public policy.

chapters, we will explore the answers to three fundamental questions: What makes a good multivitamin? How should you choose a multivitamin? Most important, do you need to take a multivitamin?

First, before answering these questions, let's step back in time and examine the history of the multivitamin, starting with the discovery of vitamins themselves. While vitamins as we know them today were not discovered until 1911, the importance of these micronutrients became clear in the modern world as early as 1747 when a Scottish naval surgeon named James Lind discovered that an unknown micronutrient found in lemons (later named vitamin C) prevented scurvy—a horrible micronutrient-deficiency disease rampant in the eighteenth century.

While James Lind may be credited for his theory that citrus fruits cured scurvy, there are records from the late 1400s that scurvy was being cured by similar means. In fact, there is a legend that tells of several Portuguese sailors on one of the voyages of Christopher Columbus who fell ill with scurvy. For religious reasons, they asked that they be dropped off to die and be properly buried on an island, rather than to be buried at sea. The sailors were put ashore on the next island en route, and Columbus sailed off expecting to never see them alive again. It is said that when he sailed by that island on his return voyage to bury them, he saw the very same sailors all in good health. This island is now called Curacao, meaning cure, and is known for its abundance of fresh fruits—packed with vitamin C.

Additionally, in 1601, British Captain James Lancaster unintentionally performed a controlled study on scurvy. He sailed his vessel among a large fleet of ships. Every morning he served each of his men three teaspoons of lemon juice, which had a reputation for warding off scurvy. Unlike all of the other vessels in the fleet, which had been devastated by scurvy, all of his men arrived to their destination in good health.

Scurvy is just one micronutrient-deficiency disease. The fact is, micronutrient deficiency has been the cause of disease throughout the ages. In the late 1800s a Dutch physician named Christiaan Eijkman made a groundbreaking discovery concerning another micronutrient deficiency, due to a fortunate mistake. Having run out of inexpensive, unpolished (unprocessed) rice to feed to his laboratory chickens, Eijkman temporarily switched to feeding them polished (processed) rice, usually reserved for human consumption. After a short period of time, he noticed that the chickens fell very ill. He discovered that the chickens had developed a paralyzing disease known as beriberi, typically only found in humans.

The word *beri* means weakness in Singhalese, a language in Sri Lanka, where beriberi was widespread. Eijkman witnessed that switching chicken feed from unpolished rice to polished rice brought about beriberi in the chickens. He theorized that switching polished rice for unpolished rice in the human diet could prevent this disease. As we learned earlier in Chapter 5, food processing is an EMD that can strip essential micronutrients from our foods. Serving the chickens processed, polished rice caused the chickens to become deficient in essential micronutrients. They had literally processed the micronutrients out of the rice and caused a micronutrient-deficiency disease.

Eijkman experimented endlessly in his laboratory to uncover what part of the rice had this medicinal effect. In one such experiment, he noted that when the temperature of the rice was raised to 120 degrees Celsius (248 degrees Fahrenheit), the unpolished (unprocessed) rice no longer prevented the beriberi. Were you able to recognize the EMD? This experiment supports our earlier Naked Fact #5, which states that food preparation methods, in this case heating at a high temperature, can cause large percentages of many essential micronutrients to be depleted.

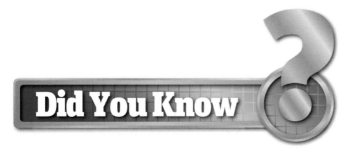

According to Martha Stewart, a 250-degree oven is considered a cool oven. A moderate oven temperature is 375 degrees, and a very hot oven is 475 degrees. This makes a cool oven hot enough to cause depletion to occur.

In 1905 William Fletcher, an English physician, decided to take Eijkman's rice study to Malaysia, then a British colony, to try for the first time to treat the lethal disease beriberi. Fletcher had great success treating and curing inmates with the unpolished rice. The story continues seven years later when a Polish chemist, named Casimir Funk, began working in Eijkman's meticulously preserved laboratory in London. Funk is the scientist who ultimately coined the word *vitamin*.

Casimir Funk was captivated by Fletcher's success in curing beriberi, so he decided to examine the husks from the rice that had been fed to the men in Malaysia. It was determined that there was

VITALIS + AMINE = VITAMIN

a "factor" in the unpolished rice that had cured beriberi. These "factors," responsible for curing diseases such as beriberi and scurvy, were renamed "vitamins." The word *vitamine* was derived from the Latin *vitalis,* meaning vital, and *amine,* a type of nitrogen-containing compound originally thought to be in all of the "factors." These vital amines, or vitamins, were realized by Funk to be essential for proper body function.

Meanwhile, Sir Frederick Hopkins, a British biochemist and one of the founders of biochemistry, experimented by feeding mice a synthetic diet. He discovered that this diet reduced bone growth in the mice. However, when he supplemented this same diet with milk, the growth pattern returned to that of a normal rodent. He hypothesized "additional food factors," as he called them, found in the milk were responsible.

When Funk and Hopkins came together in 1912, they proposed the *Vitamin Hypothesis of Disease,* stating that certain diseases are caused by a dietary lack of specific vitamins. Does it seem odd to you that as far back as 1912 science already associated micronutrient deficiencies with disease? If they knew it back then, why has it taken so long for science to discuss whether or not micronutrient sufficiency could bring about health? Isn't it about time for a revival of this theory?

In 1913, Elmer McCollum, Ph.D., and Marguerite Davis of Yale University were the first to isolate one of these "additional food factors" now referred to throughout the scientific world as vitamins. Being the first of its kind, it was called vitamin A. All the vitamins were originally named with only letters. (The numerous B vitamins were later discovered to be a subset of the originally discovered vitamin B, so that is why they include letters and numbers such as B_1, B_2, B_3, etc.)

Interestingly enough the third vitamin to be named, vitamin C, is not an amine. However, by this time scientists were so comfortable with the word *vitamin* that it just stuck regardless of whether the requirement for being an amine was met. Vitamin C is also referred to as ascorbic acid. This name comes from the final revelation that it was the vitamin C in the citrus that was anti-scurvy—or anti-scorbic, and finally just ascorbic.

In 1922, working in his new post at Johns Hopkins University, Dr. McCollum was finally able to "catch," as it was then termed, or "isolate" vitamin D, which he found aided in bone growth as well as prevented the disease called rickets.

In 1924, a group at the University of California furthered Sir Frederick Hopkins's earlier research on mice and milk. They found that while the mice that were fed milk appeared healthy, none of them could breed. This brought them to the discovery of vitamin E, which they were able to isolate in wheat and green leaves. You may notice on your multivitamin, if you take one, that vitamin E may be listed as tocopherols. The word *tocopherols* comes from the Greek words *tokos,* meaning childbirth, and *phero,* meaning to bring forth, thus making tocopherol the most appropriate name for a vitamin that reversed infertility. Throughout the beginning of the twentieth century the vitamin discoveries just kept coming. By the end of the 1930s all of our modern-day vitamins had been identified, and each of these vitamins was curing diseases.

The Invention of the Multivitamin

SO, WHO ACTUALLY INVENTED THE MULTIVITAMIN? Well, while all this research was going on, a man named Carl F. Rehnborg was in China from 1915 to 1927, working as a salesperson for Colgate. While there, he observed that urban dwellers were suffering from malnutrition and diseases like scurvy and beriberi, but that these conditions were not as widespread among the poorer people living in the more remote rural areas. He began to study the relationship between what these two groups were eating and their overall health and found that the people in the remote areas had access to fresh fruits and vegetables and were much healthier than the city dwellers. This is similar to what we witnessed on the Calton Project.

During a time of political unrest in Shanghai when many were forced into isolation, Rehnborg conceived of an idea to use nutritional elements to protect himself and his friends from developing scurvy and beriberi and maintain their health. He supplemented their daily soup with local herbs, grasses, vegetables, rusty nails (for iron), limestone (for calcium and magnesium), and ground-up animal bones (also for calcium). He shared his ill-tasting broth with his friends, and months later when the political unrest finally ended, Rehnborg and his friends emerged from their confinement much healthier than those who had not eaten his broth. This gave Rehnborg the revolutionary idea to create a single pill that would contain all the newly discovered vitamins,

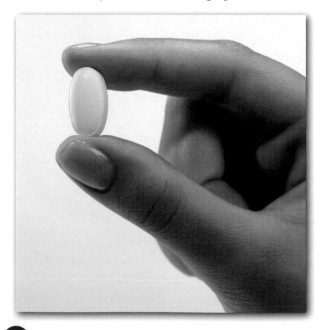

as well as minerals, in one easy-to-take product. Upon his return to California he did just that, and in 1934 Carl F. Rehnborg produced one of the world's first multivitamin/multi-mineral food supplements under the name California Vitamins.

You may have noticed what a relatively new science the study of micro-nutrients is. When you think about it, it's pretty surprising. After all, some of you might have already been born when the first vitamins were discovered—if not you, your parents or your grandparents.

Each day, science is uncovering new insight as to how the individual micronutrients within the multivitamins themselves really work. These recent scientific discoveries concerning multivitamins may help to decipher why participants in the *British Journal of Nutrition* study didn't receive all of the antiobesity benefits when taking their multivitamins. If you remember at the end of the last chapter we discovered that when scientists put overweight individuals on a calorie-restricted diet with one group taking a multivitamin and a second group taking a placebo, two interesting results were observed. Let's review their findings here:

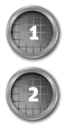

1 Those subjects who took the multivitamins and minerals reported a natural appetite-suppressing effect and felt more satisfied with the diet's smaller portions for longer periods of time.

2 Both of the groups had lost the same amount of weight.

This study revealed that while the multivitamin showed some benefit, in this case it naturally suppressed the subject's appetites, the individuals supplementing with a multivitamin did not lose more weight than those without supplementation. Why didn't the subjects taking multivitamins get all of the fantastic weight-loss benefits that we had seen in the earlier studies when isolated micronutrients were administered?

• • • • • • • • • • • • •

The ABCs of Optimal Supplementation

IN ORDER TO GET TO THE BOTTOM OF THIS QUESTION we now introduce to you some of the most vital, cutting-edge information in this book—which can finally unlock the full power and potential of the micronutrient. We call it the ABCs of Optimal Supplementation. This easy-to-remember acronym stands for the four elements you need to consider when choosing an effective dietary supplement, especially a multivitamin:

Absorption
Beneficial Quantities
Competition
Synergy

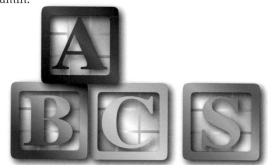

While at first glance the concepts of Absorption, Beneficial Quantities, Competition, and Synergy may not seem all that earth-shattering, understanding these four factors (especially the third factor, Competition) will completely alter the way you perceive and take micronutrients. Unlike individual *superheroes* that act independently of one another to protect us from a specific condition or disease, micronutrients interact with each other in a highly complex dance, each having their own personal traits and unique likes and dislikes. Back in Chapter 3, we introduced you to the House of Optimal Health (HOH). We explained that vitamins are like skilled workers building a house. They worked alongside the architects and foremen (minerals), independent contractors (essential fatty acids—EFAs), and assistants (accessory micronutrients), which all need to be present in sufficient quantities and at the right times for the House of Optimal Health to be built well.

Expanding on this analogy will help us to better understand how the ABCs can be used to achieve optimal health. We start with this premise: *In order for optimal health to occur, your House of Optimal Health needs be built perfectly, every day.* All of the builders, painters, foremen, roofers, independent contractors, architects, and electricians must all do their jobs efficiently on a daily basis if your house is going to be completed properly and punctually.

If this does not occur, then one of two things may eventually happen:

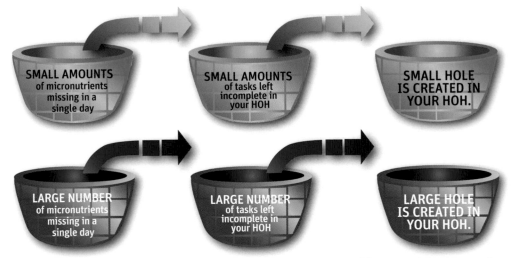

As we stated in our Naked Fact #3, a deficiency in one or more of the essential micronutrients may ultimately cause a health-related condition or disease. The extent to which your HOH is left unfinished each day (the size of the hole) and the length of time (i.e., days, weeks, or years) that these holes continue to be present can directly affect the severity and/or type of health condition or disease from which you may be suffering. Let's say, for example, that you devoured a bowl of Halloween candy someone brought to your office, and then skipped lunch because you were just too full to eat. This singular experience may cause a small hole, as these *poor foods* filled with naked calories rob you of the micronutrients needed to build your HOH. But unless repeated frequently, this will more than likely not cause any actual health conditions.

If, however, you always skip breakfast, drink black coffee all morning, and eat only micronutrient-poor meals, you may be causing a large hole in your HOH on a daily basis. These larger holes, over time, will have a high likelihood of expanding into a chronic health condition or disease such as obesity, diabetes, cardiovascular disease, osteoporosis, or even cancer. According to Robert Heaney, M.D., Professor of Medicine at Creighton University, "Inadequate intakes of many nutrients are now recognized as contributing to several of the major chronic diseases that affect the populations of the industrialized nations. Often taking many years to manifest themselves, these disease outcomes should be thought of as long-latency deficiency diseases." It's important to note that each micronutrient is so specialized that the hole created by its absence can only be filled by the presence of that one specific micronutrient.

For example, the disease caused by a deficiency of vitamin C (scurvy) cannot be cured by becoming sufficient in any other micronutrient. Only vitamin C will work. In our House of Optimal Health each essential micronutrient, represented by our construction crew, must all be present every day in order to keep all holes, both large and small, from being created.

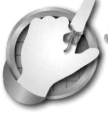

Remember

The more holes you have and the longer their duration directly affect the severity of the health conditions or diseases that may result.

- - - - - - - - - - - - - -

Micronutrient Depletion: A State of Emergency

WHILE IT MAY BE A BIT OVERSIMPLIFIED, we can now all understand how the "holes in the house" theory explains deficiency and disease. *However, if our bodies are creating these holes, why don't we feel them? If the vast majority of us have micronutrient deficiencies, then why aren't we all falling down and dying from these deficiency holes? How are our bodies all managing to function with this scarcity of micronutrients?* In order to understand this we must first understand something called the "triage" hypothesis. Triage is defined as "the determination of priorities for action in an emergency." We are most familiar with the term in battlefield or catastrophe settings where a doctor must figure out which patient needs to be treated first. Doctors, during a state of emergency, might choose to attend to the person with the most critical injury; they might also consider saving the most important person affected. In the case of the essential micronutrients, triage explains how the body prioritizes the use of a specific supplied micronutrient when there is a deficiency of this micronutrient.

Your body's first priority is short-term self-preservation. Therefore, the triage hypothesis states that your body will first use ingested micronutrients to perform the functions necessary to ensure short-term survival and last for the regulation and repair of cellular DNA and proteins that increase longevity. In a report published in the *Proceedings of the National Academy of Sciences (PNAS)*, Dr. Bruce N. Ames explains his triage hypothesis like this: "I hypothesize that short-term survival was achieved by allocating scarce micronutrients by triage . . . If this hypothesis is correct, micronutrient deficiencies that trigger the triage response would accelerate cancer, aging, and neural decay but would leave critical metabolic functions, such as ATP production, intact."

Dr. Ames states that the body already works on the triage principle. For example, if oxygen delivery is inadequate, the body prioritizes its use and insures blood flow to the top-ranked organs—the heart and brain. As you can see, it would make sense that your body views micronutrient allocation the very same way. This means that when in a state of micronutrient deficiency, our bodies are choosing which functions are of high priority and allocating our scarce micronutrients to these functions. However, this leaves many functions of lower priority ignored, making us susceptible to chronic lifestyle diseases. This explains why we can walk around so completely unaware of these deficiencies. The holes created begin in micronutrient activities of lesser importance. It is not until these unrealized holes expand over time that long-latency diseases set in, and by the time they are discovered, it is often too late.

• • • • • • • • • • • • • • • •

"A" Is for Absorption

IF YOU'VE EVER INQUIRED about taking a multivitamin you may have heard one of these two statements: "You can get all of your vitamins and minerals by eating a healthy diet," or "All you get when taking a multivitamin is expensive urine." Well, we now know, based on the evidence we have examined thus far, including published scientific studies and the USDA's research, that micronutrient deficiency is a pandemic and that no diet, random or structured, has been shown to supply the minimum Reference Daily Intake (RDI) requirement of essential micronutrients from food alone.

Nevertheless, if your multivitamin supplement is not properly formulated, there may be truth to the second statement—about expensive urine. Registered and licensed dietitian, Joanne Larsen, founder and editor of dietitian.com agrees. She writes, "Remember that the human body absorbs only about 10 to 15 percent of a vitamin pill and excretes the rest in urine and feces. Pretty expensive urine for some!"

As it turns out, it may be very difficult to absorb the vitamins and minerals within many of today's most popular multivitamins due to a variety of limiting factors, and if your body does not absorb them, they will simply pass right through it. In fact, one of the most common limiting factors blocking our body's ability to utilize the micronutrients we ingest in our multivitamin tablets and capsules is poor disintegration—its inability to break down and release the micronutrients for absorption.

According to a study published in the *Journal of Pharmacy and Pharmaceutical Sciences*, Raimar Löbenberg, Ph.D., of the University of Alberta states, "Active ingredients [micronutrients] can only be absorbed if they are released into solution from the dosage form. Disintegration is the first step in this process . . . if a mineral has to be absorbed within an absorption window and the dosage form does not release its content in a timely manner, then the therapy might be compromised or fail."

Dr. Löbenberg examined forty-nine well-known commercially available multivitamins that were in either tablet (pill) or capsule form to determine if they could release their contained micronutrients within a twenty-minute time period—the time necessary for potential absorption. The results showed that out of the forty-nine multivitamins studied, twenty-five (or 51 percent) did not disintegrate. Furthermore, the *Physicians Desk Reference (PDR),* a guide to all things prescribed, indicates that the contents of both capsules and pills, which make up the majority of multivitamin sales, are only 10 to 20 percent absorbed by the body, while liquid formulas are the most absorbable at up to 98 percent.

A business associate of ours told us a humorous tale concerning disintegration that further illustrates this concern, which she cleverly called "the scoop on the poop." She shared with us a story that she had heard from her friend Stephanie. On their family farm outside of Sterling, Kansas, Stephanie's grandfather hired someone to fix the septic tank that had backed up. The workers arrived with a backhoe to dig down through the muck to fix it. To their surprise after removing the first layer, thousands of intact vitamins pills were exposed. Our colleague explained that "thousands is not an exaggeration because the septic tank had not been cleaned out in about five years, and Stephanie's grandmother and grandfather both took One-A-Day vitamins . . . well, once a day, and that amounts to 730 a year, or 3,650 over five years." Stephanie's grandfather had even used Rid-X Septic System Treatment faithfully, and everything BUT the vitamins pills had disintegrated. In fact, it was the consensus that the vitamin pills were the reason the system had backed up. After fixing the tank, her grandfather proclaimed that he had wasted a fortune and that he didn't want another one of those [expletive] vitamin pills brought into the house ever again!

As you can see, between the scientific findings and our humorous tale, due to their compromised disintegration potential there may be good reason for the negative opinions some people have about multivitamins. However, taking a multivitamin delivered in a liquid form would all but ensure micronutrient absorption. According to the American Pharmaceutical Association textbook, *The APhA Complete Review for Pharmacy,* "A drug dissolved in an aqueous [liquid] solution is in the most bioavailable [absorbable] form. Since the drug is already in solution, no dissolution [disintegration] step is necessary before systemic absorption occurs."

> *A multivitamin delivered in a liquid form would all but ensure micronutrient absorption.*

Additionally, many reputable doctors and nutritionists agree that a liquid delivery method is superior in terms of absorbency. For example,

Natasha Turner, N.D., author of the bestselling book *The Hormone Diet*, states, "Liquid vitamins or minerals are the easiest to absorb (especially for children or those who have difficulty swallowing pills)." Although she cautions, "Be sure to avoid the extra sugars or fructose often added to these mixtures to enhance the taste."

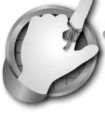

Remember

When choosing a supplement make sure they are free of artificial flavors, colors, yeast, sugar, starch, and preservatives, as well as something called excipients. Excipients, such as binders, fillers, and flow agents, can be used to either make the ingredients stick together, bulk products up to a convenient size, or allow formulas to run smoothly through manufacturers' machines. These can contribute to the poor disintegration rates for tablets (pills) and capsules.

Have you noticed that some multivitamin tablets are shiny? That's because some companies coat their multivitamins with shellac, wax, and hydroxypropylmethylcellulose, which keeps the moisture out so they will have a longer shelf life. While this may be good for the vitamin company's bottom line, it is not good for you. These excipients and coatings can decrease the solubility of a multivitamin tablet or capsule, reducing its ability to readily disintegrate.

You may have noticed, in Dr. Turner's earlier statement, that liquid multivitamins are especially good for both children and adults who have difficulty swallowing pills. A nationwide survey conducted by Harris Interactive, a global market research firm (they conduct the Harris poll), reported that 40 percent of all people surveyed have difficulty taking pills. The study reported that these individuals find swallowing pills so difficult that many delay, skip, or discontinue taking the pills or capsules altogether. They are not alone in avoiding these forms of supplementation. Individuals with specific conditions such as irritable bowel syndrome, hiatal hernias, diverticulitis, and those who have undergone bariatric surgery also have particular difficulty when taking their supplements in a pill or capsule form. According to the *Consumer Guide to Bariatric Surgery*, "Chewable and liquid multivitamins are the most easily absorbed and are recommended after all bariatric surgery procedures. They are also less likely to cause heartburn and ulcers."

While it may now appear that you should be searching for liquid multivitamins, you have some previously acquired knowledge that may affect this option. Back in Chapter 5 you learned that environmental elements such as temperature, light, and air deplete micronutrients from food as they travel to your table. Well, these same elements can deplete micronutrients from a premade liquid vitamin as well. In fact, those vitamin-enhanced waters that sit on the store's shelf are allowing light to degrade the very micronutrients it is promising to supply. To add insult to injury, as these micronutrients degrade, they release antagonistic elements that further degrade other micronutrients in the same formula. For example, vitamin B_{12} in a liquid solution can break down and release a cobalt ion. This cobalt ion can then contribute to the destruction of vitamins B_1 and B_6.

What Fillers and Sugars Are Hiding in Your Vitamin Pill?

Look at all of the added binders, fillers, sweeteners, preservatives, and artificial colors listed below in **red** found in a typical multivitamin pill.

INGREDIENTS:

Calcium Carbonate, Magnesium Oxide, **Cellulose**, Ascorbic Acid, Dicalcium Phosphate, dl-Alpha-Tocopheryl Acetate, Croscarmellose Sodium, **Sucrose**, Niacinamide, Gelatin, **Polyvinyl Alcohol**, Zinc Oxide, D-Calcium Pantothenate, Silicon Dioxide, **Crospovidone**, **Maltodextrin**, **Magnesium Stearate**, **Polyethylene Glycol**, **Talc**, Manganese Sulfate, **FD&C Yellow #5 (tartrazine) Lake**, Pyridoxine Hydrochloride, Cupric Sulfate, **Modified Corn Starch**, Riboflavin, Thiamine Mononitrate, **Titanium Dioxide (color)**, Calcium Silicate, **Hydroxypropyl Methylcellulose**, **Glucose**, **FD&C Blue #1 Lake**, Vitamin A Acetate, **FD&C Red #40**, Chromium Chloride, Folic Acid, Beta-Carotene, **FD&C Blue #2**, Biotin, Sodium Selenate, **FD&C Yellow #6**, Cholecalciferol, Phytonadione, Cyanocobalamin, Tricalcium Phosphate, **BHA**, **BHT**.

What can you find listed on your multivitamin supplement?

It's not only the light that causes these depletions. If your liquid multivitamin comes in a large, multiserving container, every time you open the bottle to take your daily dose you expose your micronutrients to air (oxidation). So how do we get the benefits of a liquid multivitamin while protecting the micronutrients from these destructive elements? The best answer may be a single-serving, powdered multivitamin. Then, when you rip open the foil packet (that protects the micronutrients from both light and air) and pour the micronutrients into water, you will have a highly absorbable liquid multivitamin with limited exposure to destructive elements. This brings us to **Naked Fact #13.**

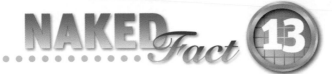
Single-serving, powdered multivitamins delivered in liquid form are more suitable to a large percentage of the population, are readily available for absorption, and are protected from micronutrient-depleting elements.

Absorption in Your House of Optimal Health

Let's examine how absorption affects our House of Optimal Health. Remember that our HOH must be built well and on time each day in order for optimal health to be possible. For the purposes of this example we are going to say that the total number of qualified construction crew members, or "micronutrients," we need to build our HOH is one hundred. They include all of the vitamins, minerals, EFAs, and accessory micronutrients that act as the architects, cement workers, framers, painters, plumbers, electricians, assistants, and all the other imperative members of the construction crew. Based on our previous absorbability rate statistics, if we take a multivitamin in the form of a tablet (pill) or capsule, you may only have between ten and twenty of your required one hundred workers show up to work. Based on absorbability alone it would be impossible for them to get all of the work done on time and more than likely the crew members that did show up wouldn't have half of the skills necessary to complete the HOH well. Small holes would be inevitable, and large holes would be likely.

However, taking single-serving, powdered multivitamins delivered in liquid form would bring far more, perhaps up to ninety-eight of these qualified crew members, to the job site. If we consider absorbency based on transport system alone, these workers will have a good chance at achieving the HOH requirements. You can now see how imperative proper absorption is to the completion of your HOH.

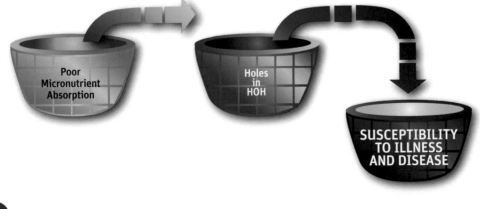

Poor Micronutrient Absorption

Holes in HOH

SUSCEPTIBILITY TO ILLNESS AND DISEASE

"B" Is for Beneficial Quantities

THE B IN THE ABCS of Optimal Supplementation stands for *Beneficial Quantities*. Beneficial quantities are the amount of each of the essential micronutrients that would be beneficial for us to take in through supplementation in order to achieve optimal health. As we have already learned, the Reference Daily Intake (RDI) is a guideline outlining the minimum daily requirements of each essential micronutrient considered sufficient to prevent micronutrient-deficiency diseases. While the RDIs seem to be enough to prevent deficiency diseases, are they enough to produce optimal health? According to Shari Lieberman, Ph.D., "The RDIs are, with a few exceptions, the nutritional equivalent of the minimum wage. They are probably high enough to keep you alive—although even this is open to question. But they do not appear high enough to allow you to enjoy the best quality of life."

Regarding RDA/RDI guidelines, Albert Szent-Györgi, Ph.D., M.D., the Nobel Prize winner for his discovery of vitamin C (ascorbic acid) says, "The medical profession itself took a very narrow and very wrong view. Lack of ascorbic acid caused scurvy, so if there was no scurvy there was no lack of ascorbic acid. Nothing could be clearer than this. The only trouble was that scurvy is not a first symptom of a lack but a final collapse, a premortal syndrome and there is a wide gap between scurvy and full health."

Dr. Szent-Györgi spent much of his career lecturing on the difference between, what he referred to in Latin as *dosis optima quotidiana,* which translates to Optimal Daily Doses (ODD), and the minimum doses of the micronutrients needed to prevent deficiency diseases. He believed that while the RDA/RDI may prevent deficiency diseases, optimal health would be achieved only at doses higher than minimum requirements. Dr. Szent-Györgi's Optimal Daily Doses are what we introduced you to earlier in Chapter 3, which we defined as the amount of micronutrients needed to produce optimal health—oftentimes higher than the RDI.

So, we know that the RDIs are quantities most likely high enough to prevent deficiency diseases. That much is clear. However, as Dr. Szent-Györgi stated, preventing disease is a far cry from optimal health. Then how do we define beneficial quantities? How much of each micronutrient do we need to consume in order to achieve optimal health? To figure this out we will need to use knowledge we have previously accumulated.

We know that our diets, even those designed by nutritional experts and followed to a tee, do not provide RDI requirements. Even when we follow a nutrivore's first step and choose *rich foods* over *poor foods,* we most likely will still fall short.

Next, we must consider the micronutrients lost due to those dreaded Everyday Micronutrient Depleters. When our EMDs are accounted for we can easily see that most, if not all of us, quickly fall further below RDI requirements. If we look at these first facts together, they would look something like the chart below.

Optimal Daily Doses vary for each of us. This is because Optimal Daily Doses are dependent on biochemical individuality, which can include an individual's sex, lifestyle, genetics, medical conditions, and age. For example, calcium requirements are highest for women over forty, who are at greater risk for osteoporosis. There is also evidence that premenopausal and/or pregnant women should take an iron supplement daily. While iron is not suggested as a supplement for most men, it is recommended that both male and female athletes as well as vegans and vegetarians consider iron supplementation. For this reason, in upcoming charts we will represent Optimal Daily Doses as a range, rather than as a definitive amount.

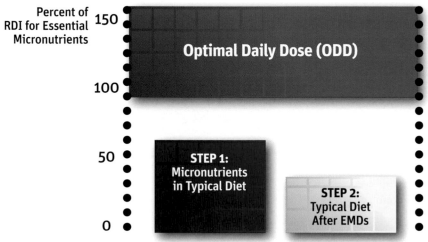

Percent of RDI for Essential Micronutrients

150 — **Optimal Daily Dose (ODD)**

100

50 — **STEP 1: Micronutrients in Typical Diet**

STEP 2: Typical Diet After EMDs

0

Both Steps 1 and 2 will leave you short of reaching RDI sufficiency.

You can see from the chart above, after steps 1 and 2, we fall short of reaching even RDI sufficiency and are a long way from reaching Optimal Daily Doses and, ultimately, optimal health. While our situation may appear grim, there is a solution—the third and final step, which we have not yet included in the chart above, is supplementation. Based on our chart so far, in order to achieve optimal health, we will need to take a supplement to ensure Optimal Daily Doses.

What amount of micronutrients, if added through supplementation, would all but guarantee that we reach this goal? We believe that this could be achieved by taking a supplement that delivers close to 100 percent of the RDI for each essential micronutrient. We define this quantity as beneficial quantities.

By stacking a multivitamin containing beneficial quantities (with approximately 100 percent of the RDI) on top of the micronutrients remaining from your *rich food* diet after the EMDs are accounted for, we are all but guaranteed to reach Optimal Daily Doses.

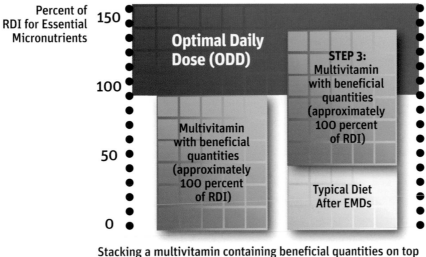

Stacking a multivitamin containing beneficial quantities on top of the micronutrients remaining from your diet (after the EMDs are accounted for) all but guarantees reaching Optimal Daily Doses (ODD).

You can see how a multivitamin that delivers beneficial quantities is a vital tool in obtaining Optimal Daily Doses. However, most multivitamins do not contain even the minimum required amounts of certain micronutrients. This could be because it is costly to do so. It might also be because some of the bulkier minerals, such as calcium and magnesium, wouldn't fit neatly into one little pill (another reason a powder/ liquid supplement is beneficial). When we put all of this information on beneficial quantities together, we can agree on **Naked Fact #14.**

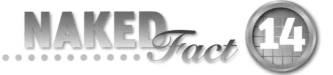

Combining a multivitamin that contains beneficial quantities (with approximately 100 percent of the RDI) with a micronutrient-rich diet all but guarantees Optimal Daily Doses (ODD).

Timing Is Everything

Do you remember earlier in the chapter when we stated that in order for the House of Optimal Health to be built well, all of the essential micronutrients need to be present in sufficient quantities at the right times? Well, you have just defined the "sufficient quantities" portion of that statement. We must now examine how timing plays a key role in the beneficial quantities equation. When discussing timing we are actually referring to the need for multiple doses. Taking a one-a-day multivitamin has a glaring flaw. Do you remember the two types of vitamins, water-soluble and fat-soluble? Water-soluble vitamins move through the body very quickly. Because of this, many physicians and nutritionists, including Dr. Oz, suggest taking several of the water-soluble micronutrients in separate doses.

"You want to give your body the right amount of fuel for when you need it," says Dr. Oz. "Vitamins have water-soluble elements to them so they are quickly moved through your system." Dr. Oz recommends splitting your multivitamin into a.m. and p.m. doses because, "By taking half your multivitamin in the morning and half in the evening, you're guaranteeing that your body can absorb all the nutrients it can."

It was first reported back in 1994, on page one of *USA Today* that vitamin C, a water-soluble vitamin, is absorbed and excreted from the body in a twelve-hour period. The story quoted the researcher who made the discovery as saying, "If vitamin C really does work as an antioxidant, then taking a supplement once a day might be like wearing a condom half the time."

According to a study in the *Journal of American Aging Association,* the true benefits of vitamins C and E will not be realized until clinical trials provide vitamin C to participants twice a day. If optimal health is your goal, then a once-a-day multivitamin is likely to leave you short.

The second reason that some micronutrients need to be taken multiple times over the period of a day is limited absorption capacity. Although the RDI recommends that healthy adults take in 1,000 mg of calcium a day, and women over the age of fifty take 1,200 mg, science suggests that calcium can only be absorbed at increments of no more than 600 mg at one time. In order to ensure either of these quantities, one would be required to take in calcium multiple times during a day whether in supplement form or through food. We can see that due to both water solubility and the body's limited absorption capacity, it is essential that we take a multivitamin that supplies micronutrients at multiple times every day, if optimal health is to be achieved. This leads us to our **Naked Fact #15.**

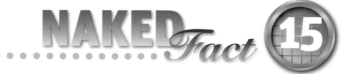

Multivitamin supplements should be taken multiple times throughout the day, due to water solubility and our body's limited absorption capacity.

Supplement Facts		
	Amount Per Serving	% Daily Value (DV)
Vitamin C	60 mg	100%
Vitamin D	2000 IU	500%
Folic Acid	400 mcg	100%
Calcium	200 mg	20%
Magnesium	50 mg	13%
Vitamin B12	6 mg	100%

% DV really means what percentage of the required RDI is in the supplement.

You should look for a supplement that has 100% DV of the essential micronutrients.

Research now shows that supplementing with higher quantities of vitamin D (1,000 to 2,000 IU), quantities higher than the current RDI of vitamin D (400 IU), may be beneficial in the fight against cancer, obesity, and Alzheimer's.

Many supplements do not contain 100% of the RDI for many of the essential minerals.

Remember, because 100% of the DV of calcium cannot be absorbed in a single dose, the DV of calcium will always be less than 100%. It should, however, be between 500 and 600 mg or 50 to 60% DV.

WARNING: Taking mega-doses of minerals can be quite toxic.

Beneficial Quantities in Your House of Optimal Health

How would our chances for successfully completing our House of Optimal Health look if we didn't take in beneficial quantities of micronutrients? Let's look at beneficial quantities independently of the aforementioned absorption factors. We will assume that absorption was at 100 percent. Remember that building our HOH will require a minimum of one hundred crew members with a wide variety of skill sets. They are all scheduled to arrive at 6 a.m. (or at the time you wake up) to get in a full day of work. At about 6:15 a.m. (right after you take your multivitamin that does not contain 100 percent of the RDI for many of the essential micronutrients), as you look around the job site you realize that only seventy-five crew members have shown up. You just don't have enough skilled workers to build your HOH in a structurally sound way by the end of the day.

To make matters worse, some of the ultra-important minerals were no-shows. Remember that without minerals, the vitamins don't know what tasks to perform and they become useless. Also, most of the crew members that did show up are only part-timers. Their contracts dictate they work half days. By the second half of the day (twelve hours later), these part timers, or water-soluble vitamins and minerals, punch out and leave the job site. This will leave you even more shorthanded than when you started. Beneficial quantities help to ensure a full crew throughout the whole day to complete your HOH.

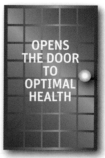

OPENS THE DOOR TO OPTIMAL HEALTH

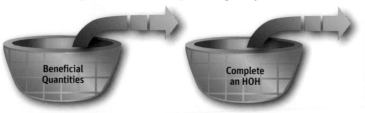

Beneficial Quantities

Complete an HOH

It should now be clear that the first two components of our ABCs of Optimal Supplementation—absorption and beneficial quantities—are essential to optimal health. A *rich-food* diet along with a single-serving, powdered multivitamin delivered in liquid form containing approximately 100 percent of the RDI of essential micronutrients can go a long way toward insuring your chances of receiving ODD. However, don't get too comfortable because you have only learned half of the story. The biggest threat to your chances of achieving ODD is yet to be discussed. In Chapter 10 we will finally introduce you to both the C and S in our Optimal Supplementation acronym.

We will take an in-depth look at the concepts of *competition,* the treacherous villain in your ODD quest, that can trap and block any micronutrient benefit you may have thought you secured; and *synergy,* the dynamic hero, capable of releasing and enhancing health benefits you may never have thought possible.

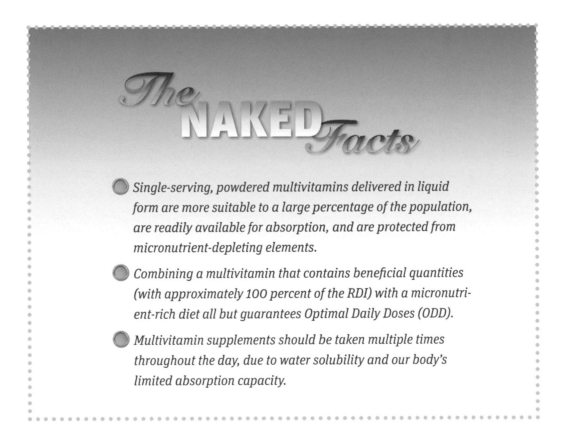

The NAKED Facts

- Single-serving, powdered multivitamins delivered in liquid form are more suitable to a large percentage of the population, are readily available for absorption, and are protected from micronutrient-depleting elements.

- Combining a multivitamin that contains beneficial quantities (with approximately 100 percent of the RDI) with a micronutrient-rich diet all but guarantees Optimal Daily Doses (ODD).

- Multivitamin supplements should be taken multiple times throughout the day, due to water solubility and our body's limited absorption capacity.

Chapter Ten

The Web of Competition and the Dynamic Duos of Synergy

The ABCs Continued

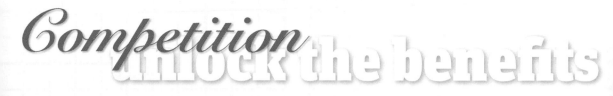

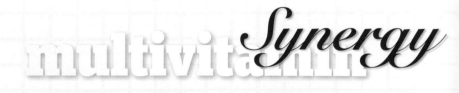

"When spider webs unite, they can tie up a lion.**"**
—Ethiopian Proverb

In the last chapter we witnessed Sara, our culinary student, struggle with whipping her egg whites into meringue. She had no idea that the egg was as complicated as Chef Marie had described. However, after learning all the rules and examining how the egg's different parts played intricate and sensitive roles in the whipping process, Sara never made the same mistakes again. The same holds true for all of you. Just as Chef Marie's rules for whipping egg whites worked to perfect Sara's meringue, our rules for choosing a well-formulated supplement will teach you to identify a maximally beneficial multivitamin.

We have just completed our introduction and examination of the first two letters of our ABCs of Optimal Supplementation—*absorption* and *beneficial quantities*—and explored how they can affect our ability to successfully complete our House of Optimal Health (HOH). But how might these first two elements factor into the overall effectiveness of a multivitamin?

Based on what we learned in Chapter 9, there is a good chance that both absorption and beneficial quantities contributed to the limited success of the *British Journal of Nutrition* multivitamin study. Maybe if the participants had taken single-serving, powdered multivitamins delivered in liquid form, the micronutrients would have been better absorbed. Perhaps then, they would have seen a weight-loss benefit. It is also probable that the study's multivitamin and mineral supplement did not contain *beneficial quantities* of each micronutrient, and unlikely that the scientists supplied important water-soluble vitamins and minerals twice a day, not taking into account their part-time personalities. These factors could all have hindered the multivitamins' ability to work their "antiobesity" magic.

We now uncover the next two components: *competition* (C) and *synergy* (S). When A and B are combined with C and S, we have the ability to "unlock" the benefits of each micronutrient within a multivitamin.

● ● ● ● ● ● ● ● ● ● ● ● ● ● ●

"C" Is for Micronutrient Competition

THE ABCS OF OPTIMAL SUPPLEMENTATION'S last two letters, C and S, stand for Competition and Synergy. As we mentioned in Chapter 3, competition is the "villain" and synergy the "hero" in our micronutrient-sufficiency story. Our tale's "villain" is perhaps the most overlooked factor contributing to poor availability of micronutrients in all nutritional supplements today. Much of what we know about micronutrient competition is often hidden away in obscure journal studies, or only briefly mentioned in extensive research findings. Dr. Joseph Mercola illuminates this fact in an article discussing the micronutrient competition between vitamins A and D. He states, "Hidden on page 8 of the paper was one sentence and a small table showing that the benefits of vitamin D are almost entirely negated in those with the highest vitamin A intake." He further states that the study, published in 2010 by the *British Medical Journal,* "is the largest study to date showing vitamin A blocks vitamin D's effects." With micronutrient competition becoming one of the hottest topics in emerging health science, isn't it time you become acquainted with the concept of competition?

In our brief discussion of competition in Chapter 3, we told you that many of the essential micronutrients your body needs for good health actually compete for absorption pathways (receptor sites), resulting in the absorption of one at the expense of the other. We explained that micronutrient competition is like the many famous rivals you have heard about—David Letterman and Jay Leno, the republicans and the democrats, or the NY Giants and the Dallas Cowboys. We explained that certain micronutrients, such as copper and zinc, duke it out for domination of the receptor site. Of course, micronutrient competition isn't as simple as that. In fact, there are four types of competition that can occur between micronutrients. Let's take a closer look:

 CHEMICAL COMPETITION takes place during the manufacturing of a multivitamin or nutritional supplement. Manufacturers combine competing micronutrients in one formulation and a chemical battle ensues within the formulation itself, leaving the competing micronutrients unable to be absorbed. An example of this is that zinc forms an insoluble complex with folic acid (vitamin B_9) when they are put together in a nutritional supplement or multivitamin. When this happens, neither will be absorbed.

BIOCHEMICAL COMPETITION happens after the body has ingested the micronutrients in the multivitamin, but before the micronutrients have been absorbed. The micronutrients compete for a common receptor site for absorption or transport pathways, as is the case between lutein and beta-carotene.

PHYSIOLOGICAL COMPETITION occurs after the micronutrients have been absorbed; when one or both of the two competing micronutrients may cause decreased utilization, even after absorption has taken place. For instance, in some studies copper has been shown to reduce the activity of pantothenic acid (vitamin B_5).

CLINICAL COMPETITION takes place when the presence of one micronutrient masks the deficiency of another, making it difficult to detect deficiency. The classic example here is folic acid (vitamin B_9) and vitamin B_{12}. Folic acid can mask B_{12} anemia, a condition of inadequate red blood cells that can lead to depression, dementia, and the inability to carry oxygen throughout the body.

Don't worry, we don't want you to get hung up on the names of these four types of micronutrient competition. We have separated them here so you can see that they can occur multiple times along a micronutrient's journey—from the manufacturing of a nutritional supplement, all the way through to utilization. With so many opportunities for competition to occur, the number of competitive reactions taking place between the micronutrients can quickly spiral into a complicated web. In fact, we have coined this "The Web of Competition" (see Figure 10.1). This web depicts the number of micronutrient competitions that may occur within a typical multivitamin.

Both of the columns in Figure 10.1 have the same list of micronutrients that are often included in popular nutritional supplements, including multivitamins and fortified foods. Fortified foods, by the way, are another form of a nutritional supplement. Micronutrients are added during the manufacturing of these foods, so if you eat fortified foods such as bread, milk, cereal, pasta, and rice, micronutrient competition is already a very real factor in your life. Each red line indicates where a competition would take place between micronutrients if they were to be taken at the same time. This means that the presence of one inhibits the absorption or utilization of the other. After examining "The Web of Competition," take a moment to consider its far-reaching ramifications.

Does the number of competitions that exist between micronutrients surprise you? How could it be that all of these benefit-robbing micronutrient competitions take place every day in our nutritional supplements, yet we have just started to hear about them? We must all remember how young the study of micronutrients really is. To put things in perspective, it has been only 100

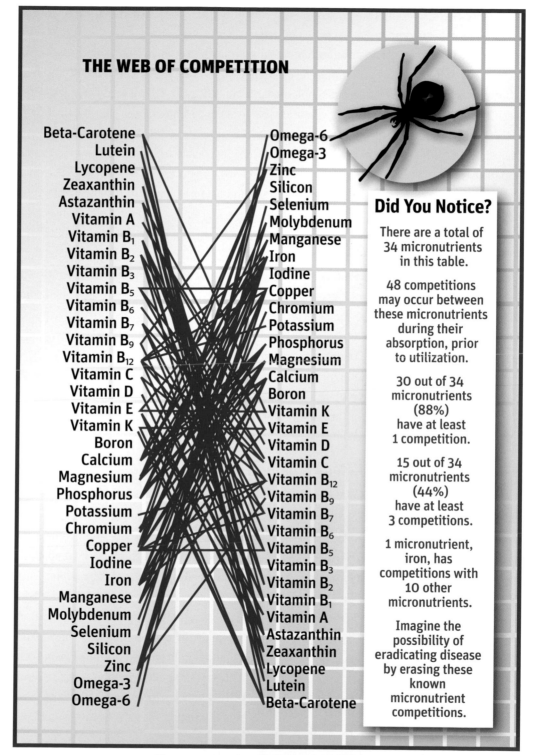

Figure 10.1. The Web of Competition

years since the first vitamin was discovered; it should not surprise us then that there are still many facets of the micronutrient yet to be realized.

However, the science of micronutrient competition is moving ahead. In 1998, a study published in *American Journal of Clinical Nutrition* revealed that "lutein negatively affected beta-carotene absorption when the two were given simultaneously." In 2002, the TOZAL study on age-related macular degeneration (AMD), an eye condition that leads to blindness, used this information to successfully reverse and prevent the progression of this disease. TOZAL developer Edward Paul, O.D., Ph.D., of the International Academy of Low Vision Specialists, called this discovery "ground shaking."

For years, scientists have known that both lutein and beta-carotene had beneficial effects on subjects with AMD. However, in this study when, for the first time, the competition between lutein and beta-carotene was accounted for, the benefits of both micronutrients were realized and micronutrient supplementation either improved or stabilized vision in 76.7 percent of patients. According to Dr. Paul this information "will really turn the way we look at nutrition on its ear." He adds that this new understanding of micronutrient competition represents a "huge paradigm shift when you consider that we had been recommending lutein be combined with other antioxidants, which is a reasonable thing to recommend. But when these two nutrients are competing for the same receptor site, they're only neutralizing one another."

Could this be correct? Could accounting for a single micronutrient competition actually reverse or prevent the progression of disease? It seems to be true. Take a look again at "The Web of Competition." Can you imagine how many other diseases may be prevented, or reversed, if we could simply erase all of those red lines?

Anti-Competition Technology Eliminates the Competition

It is important for us to point out here that while absorption and beneficial quantities are crucial factors in obtaining Optimal Daily Doses (ODD), if the micronutrients in a multivitamin are still competing, their benefits will not be realized. This makes micronutrient competition perhaps the most important component of the ABCs of Supplementation. Think of it this way: If competition blocks the availability of each micronutrient, then what we need is a little *"anti-competition."* Just as antibiotics kill bacteria, Anti-Competition Technology (ACT) can eliminate the negative effects of micronutrient competition. The charts on the following page demonstrate how taking a multivitamin with Anti-Competition Technology is imperative in your quest to reach ODD. It may be the crucial factor that makes your micronutrients ACT as they should.

Just as antibiotics kill bacteria, Anti-Competition Technology (ACT) can eliminate the negative effects of micronutrient competition.

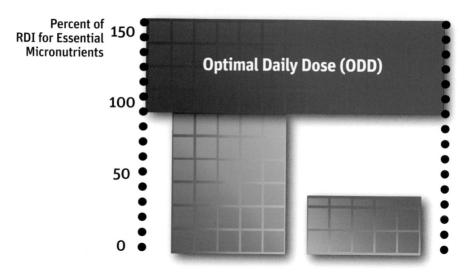

Percent of RDI for Essential Micronutrients

150

100

50

0

Optimal Daily Dose (ODD)

A multivitamin containing 100 percent of the Reference Daily intake (RDI) prior to accounting for micronutrient competition.

The reduced amount of micronutrients actually available in that same multivitamin due to micronutrient competition.

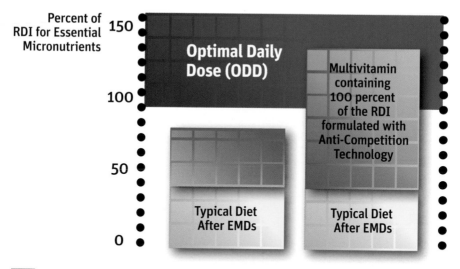

Percent of RDI for Essential Micronutrients

150

100

50

0

Optimal Daily Dose (ODD)

Multivitamin containing 100 percent of the RDI formulated with Anti-Competition Technology

Typical Diet After EMDs

Typical Diet After EMDs

The reduced amount of micronutrients actually available in that same multivitamin due to micronutrient competition.

Multivitamin containing 100 percent of the RDI formulated with Anti-Competition Technology.

Stacking a multivitamin containing Anti-Competition Technology on top of the micronutrients remaining from a rich diet (less EMDs) makes it possible to reach Optimal Daily Doses (ODD).

Competition in Your House of Optimal Health

Can you see how micronutrient competition might affect our ability to complete our HOH well and on time? Even though we might think we have absorption and beneficial quantities in place, when competition is present it greatly diminishes the ability of the individual micronutrients either to be absorbed or to be properly utilized. A good way to understand competition in terms of our House of Optimal Health is to imagine that the workers (micronutrients) all arrive at the job site with their hands tied behind their backs, making it impossible for them to work. By untying these workers' hands (utilizing Anti-Competition Technology), the workers are able to finish the HOH well and on time.

Eliminating the competition between micronutrients in our nutritional supplements would lead to a greater chance of completing our HOH on a daily basis and achieving optimal health. This would allow the full benefits of individual micronutrients to be realized. According to the late Derek H. Shrimpton, Ph.D., scientific advisor to the European Federation of Health Product Manufacturers, the benefits of a multivitamin "may not be fully realized in those instances where the possibility of micronutrient interaction [competition] has been ignored." Let's make this our **Naked Fact #16.**

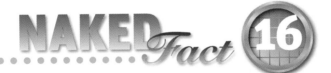

The elimination of micronutrient competition allows the full benefits of each micronutrient to be realized. The more benefits realized, the closer we are to optimal health.

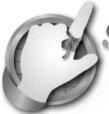

Remember

Just like children, micronutrients can sometimes be naughty. Separating two quarrelsome kids may be the only way to get them to stop fighting. Competing micronutrients must also be separated using Anti-Competition Technology in order to eliminate competition.

• • • • • • • • • • • • • • • • • •

"S" Is for Micronutrient Synergy

THE FINAL FACTOR IN OUR DISCUSSION of the ABCs of Optimal Supplementation is the S, for Synergy—the flipside of competition. You may remember that we illustrated synergy in Chapter 3 with the dynamic duos of Sherlock Holmes and Dr. Watson and Lennon and McCartney. Think about how micronutrient competition has negatively affected our ability to achieve optimal health; now turn these competitions upside down, and a world of positive benefits suddenly appears. For every type of micronutrient competition, there is an equal and opposite synergy to which it relates.

 The opposite of a chemical competition is a **CHEMICAL SYNERGY.** Both take place in the nutritional supplement itself prior to ingesting. A chemical synergy occurs when two micronutrients are put into the same multivitamin to form an advantageous complex that can help to increase the absorption of either micronutrient, or possibly both. Zinc and riboflavin (vitamin B_2) share such a relationship.

 The opposite of a biochemical competition is a **BIOCHEMICAL SYNERGY.** In this case, rather than fighting for a receptor site or pathway, one micronutrient aids in the absorption of the other. This is the case when vitamin D enhances the absorption of calcium.

 The opposite of a physiological competition is a **PHYSIOLOGICAL SYNERGY.** Unlike its competitive counterpart where two micronutrients decrease each other's utilization, physiological synergy causes one micronutrient to aid in the performance of a second micronutrient. This occurs because one micronutrient needs to perform a specific function in order for a second micronutrient to do its job. For example, vitamin K needs to be available in the body when calcium arrives. It is essential in the formation of bone tissue.

 The opposite of clinical competition is **CLINICAL SYNERGY.** Clinical synergy takes place when micronutrients have been found to work together to create an observable yet unexpected beneficial change in the body. These clinical synergies have been attributed to decreasing the chances of a disease. An example of this is when folic acid (B_9) and vitamins B_{12} and B_6 are all present in adequate quantities and convert homocysteine into cysteine and methionine. This conversion lowers homocysteine, which is a known marker of coronary disease.

The Dynamic Duos of Synergy

Again, you don't need to memorize the specific ways in which micronutrient synergy can occur. We put them here simply to demonstrate to you the extent to which they can increase the effectiveness of your multivitamin. How advantageous is synergy? According to Dr. Paul, bioflavonoids, such as grape seed extract, have demonstrated a synergistic effect with vitamin C, boosting vitamin C absorption by 50 percent.

Perhaps you are curious as to how many of these incredible synergistic relationships that exist among micronutrients may be contained in your multivitamin. You can see just how many there are by examining Figure 10.2, "The Dynamic Duos of Synergy." Keep in mind that the more green lines you see, the more dependent these micronutrients are on each other. Without proper formulation, many of these advantageous synergies might never be realized.

Synergy in the House of Optimal Health

Although micronutrient synergy mirrors micronutrient competition, it cannot reverse or eliminate it. Synergy does not have that kind of power. Instead, it offers extras—or perks—in the form of enhanced utilization and absorption. Think of synergy as the icing on the ABCs of Supplementation cake. Assuming that A, B, and C are all accounted for, synergy works to enhance our results.

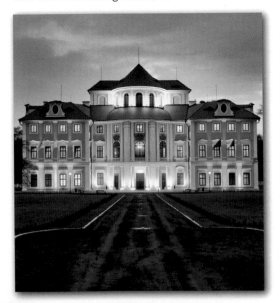

Let's take one final look at the HOH to imagine how micronutrient synergy might play its role. In this scenario, all 100 workers show up (absorption, beneficial quantities, and competition have all been accounted for). This allows synergy to work its magic. The workers (micronutrients) work so well together that not only is the HOH built well and on time, it far surpasses your expectations. Now, rather than the three thousand-square-foot home you had contracted, you find that they have built you a ten thousand-square-foot mansion, complete with swimming pool, tennis courts, and an indoor bowling alley.

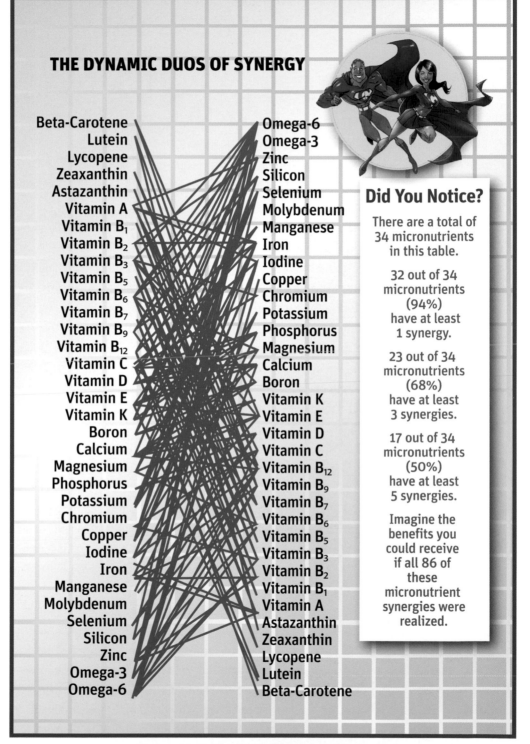

THE DYNAMIC DUOS OF SYNERGY

Beta-Carotene	Omega-6
Lutein	Omega-3
Lycopene	Zinc
Zeaxanthin	Silicon
Astazanthin	Selenium
Vitamin A	Molybdenum
Vitamin B$_1$	Manganese
Vitamin B$_2$	Iron
Vitamin B$_3$	Iodine
Vitamin B$_5$	Copper
Vitamin B$_6$	Chromium
Vitamin B$_7$	Potassium
Vitamin B$_9$	Phosphorus
Vitamin B$_{12}$	Magnesium
Vitamin C	Calcium
Vitamin D	Boron
Vitamin E	Vitamin K
Vitamin K	Vitamin E
Boron	Vitamin D
Calcium	Vitamin C
Magnesium	Vitamin B$_{12}$
Phosphorus	Vitamin B$_9$
Potassium	Vitamin B$_7$
Chromium	Vitamin B$_6$
Copper	Vitamin B$_5$
Iodine	Vitamin B$_3$
Iron	Vitamin B$_2$
Manganese	Vitamin B$_1$
Molybdenum	Vitamin A
Selenium	Astazanthin
Silicon	Zeaxanthin
Zinc	Lycopene
Omega-3	Lutein
Omega-6	Beta-Carotene

Did You Notice?

There are a total of 34 micronutrients in this table.

32 out of 34 micronutrients (94%) have at least 1 synergy.

23 out of 34 micronutrients (68%) have at least 3 synergies.

17 out of 34 micronutrients (50%) have at least 5 synergies.

Imagine the benefits you could receive if all 86 of these micronutrient synergies were realized.

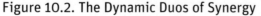

Figure 10.2. The Dynamic Duos of Synergy

A nutritional supplement that utilizes micronutrient synergy in its formulation—and harnesses these synergistic powers—can provide increased absorption and overall benefit. This is the foundation for our **Naked Fact #17.**

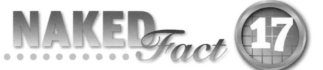

Micronutrient synergy can increase the absorption and utilization between specific micronutrients, resulting in greater micronutrient benefits. The more benefits realized, the closer we are to optimal health.

Aren't the concepts of micronutrient competition and micronutrient synergy incredible? Can you see that understanding how they work could forever change how we take supplements? Let's put them together now in an illustration we call the "Domino Effect." We begin by introducing a single micronutrient competition between vitamins A and D. You will see how this singular competition can affect numerous micronutrients in the multivitamin and ultimately wreak havoc in your body. Remember that this is *only one* of the many competitions that occur in a standard multivitamin. You may just fall over when you see how far-reaching the effects can be!

Do you see how important micronutrient synergy is to your health? What could it mean if you were able to receive all of the micronutrients without any competitions? Prior to beginning any program designed for weight loss, cancer, diabetes, hypertension, or any other condition or disease, our private clients must first become micronutrient sufficient. We have mandated that our clients utilize the same concepts we have just introduced to you, and take a supplement that is formulated with all of the ABCs of Optimal Supplementation in mind, including enhanced synergistic properties and Anti-Competition Technology. We have seen incredible results. We often find that weight loss accelerated, blood pressure normalized, and cholesterol levels dramatically improved. Sometimes, surprising health benefits are revealed that we never would have imagined.

THE **DOMINO EFFECT** OF
MICRONUTRIENT COMPETITION

STEP ONE

Let's begin by taking a standard multivitamin and mineral supplement containing both vitamins A and D. These two vitamins compete for receptor sites for absorption. Therefore, when vitamin A gets absorbed, vitamin D may not. Assuming this happens, you may develop a vitamin D deficiency.

D   A

REMEMBER: Vitamin D maintains healthy bones, aids in immunity, and works as an anti-inflammatory. Low levels of vitamin D have also been scientifically linked to excess body weight.

STEP TWO

A vitamin D deficiency would affect your calcium (Ca) levels. This is because vitamin D is synergistic with calcium and is needed to make the calcium-binding protein essential for the calcium's absorption. The end result is compromised calcium absorption, potentially leading to a deficiency in calcium.

Ca   D   A

REMEMBER: Calcium's chief functions in the human body are the mineralization of bones and teeth, muscle contractions and relaxations, nerve functioning, blood clotting, blood pressure, and immune defense. All of these functions have now been jeopardized.

STEP THREE

Reduced calcium levels may create another problem. Since the proper absorption of vitamin B_{12} is dependent on calcium, your reduced calcium levels may result in reduced B_{12} levels.

B_{12} Ca   D   A

REMEMBER: A slight deficiency of vitamin B_{12} can lead to anemia, fatigue, mania, and depression, while a long-term deficiency can potentially cause permanent damage to the brain and central nervous system.

STEP FOUR

Vitamin B_{12} is part of a close-knit, intimately involved family of B vitamins. A lack of vitamin B_{12} may put

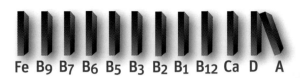

Fe B_9 B_7 B_6 B_5 B_3 B_2 B_1 B_{12} Ca   D   A

the absorption and/or utilization of vitamin B_1 (thiamine), vitamin B_2 (riboflavin), vitamin B_3 (niacin), vitamin B_5 (pantthenic acid), vitamin B_6, vitamin B_7 (biotin), vitamin B_9 (folic acid), as well as iron (Fe) at risk.

Just imagine what might happen if we started this domino effect with all of the villainous micronutrient competitions.

Meet Mabel

Mabel, a client of ours in her mid-fifties, came to us to lose weight. She was active, engaged to be married, and traveling around the world with her fiancé. We designed a program to help Mabel regain the thinner body of her youth that didn't keep her from enjoying the many exotic places on her itinerary. Some time had passed when we finally caught up with Mabel face-to-face. (Thanks to technology, we often follow a client's progress via telephone, email, or Skype.) At first sight, she looked incredible. The 30 pounds she had taken off her five-foot, four-inch frame had made a dramatic difference. She was literally bouncing with excitement as she entered the room, eager to show us her fabulous new figure.

Mabel had always been a late riser and she spilled over with joy as she explained how our program had energized her so much that she now awoke eagerly at 7 a.m. every day to walk off a few calories. There was something else that seemed different about her, but we just couldn't place it; then it hit us—Mabel was reading and reviewing her personal weight-loss journal without her glasses. When we asked her about this, she almost jumped out of her seat. She had forgotten to mention an unexpected side effect of the program. The micronutrients that she was taking in, in our anti-competition format, had reversed her eye condition. During her last appointment with her eye doctor, he made her retake the eye exam numerous times because he did not believe his own readings.

With Mabel, the desired effect of her program was weight loss. However, one of the unexpected surprises was that her eyesight had improved. She had never considered that her poor vision was a simple manifestation of a micronutrient deficiency. She had always taken multivitamins, but she had never been able to absorb key micronutrients because of their inherent competitions. As it turns out, by implementing our three-step plan of eating a rich-food diet, reducing EMDs, and creating micronutrient sufficiency with anti-competition supplementation, Mabel was able to achieve her goal of weight loss and receive an unexpected health benefit. If Mabel was able to improve her poor eyesight by overcoming her micronutrient deficiencies, imagine the great and unexpected benefits that await you as well. Remember, micronutrient deficiencies manifest themselves differently in each individual. Mabel's improved vision could be your improved sleep pattern or reduced arthritic pain. Can you now see why the multivitamin in the *British Journal of Nutrition* study from our last chapter failed to show any weight-loss benefit from taking a multivitamin, even though the micronutrients in the multivitamin on their own had been scientifically shown to produce weight loss? In our opinion, it all comes down to the ABCs of Optimal Supplementation, especially micronutrient competition.

By realizing the competitive potential of micronutrients, we can separate these competitors and effectively "unlock" the power of the individual micronutrients. After all, when the competitive aspects of just two micronutrients were accounted for (lutein and beta-carotene), stabilization or improvement in age-related macular degeneration (AMD) was realized in 76.7 percent of patients. Imagine what would happen if the scientifically proven weight-loss benefits from micronutrients like zinc, CoQ_{10}, and vitamins A, C, and E (highlighted in Chapter 8 for their antiobesity abilities) could be realized. By applying the ABCs of Optimal Supplementation, your daily multivitamin may prevent debilitating health conditions and diseases, offer unexpected benefits, and be the safest and most effective fat burner on the market today.

● ● ● ● ● ● ● ● ● ● ● ● ● ● ● ● ●

Is a Multivitamin Right for You?

OUR LIVES, AND THE LIVES OF OUR CLIENTS, are no different from many of yours. We work hard and face stressful situations daily. Every day we hit the gym to build strong muscles, increase bone density, and keep aerobically fit. We eat out a few times a week, love spinach salads, and have been known to enjoy wine on occasion. While we have eliminated sugar, HFCS (high fructose corn syrup), and white flour from our diets at home, we do enjoy the occasional splurge from time to time. It is our awareness of the naked calories in our foods as well as all the Everyday Micronutrient Depleters (EMDs) in our lives that make it prudent for us to take a multivitamin. We believe that it is the right solution for us—a solution that fills the nutritional gap between where our diet leaves off and where micronutrient sufficiency is achieved.

You now have all the information you need to decide for yourselves if taking a multivitamin is right for you. You have witnessed the effects of mineral depletion causing sick soil and the numerous EMDs from the farm to the fork. We have shown the balanced diet to be nothing more than a myth, a fictional urban legend that we had once thought to be true. You have identified the lifestyle EMDs that you encounter daily, robbing you of health-promoting micronutrients. With all of your new knowledge, you should now realize that your chances at micronutrient sufficiency seem pretty slim without supplementation. Although you may have made up your mind and have determined that supplementation is right for you, as with any big life decision a second opinion is always helpful. Here are the opinions of some of the world's most prominent physicians, scientists, and organizations concerning the importance of multivitamin supplementation.

> **"**I think all Americans—adults, teenagers and children—should be taking a multivitamin. Period.**"**
> —Jeffrey Blumberg, Ph.D., Professor, Friedman School of Nutrition Science and Policy at Tufts University

> **"**Trying to follow all the studies on vitamins and health can make your head swirl. But, when it's all boiled down, the take-home message is actually pretty simple: A daily multivitamin, and maybe an extra vitamin D supplement, is a great way to make sure you're getting all the nutrients you need to be healthy.**"**
> —Harvard School of Public Health

66I think of multivitamins as an insurance policy against an imperfect diet.**99**

—Michael Roizen, M.D., Chairman of Cleveland Clinic's Wellness Institute

66It's not a substitute for getting your vitamins from fruits and vegetables, but everyone should take them as more of an insurance policy.**99**

—David Katz, M.D., Director of the Yale-Griffin Prevention Research Center

66If you want to age faster, a good way to do it is to be short of some vitamin or mineral. I think everyone in the world should take a multivitamin as insurance. I take one daily. Nutritionists don't like the idea of telling people to take pills. They want people to eat better instead. But they've been trying for twenty-five years to change people's eating habits without much success. You need to have a good diet with lots of vitamins and minerals, but we know lots of people don't. So I say, try and eat well but take a multivitamin.**99**

—Bruce Ames, Ph.D., Professor, University of California at Berkeley

66A multivitamin is a cheap and effective genuine 'life insurance' policy. It won't make up for the sins of an unhealthy diet, but it fills in the nutritional holes that can plague even the most conscientious eater.**99**

—Walter Willett, M.D., MPH, Chair, Department of Nutrition, Harvard School of Public Health

In 2002, the American Medical Association (AMA), after reviewing extensive overwhelming evidence, overturned its longstanding position against multivitamins and advised all adults to take one multivitamin daily. This leads us to conclude our **Naked Fact #18**.

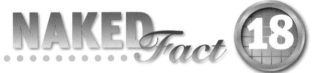

Many health experts, including the American Medical Association, recommend a daily multivitamin.

THE 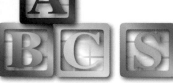 OF OPTIMAL SUPPLEMENTATION GUIDELINES

Now that we are all on the same page regarding the vital importance of a daily multivitamin to ensure micronutrient sufficiency, we offer you a few guidelines that we believe will help you purchase the best, most effective product on the market today. Can you think of anything you have learned that might help you pick the most absorbable supplement that would supply you with *beneficial quantities?* Have we given you any information that could help your micronutrients arrive without *competition* to increase availability? What knowledge could help you choose a supplement with synergies that enhance overall benefits? That's right—we can use the ABCs of Optimal Supplementation as our guide.

A Is for Absorption

 Multivitamins delivered in liquid form have the best rate of absorption with the fewest binders and fillers.

 Multivitamins delivered in liquid form are more convenient for the portion of the population that has difficulty swallowing, has undergone bariatric surgery, or suffers from specific health conditions.

 Everyday Micronutrient Depleters (EMDs) such as added sugar or HFCS (high fructose corn syrup), as well as artificial colors and flavors, should be avoided when seeking a multivitamin.

 When you take a single-serving, powdered multivitamin delivered in a liquid form, you get a highly absorbable multivitamin with limited exposure to destructive elements.

B Is for Beneficial Quantities

 Optimal Daily Doses (ODD) can best be achieved through a combination of a micronutrient-rich diet and a daily multivitamin supplying beneficial quantities (approximately 100 percent of RDI [reference daily intake] for all essential micronutrients).

 Increasing intakes above the current RDI for some micronutrients, like vitamin D, may be beneficial.

Multivitamin supplements should be taken multiple times throughout the day, due to water solubility and the body's limited absorption capacity.

C Is for Micronutrient Competition

 Look for multivitamins/supplements that remove micronutrient competition. The only way to ensure complete elimination of competitions is to separate micronutrients into multiple formulas to be taken at different times of the day.

 Products labeled with Anti-Competition Technology (ACT) have been formulated to eliminate competition. Taking a supplement that utilizes this technology is much easier than separating out your own micronutrients throughout the day.

S Is for Micronutrient Synergy

 Using the micronutrients' natural synergistic relationships can greatly increase the absorption and utilization of many essential micronutrients.

 Taking a nutritional supplement or multivitamin that is formulated to utilize these natural synergistic relationships can result in greater micronutrient benefits.

When we put the ABCs of Optimal Supplementation together, the most effective multivitamin would be a single-serving, powdered formula delivered in a liquid form that contains beneficial quantities (approximately 100 percent of the RDI for each micronutrient). In addition, certain micronutrients should be taken twice a day; in some cases, such as vitamin D, it is recommended to take in doses higher than current RDI.

Take a minute to evaluate how your multivitamin stacks up. We will show you how to find a multivitamin that satisfies the ABCs of Optimal Supplementation. Go to www.caltonnutrition. com/multivitamin-quiz

The multivitamin you choose should also utilize Anti-Competition Technology that completely separates known competitive micronutrients to ensure absorption. This will mandate that it contain at least two completely different formulations to be taken at two completely different times during the day. And last, synergistic micronutrients should be paired in each formula to enhance the potential health benefits of each micronutrient to its utmost.

We conclude Chapter 10 with **Naked Fact #19:**

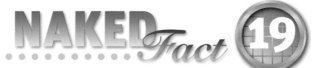

When choosing a multivitamin supplement, it is best to follow the ABCs of Optimal Supplementation guidelines and pick a single-serving, powdered multivitamin delivered in liquid form that provides beneficial quantities of essential micronutrients and is formulated to include both Anti-Competition Technology and synergy.

Universities and physicians recommend the following when choosing a multivitamin:

Dr. Oz's Ultimate Supplement Checklist

Multivitamin

Look for 100 percent of the daily value of the twelve essential vitamins and minerals—like vitamins B, C, E, and zinc.

Note: Only women who are menstruating need a multivitamin with iron.

More is not better—avoid "mega-doses." You only need 100 percent daily value, not 500 percent.

Take half in the morning and half at night to maximize absorption.

Calcium (600 mg)

Magnesium (400 mg)

Vitamin D (1,000 IU)

Fish Oil

Your daily dose must contain 600 mgs of the DHA omega-3 fatty acid.

Tufts University Health & Nutrition Letter

Calcium and Vitamin D

 "There's no question that calcium, together with vitamin D, protects bone health and helps prevent osteoporosis." Research out of Tufts Bone Metabolism Laboratory concluded that "prevention of hip fractures requires 700 to 800 milligrams of calcium per day in tandem with at least 800 International Units (IU) of vitamin D." However, Tufts feels that most multivitamins, even those touting bone benefits, "fall short of those amounts." They add that high dose vitamin D supplementation may be associated with a reduction in the rate of breast cancer.

Vitamin B_{12}

 Tufts University agrees with the FDA's note that "older people sometimes do lose the body's natural ability to absorb vitamin B_{12} from food." They suggest taking a supplement to maintain B_{12} levels.

Iron

 Richard J. Wood, Ph.D., of the University of Massachusetts, warns that people may be taking in too much iron. He says that for most people, taking a supplement without iron is preferable.

Eye Health

 Lutein is currently being tested against age-related macular degeneration (AMD). According to Allen Taylor, Ph.D., at Tufts Laboratory for Nutrition and Vision Research, for lutein to be effective for AMD, "it probably requires about 6 milligrams per day." This is far more than most multivitamins contain, even those claiming "lutein for eye health."

Harvard School of Public Health

5 Quick Tips for Getting the Right Vitamins:

Eat a healthy diet.

Take a multivitamin daily as an inexpensive nutrition insurance policy.

Think about vitamin D. Aim for 1,000 to 2,000 IU a day.

Say no to mega-dose vitamins and mega-fortified foods.

Avoid "super" supplements.

University of Maryland Medical Center

A good rule of thumb when selecting a multivitamin is to look for one that includes 100 to 300 percent of the daily value for all essential vitamins and minerals. You should also look for supplements that are designed to be taken two to four times daily to get these amounts, as opposed to one-a-day varieties. Check with a knowledgeable health-care provider if you are considering supplement doses higher than twice the daily value.

Dr. Mark Hyman, Founder and Medical Director of the Ultra Wellness Center

A high-quality multivitamin and mineral that should contain:

 mixed carotenoids, which include lutein and zeaxanthin

at least 400 mcg of folate

a mixed B-complex vitamin

Calcium-magnesium

 at least 600 mg of calcium and 400 mg of magnesium

Vitamin D3

 1,000 to 2,000 IU a day (people who are deficient in vitamin D will need more)

Omega-3 fatty acids

 should contain the fats EPA and DHA, 1,000 to 2,000 mg a day

The third and final step that a nutrivore takes to achieve micronutrient sufficiency is supplementation. Choosing to follow our Rich Food, Poor Food philosophy (Step One) and avoiding or eliminating most of the Everyday Micronutrient Depleters in your life (Step Two) can greatly enhance your overall chances of achieving micronutrient sufficiency, but supplementing with a daily multivitamin that meets the ABCs of Optimal Supplementation guidelines (Step Three) ensures that sufficiency is met. Although it is in no way mandatory to use supplements in order to be a nutrivore, we have found that the ability to achieve and/or sustain daily micronutrient sufficiency from food alone is simply not realistic for the majority of individuals.

We believe, as do many health experts, that a properly formulated multivitamin is a prudent addition to a micronutrient-rich diet. Consider it a daily health-insurance policy for your most valuable asset—your health.

• • • • • • • • • • • • • • • •

Nutreince™—The Multivitamin Reinvented

AFTER READING ALL THIS NEW INFORMATION about absorption, beneficial quantities, competition, and synergy, you may be left scratching your head, wondering where you can find a multivitamin that meets the ABCs of Optimal Supplementation Guidelines. Well, you're not alone; so were we. After all, this is the very same information we discovered in our research to reverse Mira's advanced osteoporosis. We too were left wondering where we were going to find a multivitamin that would offer superior absorption or that contained the 600 mg of calcium, 400 mg of magnesium, 6 mg of lutein and the 1,000–2,000 IU of vitamin D most experts recommend. And sadly, none of the multivitamins we found on store shelves were formulated using Anti-Competition Technology or anything like it. Sure, the synergies were there, but remember that without getting rid of the micronutrient competitions, the synergies are all but useless.

So, what could we do? Because we hypothesized that removing the micronutrient competitions would be essential to Mira's healing, we began by purchasing each micronutrient separately and taking them in small groupings before and after each of our four meals, eight times throughout the day. Two or three pills before breakfast, three or four after, and so on until the thirty-plus pills we had to take each day were gone. Not only was this method hugely expensive, costing nearly 300 dollars for each of us per month, but it became a seemingly never-ending chore of choking down pills every time we turned around. Even Mira, who didn't have a hard time swallowing pills in the beginning, developed an aversion to them about a year and 10,000-plus pills later.

But it worked! The proof was in the DEXA scan, and after seeing Mira's incredible recovery, we were committed to sharing this knowledge with others. Soon, all of our clients, including Mabel whom you read about earlier, started on the same regimen, and client after client saw their health improve as well. However, there was a side effect to this anti-competition, pill-stacking method we had developed, and it wasn't a positive one. The regimen seemed to induce a state of extreme complaining in our clients. "Why can't you just find us something that we can take a couple times a day?" they would ask. And, as we ourselves had also swallowed enough handfuls of pills to choke a horse, we decided to do something about it.

Now, in the initial printing of *Naked Calories,* we didn't mention nutreince™, the multivitamin we personally formulated and brought to market in April 2012 to solve our supplementation dilemma. After all, this is not a book about the discovery of a multivitamin product. It is a three-step plan (beginning with food first) to reach a state of micronutrient sufficiency from which every person's health can thrive. But, due to some e-mails and reviews we received faulting us for not fully disclosing our product, we decided to mention it here. We knew that the science behind our discovery was solid—the need for a multivitamin that followed the ABCs of Optimal Supplementation guidelines, so we began to develop a product for

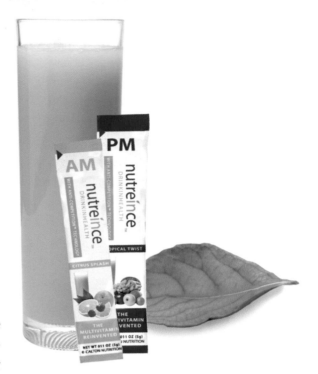

ourselves and our clients that would be easier on both our wallets and our busy schedules.

If over a period of six years, you had researched the flaws in available multivitamin supplements and discovered a means of creating something that could be administered to your loved ones and clients that reversed their poor health conditions, sped up their weight loss, and improved numerous aspects of their everyday lives, wouldn't you create it? Wouldn't you feel obligated to share your research with as many as possible?

If you have ever had a loved one who was sick, then you know what we are talking about when we say that you would do anything to help them get better. We want to be clear about one thing: if there had been even one other multivitamin, anywhere in the world, that met the ABCs of Optimal Supplementation guidelines, we would have used it. And had it worked, we would be doing everything in our power to get it into your hands right now. But there wasn't one. Our decision to manufacture nutreince was truly a labor of love, born out of desperation and necessity. Nutreince is not just a multivitamin to us; it is a part of our story—a piece of who we are. In reality, it is the natural progression of our research. We share this story with you because we want you to know why we created nutreince, and that we didn't just decide to sell a vitamin to make money. We don't think it invalidates our research; in fact, just the opposite: we think it shows our faith and commitment to our teachings. Recently, this research was validated when the US Patent and Trademark Office issued us a patent on our invention of Anti-Competition Technology (ACT).

Remember, our three-step approach you have just learned begins with food first. Our second book, *Rich Food, Poor Food,* is a testament to just how important we think high-quality micronutrient-rich food is. We also know that reducing Everyday Micronutrient Depleters (EMDs) on top of a rich food diet is an incredibly powerful second step toward optimal health. Finally, deciding if you need to supplement your diet is your third step. If you do, the ABCs of Optimal Supplementation guidelines can be used to help you choose a quality supplement, regardless of its manufacturer. If you try nutreince, great; if you use something else, that's great too. Either way, the multivitamin you choose is up to you—but at least you now have a little background on the issue and an understanding of why we felt it was important to develop nutreince.

In our final chapter we combine the Naked Facts we have gathered along our journey and reveal our "Hypothesis of Health." We will discover the vast health and financial benefits of being a nutrivore and review the three simple steps to achieving this lifestyle. Finally, when you combine all that you have learned, you will discover that you have the *potential power* to create the nutritional foundation you need to achieve optimal health.

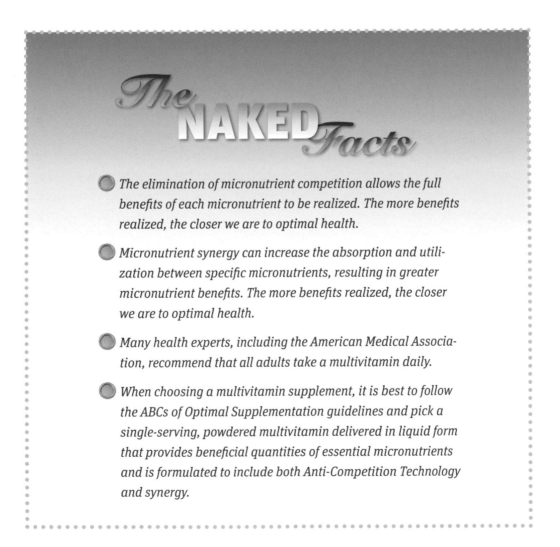

The elimination of micronutrient competition allows the full benefits of each micronutrient to be realized. The more benefits realized, the closer we are to optimal health.

Micronutrient synergy can increase the absorption and utilization between specific micronutrients, resulting in greater micronutrient benefits. The more benefits realized, the closer we are to optimal health.

Many health experts, including the American Medical Association, recommend that all adults take a multivitamin daily.

When choosing a multivitamin supplement, it is best to follow the ABCs of Optimal Supplementation guidelines and pick a single-serving, powdered multivitamin delivered in liquid form that provides beneficial quantities of essential micronutrients and is formulated to include both Anti-Competition Technology and synergy.

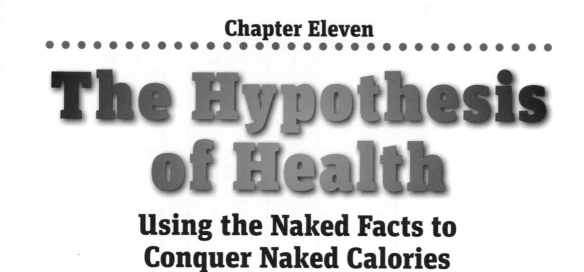

Chapter Eleven

The Hypothesis of Health

Using the Naked Facts to Conquer Naked Calories

New ideas
reality

Science and opinion
discoveries

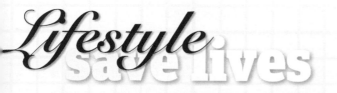

Lifestyle
save lives

> **"**Research is to see what everyone else has seen, and to think what nobody else has thought.**"**
> —Albert Szent-Györgyi, M.D., Ph.D.,
> Winner of the Nobel Prize for Medicine, 1973

Throughout history there have been those who have turned their backs on progress and refused to open their minds to the realities of new ideas, even when the new ideas were based on their own discoveries. As you may remember, in Chapter 9 we introduced you to Dutch physician Christiaan Eijkman who first discovered, due to a lack of feed for his chickens, an "anti-beriberi factor" in unpolished rice that cured the micronutrient-deficiency disease beriberi. However, there is an important part of this story we have not yet shared with you, so we will finish the tale here. Even though Eijkman was the first to recognize these "factors," he was not the one to receive credit for the discovery of the vitamin. His "anti-beriberi factor" was one of the biggest discoveries of all time, saved countless lives, and ultimately led to the discovery of vitamin B_1, yet something kept him from moving forward with his work and identifying his "factor" as vitamin B_1. Can you guess what it was? It was his inability to believe his own findings.

Eijkman was busy trying to prove that beriberi was caused by a bacterial infection, not a deficiency. It was because of this that he was not able to see the proverbial forest for the trees. The point is—Eijkman's preconceived notions would not allow him to believe what he himself had discovered.

"There are in fact two things, science and opinion; the former begets knowledge, the later ignorance."

Hippocrates said it best: "There are in fact two things, science and opinion; the former begets knowledge, the later ignorance." Eijkman refused to believe his own scientific findings. This led him to stick blindly to his guns, preventing him from discovering the true causative "factor" of beriberi and, ultimately, the discovery of the vitamin itself. Eijkman's mistake can be a valuable lesson for each of us. We must all remember to keep our minds open and trust what our own research has shown us, even if it defies what is currently thought to be true.

So what has our research shown us? Like Eijkman, you already have the information you need. Take a moment to consider the Naked Facts that we have accumulated thus far. Behind each one of these seemingly simple statements stands mounds of credible research that you personally have examined.

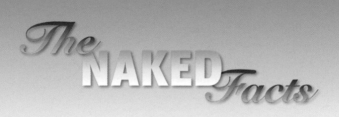

 The RDIs are daily micronutrient intake levels considered sufficient to meet the requirements of nearly all (97 to 98 percent) healthy individuals in each life-stage and gender group, while the EAR is ONLY the amount expected to satisfy the micronutrient requirements of 50 percent of the population.

 Soil and food have been studied and a micronutrient-depletion trend has been established.

 A deficiency in one or more of the essential micronutrients can ultimately cause health-related conditions or diseases.

 Collected data reveals a global micronutrient-deficiency pandemic.

 Global distribution, factory farming, food packaging, and preparation methods can cause large percentages of micronutrients to be depleted from your food *before* it reaches your plate.

 Avoiding heavily processed, Energy-Dense, Nutrient-Poor (EDNP) foods, and utilizing the Rich Food, Poor Food philosophy increases the likelihood of micronutrient sufficiency.

 Many of the foods and drinks one may choose every day can block or deplete micronutrients, thereby reducing micronutrient sufficiency.

 Prescription and over-the-counter medications deplete essential micronutrients, which can either exacerbate the same condition or initiate a new deficiency condition or disease.

 Stress, smoking, pollution, toxic chemicals, hurried lifestyle, exercise, weight loss, and lifestyle diets are all possible Everyday Micronutrient Depleters (EMDs).

10 According to published research, random, low-carbohydrate, Mediterranean, low-fat, paleo, Primal, and medically based diets from food alone have all been shown to be deficient at delivering minimum RDI levels of essential micronutrients within medically wise calorie ranges.

11 Obesity has been shown to be a condition of micronutrient deficiency.

12 Malnourishment and obesity are both conditions of micronutrient deficiency. The only thing that differs is the caloric intake.

13 Single-serving, powdered multivitamins delivered in liquid form are more suitable to a large percentage of the population, are readily available for **absorption,** and are protected from micronutrient-depleting elements.

14 Combining a multivitamin that contains **beneficial quantities** (with approximately 100 percent of the RDI) with a micronutrient-rich diet all but guarantees Optimal Daily Doses (ODD).

15 Multivitamin supplements should be taken multiple times throughout the day, due to water solubility and our body's limited absorption capacity.

16 The elimination of **micronutrient competition** allows the full benefits of each micronutrient to be realized. The more benefits realized, the closer we are to optimal health.

17 **Micronutrient synergy** can increase the absorption and utilization between specific micronutrients, resulting in greater micronutrient benefits. The more benefits realized, the closer we are to optimal health.

18 Many health experts, including the American Medical Association, recommend a daily multivitamin.

19 When choosing a multivitamin supplement, it is best to follow the ABCs of Optimal Supplementation guidelines and pick a single-serving, powdered multivitamin delivered in liquid form that provides beneficial quantities of essential micronutrients and is formulated to include both Anti-Competition Technology and synergy.

When we combine our Naked Facts, an empirical philosophy regarding the causation, prevention, and reversal of disease emerges. It may be quite a bit different from the one you had when you started this book. Unlike Eijkman, we will trust our gathered scientific facts over popular opinion. According to Hippocrates, the result will be knowledge over ignorance.

We have already established that a deficiency of one or more of the essential micronutrients is a causative factor in many of today's lifestyle conditions and diseases. We have also seen credible research showing the prevention and reversal of many of these conditions through micronutrient supplementation. Like Funk and Hopkins—the vitamin researchers from Chapter 9 who in 1912 wrote the *Vitamin Hypothesis of Disease,* stating that certain diseases are caused by a dietary lack of specific vitamins—we, too, recognize the health ramifications of micronutrient deficiency. But why stop there? Why simply point out that disease is caused by micronutrient deficiencies? It's time to take the next step.

> *A deficiency of one or more of the essential micronutrients is a causative factor in many of today's lifestyle conditions and diseases.*

Now, 100 years later, we offer a new hypothesis that not only identifies the cause of today's most prevalent health conditions and diseases, but also offers a realistic and sustainable method of preventing and reversing them. The culmination of our research, both here in *Naked Calories* and on our expeditions for the Calton Project, verify our hypothesis we share with you now. We call it the **Micronutrient Sufficiency Hypothesis of Health.** It states:

> **"**If a condition or disease can be directly linked to a micronutrient deficiency, then it can be prevented and/or reversed through sustained sufficiency of the deficient micronutrient(s).**"**

Isn't this what our research has been showing us all along? While our hypothesis is simple, we believe it is a foundation from which a mighty but obtainable vision of the future can be realized; a future where today's most common and life-threatening health conditions and diseases, such as heart disease, cancer, osteoporosis, and obesity will become as distant a memory as scurvy, beriberi, or pellagra. It's happening already. In study after study, researchers are proving that common everyday micronutrients improve health and save lives. Just as vitamin C prevented scurvy, thiamine (vitamin B_1) cured beriberi, and niacin (vitamin B_3) reversed pellagra, numerous other health conditions and diseases can be prevented and/or reversed through proper micronutrient supplementation and sufficiency. Below are some additional studies to add to our already ample list of research supporting the power of micronutrient sufficiency.

In 2011, New Zealand researchers from the Obstetrics and Gynecology Department at the University of Auckland reviewed more than thirty studies on the correlation between sub-fertile men and antioxidant supplementation. They discovered that antioxidants such as vitamins C, E, and zinc reduced infertility and increased the odds of conception more than four-fold.

In a randomized, double-blind, placebo-controlled study published in 2005 in the *Journal of the Academy of Dermatology,* women were given 10 mg daily of either silicon or a placebo. At the end of twenty weeks, the women taking silicon supplements exhibited significantly decreased skin roughness as well as increased strength of hair and nails.

Vitamin K_2, which is only found in animal sources and often deficient in the American diet, can reduce incidents of heart disease by directing calcium out of your arteries and into your bones. Researchers at Erasmus Medical Center Rotterdam in the Netherlands studied 4,807 women for over seven years and determined that supplementation with vitamin K_2 improved cardiovascular health by preventing arterial calcium accumulation, and slashed the risk of heart disease by 57 percent. Additionally, according to a 2012 study out of Haro-kopio University in Athens, vitamin K_2 serves up added bone benefits and induces positive changes in bone mass by allowing for proper utilization of calcium.

B vitamins can reduce coronary heart disease. In a 2000 study published in the *European Journal of Clinical Nutrition,* middle-aged men with the highest blood serum folate (vitamin B_9) levels were 69 percent less likely to suffer an acute coronary event than those with the lowest levels. In an additional 2004 study, researchers from the University of Verona in Italy reported vitamin B_6 also plays an important role in heart health. When researchers split the subjects into two groups based on their vitamin B_6 blood levels, they found that those individuals in the group with the lowest half of vitamin B_6 blood levels were nearly twice as likely to suffer coronary heart disease as those in the second group, which had the highest levels of vitamin B_6.

Studies out of the Arizona Cancer Center and Cornell University determined that total cancer mortality was reduced by 50 percent in those taking 200 mcg of selenium daily. The risk of prostate cancer was reduced by as much as 74 percent, colorectal cancer by 58 percent, and lung cancer by 48 percent.

In 2000, researchers from the Department of Sociology and Criminal Science at California State University reported that adolescents who received micronutrient supplementation exhibited improved brain function, which resulted in 40 percent less violent and anti-social behavior than those receiving placebos. Additionally, a Stonybrook University Medical School study reported that when learning-disabled children started a micronutrient program, all of them showed significant academic improvements within only a few weeks.

Some children gained three to five years in reading comprehension within the first year of treatment. All the children in special-education classes were mainstreamed, able to move to regular classes. However, after one year, when half of the students discontinued their micronutrient program, their new skills dropped off, while the skills of those continuing the supplementation "continued the upward trend."

According to a study in *Metabolism*, taking chromium and niacin together reduced fasting glucose (blood sugar) levels by 6.8 percent and further improved glucose tolerance, reducing insulin requirements in as many as one-third of insulin-dependent diabetics.

According to a 2008 study in the *Archives of Internal Medicine*, researchers from Johns Hopkins University and Albert Einstein College of Medicine tested 13,331 adults aged twenty years and older to determine if an association existed between low vitamin D levels and mortality rates from all causes of death (all-cause mortality). They discovered that being among those with the lowest quarter of vitamin D blood levels was associated with a 26 percent increased rate of mortality from all causes, even in those subjects who exhibited greater physical activity and healthier lifestyles.

A 2009 study published in the *American Journal of Clinical Nutrition* found that taking micronutrient supplementation might add years to your life. It revealed that people who supplemented had younger DNA. Scientists can measure "biological age" by examining the length of an individual's telomeres, with longer telomeres signifying longer life span. Think of telomeres as the protective plastic coating at the ends of your shoelaces. Telomeres protect DNA breakdown, much like the coating on your shoelaces protects the lace from fraying.

Earlier telomere studies on sixty- to seventy-five-year-old men and women showed those with short telomeres had an 800 percent higher death rate from infectious diseases, and a 300 percent higher death rate from heart disease. This latest study found that those who took multivitamins had 5.1 percent longer telomeres than non-users. The 5.1 percent longer telomeres equated to living approximately 9.6 years longer. Research shows that vitamin B_{12} supplements increase telomere length, while vitamins C and E prevent telomere shortening.

Throughout our journey, we have shared with you just a few of the thousands of studies on disease and micronutrient sufficiency that support our new Micronutrient Sufficiency Hypothesis of Health. It makes sense, doesn't it? With micronutrient deficiency a causative factor in these conditions, removing the deficiency and creating sufficiency of the same micronutrient(s) would remove the cause or basis of the respective condition or disease. The importance of micronutrient sufficiency quickly becomes evident. Not only can micronutrient sufficiency reduce chronic diseases, improve quality of life, and increase longevity, it can also save you something more tangible—money. And in today's rough economic times, money is something we can all use a little more of. Could micronutrient sufficiency also reduce health-care costs?

Health-care costs have been steadily rising for many years. Expenditures on health care in the United States surpassed $2.5 trillion in 2009, more than three times the $714 billion spent in 1990, and more than eight times the $253 billion spent in 1980. Health-care expenses climb with age, and as American baby boomers increase in age and numbers, caring for this generation will further raise costs. There will be more than 70 million Americans over the age of seventy by the year 2030, half of whom will be over the age of seventy-five. It is estimated that this will push health-care costs to nearly $16 trillion per year. That number is the equivalent of taking every dollar we currently spend on health care and multiplying it by six!

With longer life span comes a greater prevalence of chronic diseases. According to the Centers for Disease Control and Prevention, it is estimated that the costs for chronic disease treatment account for more than 75 percent of national health expenditures. Furthermore, as the baby boomers lose their independence they require more assistance, which places further financial burden on the already strained health-care system.

Do you think that micronutrient supplementation could reduce this looming financial strain? A recent study by the Lewin Group, a firm specializing in health-care policy analysis, examined

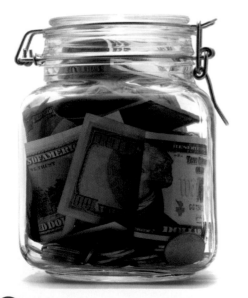

the five-year health-care cost savings of specific micronutrient supplements. The research group first had to examine the scientific evidence to prove that supplementation would reduce the risk of specific diseases that can, and do, lead to loss of independence. While we have already seen the numerous positive effects of supplementation, they limited their research to include only valid micronutrient therapies for which there is no scientific debate. Additionally, they had to develop estimates of the potential health-care expenditure savings using the congressional budget office's accounting methods.

The first micronutrient examined was omega-3 fatty acids. Although we revealed in Chapter 8 that supplementation of this essential fat drastically reduced the weight and body mass index (BMI) of obese individuals, the Lewin Group only reviewed data on omega-3 as a scientifically proven beneficial supplement for the treatment of heart disease.

Their study exposed that approximately 384,303 hospitalizations due to coronary heart disease (CHD) could be avoided in a five-year period through daily supplementation of 1,800 mg of omega-3 fatty acids (containing EPA and DHA). The Lewin Group's findings support our Micronutrient Sufficiency Hypothesis of Health in that supplementation increased micronutrient sufficiency, thus preventing disease in a large segment of the population over five years. When the researchers examined the cost benefit of this supplementation, this is what they found: Supplementation of omega-3 alone would save an estimated $3.1 billion over five years in CHD-related hospital and physician expenses. The Lewin Group, however, didn't stop with this EFA. Let's examine its findings on other micronutrients and their individual abilities to prevent disease and reduce health-care costs.

 Daily supplementation with 6 to 10 mg of lutein with zeaxanthin (antioxidants) would decrease occurrence of age-related macular degeneration (AMD). This would help 130,959 baby boomers to prevent this devastating eye condition. The supplementation provided a cost savings of $2.5 billion over five years.

 If only 10.5 million women of childbearing age took a 400 mcg folic acid supplement daily, there would be 3,000 fewer infants born with neural tube disorders. This would save $1.3 billion over the next five years.

Daily supplementation of 1,200 mg of calcium with vitamin D could prevent 734,000 hip fractures in those aged sixty-five and older. The estimated five-year net savings would be $13.9 billion.

When you add up the numbers, the five-year totals are pretty amazing. With daily supplementation of only six micronutrients, more than **1.2 million people** could avoid hospitalization, injury, visual impairment, and disease. The net savings over the same period would be more than **$20 billion.**

Each of the supplements studied proved to decrease risk of disease, allowing people like you to live healthier lives while greatly reducing the financial burden on the American government. The Lewin Group concluded, "Supplements are an inexpensive and safe way to improve health status and reduce health care costs."

Jeffery Blumberg, Ph.D., of the Friedman School of Nutrition Science and Policy at Tufts University, reviewed the Lewin Group's study and added, "As our country faces an ever-changing crisis in health care, it is important to recognize the role that dietary supplements can play in reducing our burden of disease and the costs to manage it."

It certainly appears that supplementation could save the government billions of dollars, and as we know, that saves American taxpayers money as well.

Let's take a moment to put everything together.

A deficiency in one or more of the
essential micronutrients can ultimately cause
health-related conditions or diseases.

AND

If a condition or disease can be directly linked to a
micronutrient deficiency, then it can be prevented
and/or reversed through sustained sufficiency
of the deficient micronutrient(s).

AND

Supplementation to create micronutrient sufficiency has
been proven to reverse conditions and diseases
at low cost to the individual, resulting in
huge savings for the masses.

Well, this seems like a slam dunk to us. Creating a personal state of micronutrient sufficiency should be the goal of every one of us. We believe that creating a personal micronutrient-sufficient state will be the single most important thing you do for your health and for the health of those you love. Think of it as a low-cost health-insurance program with immediate health benefits. Your own investigation has brought you to this new understanding. Now that you are aware of the everyday causes, and the health-diminishing effects of micronutrient deficiency, the question you now face is, *"What are you going to do with this knowledge?"*

You may have noticed back in Chapter 2 that we used the quote "Knowledge is power" by Sir Frances Bacon. While this is true, Napoleon Hill, the 1920's rags-to-riches success story and author of *Think and Grow Rich,* realized that Bacon was only partially right. His observations led him to discover that while many individuals throughout history were well educated, only a few went on to do extraordinary things with their knowledge. Instead, he postulated, "Knowledge is only potential power."

The truth is, no matter what you have learned about soil depletion, Everyday Micronutrient Depleters (EMDs), Energy-Dense, Nutrient-Poor (EDNP) foods, micronutrient competition, or any other topic we explored together, your knowledge will never improve your health, or the health of your loved ones, until you put it to use. It all comes down to one simple fact: knowledge is useless . . . unless we use it.

Nutrivore: As Easy as One, Two, Three

WE KNOW THAT MICRONUTRIENT DEFICIENCY equals poor health and disease, and micronutrient sufficiency is the foundation of optimal health. It is time for us all to make the decision to take control of our own health and stop blaming it on genetics or searching for it at the bottom of a prescription bottle. In the film *Forks Over Knives,* Pam Popper, N.D., Ph.D., explains, "If you go through life thinking what happens to you from a health perspective is based on your genes, you're a helpless victim."

The reality is that the health-promoting power of the micronutrient has the potential capacity to prevent and reverse countless diseases within the next century, but only if we use it. So, what are you waiting for? You are now ready to make this huge and all important change in your life. We know you can do it. The best part is, you have just learned the three simple steps to become micronutrient sufficient and live the nutrivore lifestyle. You already understand the important health benefits—it is now time for you to push ahead and incorporate the three steps of our plan into your lives.

Choose Rich Food

We are living in an exciting time, a time when old ideas about obesity and disease are falling away and a new vision of wellness based on responsible nutrition and micronutrient sufficiency is beginning. The dawn of lifestyle medicine is upon us and with it comes endless health possibilities. Medical doctors, scientists, and nutritionists are turning away from outdated nutritional advice and extolling the benefits of a micronutrient-rich lifestyle. Your first step toward micronutrient sufficiency and becoming a nutrivore is to provide your body with the richest food sources of micronutrients that you can find. After all, it's quality that counts, and we're going to demand it because we're worth it.

In America and around the world people are going out of their way to find fresh, local foods grown and raised in a safe and responsible method. These people believe, as we do, that including wild fish, grass-fed beef, locally grown fruits and vegetables, and healthful seeds and nuts in our diet is the first step toward optimal health. No longer do we believe that a healthy diet is one that starves us or is full of naked calories. It is time to put your knowledge to action by eliminating processed, energy-dense micronutrient-poor foods, and taking the time to choose quality foods based on our *Rich-Food, Poor Food* philosophy. Perhaps you are a vegan, a low-carbohydrate dieter, or gluten intolerant. It doesn't matter. Your first priority should be to choose the foods that fit into your diet profile and are the most micronutrient rich. Your food is your first line of defense against micronutrient deficiency, and you aren't going to protect yourself with low-fat, sugar-laden muffins, a bag of potato chips, or even a salad that has been sitting on the grocery store shelf for weeks . . . are you?

Buying high-quality, micronutrient-rich foods is a great first step (and one that our book, *Rich Food, Poor Food*, makes easy), but as with all quality purchases, we have to learn to care for them properly. You wouldn't wear your new Gucci shoes in the mud . . . or leave your Ferrari out in the snow overnight. Maintaining quality is just as important as choosing quality in the first place. You took the time to search out and buy quality, so why ruin it?

Prepare your high-quality foods by using responsible cooking methods to maintain their beneficial micronutrients. Don't peel your vegetables if you don't have to. Be aware of how your food is cooked. Support restaurants that go the extra mile to provide organic, local food. You will be amazed at how much better a meal can taste when it's prepared with organic, local ingredients that are fresh and bursting with flavor.

Drive Down Depletion

Choosing to eat the most micronutrient-rich foods is a fantastic first step, but it is really just that—a first step. Regardless of how jam-packed your foods are with micronutrients, there are still those treacherous little Everyday Micronutrient Depleters (EMDs) to contend with. There are no more excuses. Your health depends on your willingness to make small, but strategic changes in your life. No one can do it for you. Being a nutrivore requires that you take a good look at your life and decide which EMDs are acting as roadblocks on your highway to health. Recognize that even some of your "healthy" high-quality foods and lifestyle habits may also have leaching effects. Limit intake of these foods and challenge obvious, micronutrient-depleting habits like smoking and excessive coffee and alcohol intake. It's time to evaluate the toxins in your life and take an active approach to swiching out common, everyday products that are adding to your overall toxic load. While this includes pesticides and chemical additives in your food, it also includes numerous toxins that can be found in things like toothpaste, shampoo, sunblock, cleaning supplies, and even your cookware and food storage containers. Remember toxins are EMDs too and the more you have in your life the less likely you are to achieve a micronutrient-sufficient state.

If you currently take prescription medications, talk to your physician. Find out if he or she understands the micronutrient-depleting effects the prescribed drugs may be having. We think you will be surprised by how many medical doctors do and are willing to support your choice to protect yourself through proper micronutrient supplementation. Additionally, there are thousands of physicians out there today who are open to using nutrition to reverse many health conditions and diseases. They realize, as we do, that micronutrients are powerful tools that can and should be used instead of pharmaceutical crutches whenever possible. If your current doctor doesn't share this view, you may want a second opinion. Find an integrative practitioner who is ready to examine your condition from a new angle. And, if getting off your prescription medication isn't a feasible solution for you, then at least you are now aware of just how important it is to replenish the depleted micronutrients through proper supplementation.

Supplement

As we have stated before, choosing to take a quality supplement is like taking out a daily health-insurance plan. However, don't forget that a quality multivitamin is only a supplement and not a substitute for a healthy diet and lifestyle—its job is to help ensure minimum micronutrient sufficiency and protect you from micronutrient deficiencies when your diet or your daily actions don't always go perfectly to plan. Unlike choosing complicated car insurance or life insurance policies, choosing a supplement is easy. You want to find the policy with the best and most complete coverage. All you have to do is remember the ABCs of Optimal Supplementation guidelines.

Look for a highly absorbable single-serving, powdered multivitamin drink mix without the undesirable fillers, binders, sugars, or artificial colors and flavors. Next, choose a product with beneficial quantities (with approximately 100 percent of the RDI) that is designed to be taken more than once a day to account for water solubility and our body's limited absorption capacity. And last, embrace a supplement that is formulated with the awareness of both micronutrient competition to release micronutrient benefits and synergy to enhance them. As we mentioned earlier, take our multivitamin, nutreince, or take another—your choice; just remember that for many, this third and final step is as important as the first two when attempting to reach sufficiency.

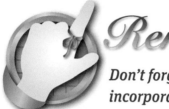

Remember

Don't forget to retake the micronutrient-sufficiency quiz after incorporating our three-step plan into your life. We think you may be surprised at just how much you have improved.

You Are Now Ready!

THE POTENTIAL POWER of all of your new knowledge is just waiting to be put into practice. You have all the tools necessary to become micronutrient sufficient, and with it, the power to create optimal health in your own life. While the three steps are simple, they are incredibly powerful. We have personally witnessed how these three steps have produced inspiring transformations in Mira and in our clients. We know that they can dramatically improve your health too! This brings us to our final **Naked Fact #20.**

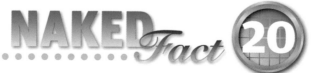

Following the three steps of the nutrivore lifestyle will put our micronutrient knowledge into practice, allowing us to achieve micronutrient sufficiency and, ultimately, optimal health.

> **❝**To maximize human health will require scientists, clinicians, and educators to abandon outdated paradigms of micronutrients that merely prevent disease, and to explore more meaningful ways to prevent chronic disease and achieve optimal health through optimal nutrition.**❞**
>
> —Dr. Bruce N. Ames

As the saying goes, no man (or woman) is an island. Together we can make a difference. While one voice can evoke change, many voices coming together behind one common goal can create a movement. We now call on people everywhere to abandon outdated paradigms and commit themselves to reaching the ultimate goal of optimal health for all.

What we have discovered on the Calton Project has forever changed our approach to health and nutrition. A micronutrient-deficiency pandemic is spreading as billions of people around the world unknowingly participate in their own demise. While we personally enjoy many aspects of modernization and progress, we must ask ourselves, *progress at what cost?* Our observations have led us to believe, as science has verified, that micronutrient deficiency is linked to all of the modern health conditions and diseases, including obesity, cardiovascular diseases, cancer, diabetes, osteoporosis, and many others. It is not simply random chance or genetic predisposition that is causing places like India and China to literally explode with obesity and diabetes, or Papua New Guineans to suddenly develop cancer. These people have known hardship, but never before have these modern diseases affected them.

The human body is an amazing thing; it adapts to its circumstances and makes do with what it has to stay alive. However, while our bodies can fight off dangerous bacterial infections and can defend us from ruthless viral attacks, it does not seem to be able to protect us from ourselves. In the end, we believe that there is one cause at the root of all modern diseases—micronutrient deficiency—and that this one cause has but one cure—micronutrient sufficiency.

Ultimately, we cannot morally afford to continue to disregard this catalyst of disease that has become so widespread. Our elected government officials, sports heroes, movie stars, doctors, scientists, nutritionists, CEOs, teachers, and parents must all stand and address the reality of the micronutrient-deficiency pandemic. Each and every one of us must come together and ask the next responsible question:

> **❝**Isn't it time to make micronutrient sufficiency the foundation of a global initiative that can protect us from the world's most devastating health conditions and diseases, and usher in an age of optimal health? **We think the answer is yes!❞**

References

Chapter 1. Micronutrient Deficiency: The Hidden Hunger

Alternative and Integral Therapies for Insomnia. Retrieved 2011, from Holistic online: http://www.holistic online. com/remedies/sleep/sleep_ins_nutrition.htm

Ames BN. Micronutrient Deficiencies: A Major Cause of DNA Damage. *Annals of the New York Academy of Sciences* 1999, 889: 87–106. doi: 10.1111/j.1749-6632.1999.tb08727.x. PMID: 10668486

Calton, J. Prevalence of Micronutrient Deficiency in Popular Diet Plans. *Journal of the International Society of Sports Nutrition* 2010, 7:24. doi:10.1186/1550-2783-7-24. PMID: 20537171. Retrieved 2010, from the National Center for Biotechnology Information: http://www.ncbi.nlm.nih.gov/ pmc/articles/ PMC2905334/

Cardiovascular disease. Retrieved 2011, from World Heath Organization (WHO): http://www.who.int/cardiovascular _diseases/en/

Dietary Supplement Fact Sheet: Selenium. Retrieved 2010, from Office of Dietary Supplements National Institutes of Health: http://ods.od.nih.gov/factsheets/selenium/

Downey L. Vitamins That Help You Sleep. Retrieved 2011, from Livestrong: http://www.live strong.com/article /110732-vitamins-sleep/

Isaacs T. Our Disappearing Minerals and Their Vital Health Role (Part 1). Retrieved 2010, from Natural News: http://www.naturalnews.com/023237_ minerals_health_soil.html

Jim Carrey says the prozac he took may have helped, but he is better off without it now –*60 Minutes Sunday*. Retrieved 2010, from CBS NEWS: http://www.cbspressexpress.com/div.php/cbs_network/ release?id=8345

Kul Gautam's remarks on VMD Global Progress Report. Retrieved 2010, from UNICEF: http://www. unicef.org/media/media_20081.html

Obesity Rates Growing Faster Than Expected. Retrieved 2010, from The Burrill Report: http://www.burrill report. com/article-2659.html

Vitamin B9 (Folic acid) Overview. Retrieved 2010, from University of Maryland Medical Center: http://www.umm. edu/altmed/articles/vitamin-b9-000338.htm

Vitamin D Linked to Lower Colorectal Cancer Risk. Retrieved 2010, from Tufts University Friedman School of Nutrition Science & Policy: http://www.tuftshealthletter.com/ShowArticle.aspx? rowId=806

Chapter 3. Nutrition 101: Understanding Nutrients

Brenna JT. "Efficiency of conversion of alpha-linolenic acid to long chain n-3 fatty acids in man." *Curr. Opin. Clin. Nutr. Metab. Care* 2002. March;5(2):127-132. doi:10.1097/00075197-20020300000002.PMID 11844977

Gerster H. "Can adults adequately convert alpha-linolenic acid (18:3n-3) to eicosapentaenoic acid (20:5n-3) and docosahexaenoic acid (22:6n-3)?" *Int. J. Vitam. Nutr. Res.* 1998. 68(3): 159–173. PMID 9637947

Zempleni J, Mock DM. Human peripheral blood mononuclear cells: Inhibition of biotin transport by reversible competition with pantothenic acid is quantitatively minor. *J Nutr Biochem.* 1999; 10(7): 427–32. PMID: 15539319

Chapter 4. The Minerals Go Missing: Micronutrient Depletion Begins

Abraham GE, Lubran MM. Serum and red cell magnesium levels in patients with premenstrual tension. *The American Journal of Clinical Nutrition* 1981, Nov: 34(11): 2364-6. PMID: 7197877

2011 Alzheimer's Disease Facts and Figures (Quick facts). Retrieved 2011, from the Alzheimer's Association: http:// www.alz.org/documents_custom/2011_ Facts_Figures_Fact_Sheet.pdf

Ames BN. Micronutrients prevent cancer and delay aging. *Toxicology Letters.* 1998;102-103:5–18. doi: 10.1016/S0378-4274(98)00269-0. PMID10022226

Attention deficit hyperactivity disorder. Retrieved 2010, from University of Maryland Medical Center: http://www.umm.edu/altmed/articles/attention-deficit-000017.htm

The Benefits of Vitamin B (video). Retrieved 2011, from *The Dr. Oz Show:* http://www.doctoroz.com/videos/benefits-vitamin-b

Bond P. Nutrition label change could pose health and sales challenge. *Natural Foods Merchandiser* 2011. Retrieved 2011, from New Hope 360: http://newhope360.com/regulation-and-legislation/ nutrition-label-change-could-pose-health-and-sales-challenge?cid=nl_360_daily

Canadian Community Health Survey (CCHS): Do Canadian Adults Meet Their Nutrient Requirements Through Food Intake Alone? Retrieved 2011, from Health Canada: http://www.hc-sc.gc.ca/fn-an/surveill/nutrition/commun/art-nutr-adult-eng.php#a1

Chocano-Bedoya PO et al. Dietary B vitamin intake and incident premenstrual syndrome. *Am J Clin Nutr* 2011 May; 93(5):1080-6. PMID: 21346091

Commonly Asked Questions (FAQs): Dietary Supplements. Retrieved 2010, from Nutrition: A service of the National Agricultural Library, USDA: http://www.nutrition.gov/nal_display/index.php?info_center=11&tax_level=2&tax_subject=393&level3_id=0&level4_id=0&level5_id=0&topic_id=2041&&placement_default=0

Davis DR et al. Changes in USDA Food Composition Data for 43 Garden Crops, 1950 to 1999. *Journal of the American College of Nutrition* 2004, 23(6): 669-682.

The developing world's new burden: obesity. Retrieved 2011, from the Food and Agriculture Organization of The United Nations: http://www.fao.org/FOCUS/E/ obesity/obes3.htm

Dirt Poor: Have Fruits and Vegetables Become Less Nutritious? Retrieved 2011, from *Scientific American:* http://www.scientificamerican.com/article.cfm?id=soil-depletion-and-nutrition-loss

Documentation: The Community Nutrition Mapping Project (CNMap): Selected Populations. Retrieved 2010, from the USDA, United States Department of Agriculture Agricultural Research Service: http://www.ars.usda.gov/Services/ docs.htm?docid=14655

Dowd J, Stafford D. *The Vitamin D Cure.* Wiley 2009. May; 1st edition: Pg.2.

Dr. Oz's Ultimate Supplement Checklist. Retrieved 2011, from *The Dr. Oz Show:* http://www.doctoroz.com/videos/dr-ozs-ultimate-supplement-checklist

Fairfield KM, Fletcher RH. Vitamins for chronic disease prevention in adults: scientific review. *Journal of the American Medical Association* 2002. Jun 19;287(23):3116-26. doi:10.1001/jama.287 .23.3116 PMID:12069675

FDA U.S. Food and Drug Administration. Federal Register Advance Notice of Proposed Rulemaking (Food Labeling) 72 FR 62149. November 2, 2007: Revision of Reference Values and Mandatory Nutrients. Retrieved 2011, from U.S. FDA: http://www.fda.gov/Food/LabelingNutrition/FoodLabelingGuidanceRegulatoryInformation/RegulationFederalRegisterDocuments/ucm073531.htm

Food Nutrition Has Been Declining! Minerals Go Down, Disease Goes Up! Retrieved 2011, from the Nutrition Security Institute: http://www.nutritionsecurity.org/PDF/Food%20Nutrition%20Decline.pdf

Fuhrman J. *Eat to Live.* Hachette Digital, Inc. 2003. Pg. 18.

Get the Facts About Cataracts. Retrieved 2011, from the American Academy of Ophthalmology: http://www.geteyesmart.org/eyesmart/eye-health-news/focus20110801.cfm

Global cancer rates could increase by 50% to 15 million by 2020. Retrieved 2010, from the World Health Organization (WHO): http://www.who.int/ mediacentre/news/releases/2003/pr27/en/index .html

Goodwin PJ, Ennis M, Pritchard KI, Koo J, Hood N. Frequency of vitamin D (Vit D) deficiency a breast cancer (BC) diagnosis and association with risk of distant recurrence and death in a prospective cohort study of T1-3, N0-1, M0 BC. *Journal of Clinical Oncology* 2008,May;20(26):511. Retrieved 2011, from American Society of Clinical Oncology: http://www.asco.org/ASCOv2/Meetings/Abstracts?&vmview=abst_detail_view&confID=55&abstractID=31397

Health Conditions-Cancer. Retrieved 2011, from the Vitamin D Council: http://www.vitamindcouncil.org/health-conditions/cancer/

Health Conditions: Cardiovascular Diseases. Retrieved 2011, from Vitamin D Council: http://www.vitamind council.org/health-conditions/cardiovascular-diseases/

Holick MF. Vitamin D and Sunlight: Strategies for Cancer Prevention and Other Health Benefits. *Clinical Journal of the American Society of Nephrology* 2008, Sep;3(5):1548-54. PMID: 18550652

How Dietary Supplements Reduce Health Care Costs. Retrieved 2011, from Dr. Mark Hyman: http://dr hyman.com/how-dietary-supplements-reduce-health-care-costs-3250/

Human Nutrition Products and Services: Nutrient Intakes: Florida: All U.S. Retrieved 2011, from the USDA, United States Department of Agriculture Agricultural Research Service: http://www.ars.usda.gov/Services/docs.htm?docid=15677

IMMPaCt-International Micronutrient Malnutrition Prevention and Control Program. Retrieved 2010, from Centers for Disease Control and Prevention (CDC): http://www.cdc.gov/immpact/index.html

Kivipelto M, Annerbo S, Hultdin J, Backman L, Viitanen M, Fratiglioni L, Lokk J. Homocysteine and holo-trans-cobalamin and the risk of dementia and Alzheimer's disease: a prospective study. *European Journal of Neurology* 2009. Jul;16(7):808-13. PMID: 19453410

Lack of Potassium Linked to High Blood Pressure. Retrieved 2010, from *The Washington Post*: http://www.washingtonpost.com/wp-dyn/content/article/2008/11/09/AR2008110900862.html

Langsjoen PH, Vadhanavikit S, Folkers K. Response of patients in classes III and IV of cardiomyopathy to therapy in a blind and crossover trial with coenzyme Q10. Proc Natl Acad Sci USA 1985, Jun;82(12):4240-4. PMID: 3858877

Lieberman N, Burning N. *The Real Vitamin and Mineral Book*. Avery 2003.3rd edition; Pg.19.

Marler J, Wallin J. Human Health, the Nutritional Quality of Harvested Food and Sustainable Farming Systems. Retrieved 2010, from the Nutrition Security Institute: http://www.nutritionsecurity.org/PDF/NSI_White%20Paper_Web.pdf

Meat and Dairy: where have the minerals gone? Retrieved 2010, from *Food Magazine:* http://www.food magazine.org.uk/articles/meat_and_dairy/

Modern Miracle Men. U.S Senate Document No. 264, 1936; 18(48): 1-2.

Moshfegh A, Goldman J, Cleveland L. 2005. *What We Eat in America,* NHANES 2001-2002: Usual Nutrient Intakes from Food Compared to Dietary Reference Intakes. U.S. Department of Agriculture, Agricultural Research Service.

Muller MF. *Colloidal Minerals and Trace Elements*. Healing Arts Press 2005.1st edition:Pg.14.

Multivitamin: Should you buy this insurance? Retrieved 2010, from The Harvard Medical School Family Health Guide: http://www.health.harvard.edu/fhg/updates/ update0906d.shtml

Nutrient Index. Retrieved 2010, from the Linus Pauling Institute at Oregon State University: http://lpi.oregon state.edu/infocenter/contentnuts.html

Roger VL, et al. Heart Disease and Stroke Statistics—2011 Update: A Report From the American Heart Association. *Circulation* 2011, 123:e18-e209: originally published online December 15, 2010 doi: 10.1161/CIR.0b013e3182009701

Ruston D, et al. The National Diet & Nutrition Survey: adults aged 19 to 64 years, volume 4. Retrieved 2011, from the Food Standards Agency: http://www.food.gov.uk/multimedia/pdfs/ ndnsv3.pdf

Schneider A. Taste, nutrients decline as size of crops grows. *Seattle Post-Intelligencer* 2007: http://www.seattlepi.com/default/article/Taste-nutrients-decline-as-size-of-crops-grows-1249451.php

Thomas, D. A Study On The Mineral Depletion Of The Foods Available To Us As A Nation Over The Period 1940 To 1991. *Nutr Health.* 2003;17(2):85-115. PMID: 14653505

Vitamin and Mineral Nutrition Information System (VMNIS): Global prevalence of vitamin A deficiency in population at risk: 1995-2005. Retrieved 2010, from the World Health Organization (WHO): http://www.who.int/vmnis/vitamina/ prevalence/report/en/

What We Eat In America: Data Tables: Nutrient Intakes: From Food by Gender and Age 2001-2008. Retrieved 2010, from the USDA, United States Department of Agriculture Agricultural Research Service: http://www.ars.usda.gov/Services/ docs.htm?docid=18349

Chapter 5. Everyday Micronutrient Depleters From Farm to Fork: The Bank Account Goes Bust

Allen GJ, Albala K, ed. *The business of food: encyclopedia of the food and drink industries* 2007. ABC-CLIO. p. 288. ISBN 9780313337253.

Americans Still Consume One-Third Of Calories From Low-Nutrient "Tip Of The Pyramid" 2000. Retrieved 2010, from Science Daily: http://www.sciencedaily.com/releases/2000/09/000929 073225.htm

Barr SB, Wright JC. Postprandial energy expenditure in whole-food and processed-food meals: implications for daily energy expenditure. *Food & Nutrition Research,* vol 54(2010) incl Supplements. Retrieved 2011, from food & nutrition research: http://www.foodandnutritionresearch.net /index.php/fnr/article/view/5144/5755

Beltrán-González F, Pérez-López AJ, López-Nicolás JM, Carbonell-Barrachina ÁA. Effects of agricultural practices on instrumental colour, mineral content, carotenoid composition, and sensory quality of mandarin orange juice 2008, cv.

Benbrook C, Zhao X, Yanez J, Davies N, Andrews P. State of Science Review: Nutritional Superiority of Organic Foods, New Evidence Confirms the Nutritional Superiority of Plant-Based Organic Foods 2008. Retrieved 2010, from The Organic Center: http://organic-center.org/science.tocreports.html

Excerpt from T*he Benefits and Risks of Vitamins and Minerals: What You Need to Know,* SHR February 2003: Protect and serve: Tips for maximizing the nutritional value of your food. Retrieved 2011, from Harvard Health Publications Harvard Medical School: http://www.health.harvard.edu/newsweek/Benefits_and_Risks_of_Vitamins_and_Minerals.htm

Block G. Foods contributing to energy intake in the US: data from NHANES III and NHANES 1999-2000. *Journal of Food Composition and Analysis* 2004. June-August;17(3-4): 439-47. doi:10.1016/j.jfca .2004.02.007. Retrieved 2011, from Science Direct: http://www.sciencedirect.com/science/article/pii/ S0889157504000328

A Brief History of Raw Milk's Long Journey...Retrieved 2011, from Raw-Milk-Facts: http://www .raw-milk-facts.com/milk_history.html

Building Strong Bones: Calcium Information for Health Care Providers. Retrieved 2011, from the National Institutes of Health, Eunice Kennedy Shriver National Institute of Child Health & Human Development: http://www.nichd.nih.gov/publications/pubs/upload/NICHD_MM_HC_FS.pdf

Devlin K. Organic milk is healthier, says study. Retrieved 2010, from *The Telegraph:* http://www.telegraph .co.uk/news/uknews/2039183/Organic-milk-is-healthier-says-study.html

Duckett SK, Neel JPS, Fontenot JP, Clapham WM. Effects of winter stocker growth rate and finishing system on: III. Tissue proximate, fatty acid, vitamin, and cholesterol content 2009. *J ANIM SCI.* June; 87:2961-2970. doi: 10.2527/jas.2009-1850. Retrieved 2011, from *Journal of Animal Science:* http://jas.fass.org/content/87/9/2961.full.pdf+html?sid=916be96d-815b-4aaa-a07a-5191c432283f

Dufault R, LeBlanc B, Schnoll R, Cornett C, Schweitzer L, Wallinga D, et al. Mercury from chlor-alkali plants: measured concentrations in food product sugar. *Environ Health.* 2009;8:2. PMCID: PMC2637263

EWG's 2011 Shopper's Guide to Pesticides in Produce: Executive Summary. Retrieved 2011, from the Environmental Working Group: http://www.ewg.org/ foodnews/summary/

Farmed Salmon and Human Health. Retrieved 2011, from the Pure Salmon Campaign: http:// www.pure salmon.org/human_health.html

Fletcher RH, Fairfield KM. Vitamins for Chronic Disease Prevention in Adults, Clinical Applications. *The Journal of* the American Medical Association 2002. 287(23):3127-29. Retrieved 2010, from *The Journal of the American Medical Association:* http://jama.ama-assn.org/content/287/23/3127.full?sid=73122e66-a912-4b32-b0ed-d7b7559f5e9a

Food Irradiation—the problems and concerns: Position Statement of The Food Commission—July 2002. Retrieved 2010, from The Food Commission: http://www.foodmagazine.org.uk/campaigns/irradiation_concerns/

Food Irradiation Q&As. Retrieved 2011, from Mercola: http://www.mercola.com/article/irradiated/irradiation.htm

Food Irradiation and Vitamin Loss 2007. Retrieved 2010, from Food and Water Watch: http://www.food andwater-watch.org/factsheet/food-irradiation-and-vitamin-loss/

Graham J. 4 Ways to Eat Better and Spend Less. Retrieved 2011, from *Reader's Digest,* Health: http://www.rd.com/health/4-ways-to-eat-better-and-spend-less-on-groceries/

Halweil B. Critical Issue Report: Still No Free Lunch: Nutrient levels in U.S. food supply eroded by pursuit of high yields 2007. Retrieved 2010, from The Organic Center: http://organic-center.org/science.tocreports .html

The Hard Facts About Flavored Milk. Retrieved 2011, from Jamie Oliver's Food Revolution: http://www.jamieoliver.com:81/us/foundation/jamies-food-revolution/facts/JOFR_milkfactsheet_6.3.pdf

Harvie A, Wise TA. "Sweetening the Pot: Implicit Subsidies to Corn Sweeteners and the U.S. Obesity Epidemic," GDAE Policy Brief 09-01, Medford, Mass.: Global Development and Environment Institute, Tufts University, February 2009. Retrieved 2010, from Tufts University: http://www.ase.tufts.edu/gdae/Pubs/rp/ PB09-01SweeteningPot-Feb09.pdf

Healthy and Sustainable Food: "Is Local More Nutritious?" It Depends. Retrieved 2010, from Harvard Medical School Center for Health and the Global Environment: http://chge.med.harvard.edu/programs/food/nutrition.html

Hernandina. *Journal of the Science of Food and Agriculture,* 88(10): 1731–1738. doi: 10.1002/jsfa.3272

Hightower J. When Salmon Go Wrong 2003. Retrieved 2011, from Jim Hightower: http://www.jimhightower.com/node/5000

Kant AK. Consumption of energy-dense, nutrient-poor foods by adult Americans: nutritional and health implications. The third National Health and Nutrition Examination Survey, 1988-1994. *The American Journal of Clinical Nutrition* 2000. Oct;72(4):929-36. PMID: 11010933.

Keough J. Multivitamins 1999. *Natural Solutions* Magazine. Retrieved 2011, from *Natural Solutions* Magazine: http://local.naturalsolutionsmag.com/ Multivitamins_Boston_MA-r1313750-Boston_MA.html

Kewalramani N, Dhiman TR. Conjugated linoleic acid—A milk fat for cancer prevention 2001. *Ind. Dairyman* 53 (8):39-43. http://www.grassfedexchange.com/ dr-tilak-dhiman

Kilshaw PHJ, Heppell LMJ, Ford JE. Effects of heat treatment of cow's milk and whey on the nutritional quality and antigenic properties1982. *Archives of Disease in Childhood.* 57(11): 842-7. doi:10.1136/ adc.57.11.842. Retrieved 2011, from the National Center for Biotechnology Information: http://www.ncbi .nlm.nih.gov/pmc/articles/PMC1628049/pdf/archdisch00752-0036.pdf

Long C, Alterman T. Meet Real Free-Range Eggs 2007. Retrieved 2011, from *Mother Earth News:* http://www.motherearthnews.com/Real-Food/2007-10-01/Tests-Reveal-Healthier-Eggs.aspx

Marchello MJ, Driskell JA. Nutrient Content of Bison Meat from Grass-and Grain-Finished Bulls. Retrieved 2011, from North Dakota State University Agriculture: http://www.ag.ndsu.edu/archive/carringt/bison/nutrients_in_meat.htm

Organic Grass-Fed Beef—Richer in Omega 3 Fatty Acids. Retrieved 2011, from Mercola: http://products .mercola.com/organic-beef/

Pandrangi S, LaBorde LF. Retention of Folate, Carotenoids, and Other Quality Characteristics in Commercially Packaged Fresh Spinach. *Journal of Food Science* 2004. 69(9): C702–C707. doi: 10.1111/j.1365-2621.2004.tb09919.x. Retrieved 2011, from Penn State University, College Of Agricultural Sciences: http://extension.psu.edu/food-safety/publications/laborde-folate.pdf/view

Parker H. A sweet problem: Princeton researchers find that high-fructose corn syrup prompts considerably more weight gain. March 2010. Retrieved 2011, from Princeton University: http://www.princeton.edu/main/news/archive/S26/91/ 22K07/

Pirog R, Benjamin A. Checking the food odometer: Comparing food miles for local versus conventional produce sales to Iowa institutions 2003. Retrieved 2011, from the Leopold Center for Sustainable Agriculture: http://www.leopold. iastate.edu/pubs/staff/files/food_travel072103.pdf

Poulter S. Why frozen vegetables are fresher than fresh, March 2010. Retrieved 2010, from *Daily Mail:* http://www.dailymail.co.uk/health/article-1255606/Why-frozen-vegetables-fresher-fresh.html

Puupponen-Pimiä R, Häkkinen ST, Aarni M, Suortti T, Lampi AM, Eurola M, Piironen V, Nuutila AM, Oksman-Caldentey KM. Blanching and long-term freezing affect various bioactive compounds of vegetables in different ways. *Journal of the Science of Food and Agriculture* 2003, 83: 1389–1402. doi: 10.1002/jsfa.1589. Retrieved 2011, from Wiley Online Library: http://onlinelibrary.wiley.com/doi/ 10.1002/jsfa.1589/ abstract

Rickman JC, Barrett DM, Bruhn CM. Nutritional comparison of fresh, frozen and canned fruits and vegetables. Part 1. Vitamins C and B and phenolic compounds: Review. *Journal of the Science of Food and Agriculture* 2007. 87: 930-944. Doi: 10.1002/jsfa.2825. Retrieved 2011, from University of California Agriculture and Natural Resources: http://ucce.ucdavis.edu/files/filelibrary/1214/36517.pdf

Rickman JC, Barrett DM, Bruhn CM. Nutritional comparison of fresh, frozen and canned fruits and vegetables II. Vitamins A and carotenoids, vitamin E, minerals and fiber: Review. *Journal of the Science of Food and Agriculture* 2007. 87: 1185–1196.. DOI: 10.1002/jsfa.2824. Retrieved 2011, from University of California Agriculture and Natural Resources: http://ucce.ucdavis.edu/files/ filelibrary/1214/36518.pdf

Rickman JC, Barrett DM, Bruhn CM. Nutritional comparison of fresh, frozen, and canned fruits and vegetables: Executive Summary. Retrieved 2011, from the Steel Market Development Institute:http://www .smdisteel.org/~/media/Files/SMDI/Containers/Container%20%20UC%20Davis%20Executive%20Summary.ashx

Salmon: Factory Farm vs. Wild. Retrieved 2011, from Mark's Daily Apple Primal Living in the Modern World: http://www.marksdailyapple.com/salmon-factory-farm-vs-wild/

Searles S. Armstrong JG. Vitamin E, Vitamin A, and Carotene Contents of Alberta Butter 1970. *Journal of Dairy Science.* Feb;53(2): 150-4. PMID: 5413655. http://download.journals.elsevierhealth.com/pdfs/journals/0022-0302/PIIS0022030270861720.pdf

Selman JD. Vitamin retention during blanching of vegetables. *Food Chemistry* 1994. 49)2):137–47.doi:10.1016/0308-8146(94)90150-3. Retrieved 2010, from Science Direct: http://www.sciencedirect.com/science/article/pii/ 0308814694901503

Shaver RD. By-Product Feedstuffs in Dairy Cattle Diets in the Upper Midwest. Retrieved 2011, from University of Wisconsin-Extension: http://www.uwex.edu/ces/dairynutrition/documents/byproductfeeds revised2008.pdf

The Stop Food Irradiation Campaign Student Activist Kit, Retrieved 2011, from Public Citizen: http://citizen .org/documents/studentkit.pdf

Tolan A, Robertson J, Orton CR, Head MJ, Christie AA, Millburn BA. Studies on the composition of food. *British Journal of Nutrition* 1974, 31, pp 185-200 doi:10.1079/BJN19740024. Retrieved 2011, from *Cambridge Journals:* http://journals.cambridge.org/action/displayAbstract?fromPage=online&aid=836244&fulltextType=RA&fileId =S0007114574000250

Top Twelve Reasons to Eat Locally. Retrieved 2011, from Locavors: http://www.locavores.com/how/why.php

USDA. Report of the Dietary Guidelines Advisory Committee on the Dietary Guidelines for Americans, 2010. Retrieved 2011, from USDA, Centers for Nutrition Policy and Promotion: http://www.cnpp .usda.gov/dgas2010-dgacreport.htm

Vallejo F, Tomás-Barberán F, García-Viguera C. Phenolic compound contents in edible parts of broccoli inflorescences after domestic cooking. *Journal of the Science of Food and Agriculture* 2003, 83: 1511–1516. doi: 10.1002/jsfa.1585. Retrieved 2011, from Wiley Online Library: http://onlinelibrary.wiley.com/doi/10.1002/jsfa.1585/abstract

Worthington V. Nutritional Quality of Organic Versus Conventional Fruits, Vegetables, and Grains *The Journal of Alternative and Complementary Medicine*. April 2001, 7(2): 161-173. doi:10.1089/ 107555301750164244. Retrieved 2011, from Liebert Online: http://www.liebertonline.com/doi/abs/10.1089/ 107555301750164244

Chapter 6. Everyday Micronutrient Depletion Continues: Don't Count Your Chickens Before They Hatch

Alberg AJ., et al. Household exposure to passive cigarette smoking and serum micronutrient concentrations. *American Journal of Clinical Nutrition* 2000. December;72(6):1576-82. Retrieved 2011, from *The American Journal of Clinical Nutrition:* http://www.ajcn.org/content/72/6/1576.full?sid=c9592b93-582a-45e9-90e8-29f66d976749

Alcohol & Nutrition. Retrieved 2011, from the Life Enhancement Office Morehead State University: http://www2.moreheadstate.edu/files/units/leo/ alcoholandnutrition.pdf

Position of the American Dietetic Association and Dietitians of Canada: Vegetarian diets. *Journal of the American Dietetic Association* 2003. June;103(6):748-65. Retrieved 2010, from the *Journal of the American Dietetic Association:* http://www.adajournal.org/article/PIIS0002822303002943/fulltext

Ames BN. The Metabolic Tune-Up: Metabolic Harmony and Disease Prevention. *The Journal of Nutrition* 2003. May;133:1544S-1548S. Retrieved 2010, from *The Journal of Nutrition:* http://jn.nutrition.org/content/133/5/1544S.full

Antacids—Aluminum, calcium, and Magnesium-containing preparations. Retrieved 2011, from the University of Maryland Medical Center: http://www.umm.edu/altmed/articles/antacids-aluminum-000176 .htm

Association recommends reduced intake of added sugars, August 24, 2009. Retrieved 2010, from the American Heart Association, Newsroom: http://newsroom.heart.org/pr/aha/800.aspx

Blancett J. Sugar in medicine: children's teeth at risk. *Pediatrics for Parents* 1990. Retrieved 2010, from CBS Interactive Business Network, BNET: http://findarticles.com/p/articles/mi_m0816/is_n10_v11/ai_9216622/

Executive Interview: Q&A with Jeffrey Blumberg, PhD. Natural and Nutritional Products Industry Center, Sep. 7, 2006. Retrieved 2010, from Newhope 360: http://newhope360.com/executive-interview-qa-jeffrey-blumberg-phd

Can you tell me what oxalates are and in which foods they can be found? Retrieved 2010, from The George Mateljan Foundation, The Worlds Healthiest Foods: http://www.whfoods.com/genpage.php? tname=george&dbid=48

Cass H. Supplement Your Prescription: What Your Doctor Doesn't Know About Nutrition. *Total Health Magazine* 2010, August; 1(3):40-44. Retrieved 2011, from *Total Health Magazine:* http://totalhealthmagazine.com/KatJames/

Cassady BA., et al. Mastication of almonds: effects of lipid bioacessibility, appetite, and hormone response. *American Journal of Clinical Nutrition* 2009. January;89(3):794-800. Retrieved 2010, from *The American Journal of Clinical Nutrition:* http://www.ajcn.org/content/89/3/794.full

Christianson A. 10 for the Road: Essential Nutrients for Endurance Athletes. Nutrition Science News May 1999. Retrieved 2010, from New Hope: http://www.newhope.com/nutritionsciencenews/NSN_backs/ May_99/10for_road.cfm

Cordova A, Navas FJ. Effect of training on zinc metabolism: Changes in serum and sweat zinc concentrations in sportsmen. *Annals of nutrition and metabolism* 1998. 42(5):274-82. Retrieved 2011, from Refdoc: http://cat.inist.fr/?aModele= afficheN&cpsidt=2427793

Couzy F., et al. "Nutritional Implications of the Interaction Minerals," *Progressive Food and Nutrition Science/* 1933.17(1):65-87. PMID: 8502756

Dietary Supplement Fact Sheet: Calcium. Retrieved 2010, from the Office of Dietary Supplements, National Institutes of Health: http://ods.od.nih.gov/ factsheets/calcium/#en12

Dietary Supplement Fact Sheet: Zinc. Retrieved 2011, from the Office of Dietary Supplements, National Institutes of Health: http://ods.od.nih.gov/factsheets/Zinc-HealthProfessional/

Digestion and Absorption of Food. The Human Physiology: Tutorials. Retrieved 2011, from Biology online: http://www.biology-online.org/9/ 16_digestion _ absorption_food.htm

Drug-Induced Nutrient Depletion. Chart. Retrieved 2011, from InVite Health: http://www.invitehealth.com/drug-induced-nutrient-depletion.html

Drugs that Deplete: Coenzyme Q10. Retrieved 2011, from the University of Maryland Medical Center: http://www.umm.edu/altmed/articles/coenzyme-q10-000706.htm

Drugs that Deplete: Vitamin B9 (Folic Acid). Retrieved 2011, from the University of Maryland Medical Center: http://www.umm.edu/altmed/articles/vitamin-b9-000722.htm

Drugs that Deplete: Zinc. Retrieved 2011, from the University of Maryland Medical Center: http://www .umm.edu/altmed/articles/zinc-000728.htm

Energy drink explosion hits food. Mintel Press Release Aug 2008. Retrieved 2010, from Mintel, Press Centre: http://www.mintel.com/press-centre/press-releases/268/energy-drink-explosion-hits-food

Etzioni A, Levy J, Nitzan M, Benderly A. Systemic carnitine deficiency exacerbated by a strict vegetarian diet. *Arch Dis Child* 1984. Feb;59(2):177-9. PMCID: PMC1628441.

Fields M., et al. Effect of Copper Deficiency on Metabolism and Mortality in Rats Fed Sucrose or Starch Diets, *Journal of Clinical Nutrition* 1983. July;113(7):1335-45. Retrieved 2011, from The Journal of Nutrition: http://jn.nutrition.org/content/113/7/1335.short

Fitzgerald M. Avoiding Nutrient Deficiencies. *Active.* Retrieved 2009, from *Active:* http://www.active.com/running/Articles/Avoiding_nutrient_deficiencies_21642.htm

Ford JA, Colhoun EM, McIntosh WB, Dutnnigan MG. Biochemical Response of Late Rickets and Osteomalacia to a Chupatty-free Diet. *British Medical Journal* 1972, 3, 446 447. Retrieved 2011, from the National Center for Biotechnology Information:http://www.ncbi.nlm.nih.gov/pmc/articles/PMC1786011/ pdf/brmedj02218-0026.pdf

Gahche J., et al. Dietary Supplement Use Among U.S. Adults Has Increased Since NHANES III (1988–1994). NCHS Data Brief. No. 61, April 2011. Retrieved 2011, from Centers for Disease Control and Prevention, National Center for Health Statistics: http://cdc.gov/nchs/data/databriefs/db61.pdf

Gong K, Gagner M, Pomp A, Almahmeed T, Bardaro SJ. Micronutrient deficiencies after laparoscopic gastric bypass: recommendations. *Obesity Surgery* 2008. Sep;18(9):1062-6. Epub 2008 Jun 6. PMID: 18535863

Gu Q, Dillion CF, Burt VL. Prescription Drug Use Continues to Increase: U.S. Prescription Drug Data for 2007–2008. NCHS Data Brief, September 2010;42. Retrieved 2011, from Centers for Disease Control and Prevention: http://www.cdc.gov/nchs/data/databriefs/db42.htm

Handelman, GJ, Packer L, Cross CE. Destruction of tocopherols, carotenoids, and retinol in human plasma by cigarette smoke. *American Journal of Clinical Nutrtion* 1996. April;63(4):559–65. Retrieved 2010, from *The American Journal of Clinical Nutrition:* http://www.ajcn.org/content/63/4/559.abstract

Health Concerns: Asthma. Retrieved 2011, from Life Extension: http://www.lef.org/protocols/respiratory/asthma_01.htm

Heaney RP, Rafferty K. Carbonated beverages and urinary calcium excretion. *American Journal of Clinical Nutrition* 2001. Sep;74(3):343-7. PMID: 11522558

High Fructose Corn Syrup: A Not So Sweet Surprise. *Organic Lifestyle Magazine* 2008. Oct/Nov;51:44-49. Retrieved 2011, from Organic Lifestyle Magazine: http://www.organiclifestylemagazine.com/issue-5/high-fructose-corn-syrup-not-so-sweet-surprise.php

Hipkiss AR. Glycation, ageing and carnosine: are carnivorous diets beneficial? *Mech Ageing Dev.* 2005 Oct;126(10):1034-9. PMID: 15955546.

The History of Coffee. Retrieved 2011, from PBS, Frontline World: http://www.pbs.org/frontlineworld/stories/guatemala.mexico/facts.html#top

Hokin BD, Butler T. Cyanocobalamin (vitamin B-12) status in Seventh-day Adventist ministers in Australia. *Am J Clin Nutr* 1999; 70(suppl): 576S-8S 1999. PMID: 10479234

Holick MF. Resurrection of vitamin D deficiency and rickets. *J Clin Invest.* 2006;116(8):2062–2072 doi:10.1172/JCI29449. PMID: 16886050

Houtkooper L, Farrell VA. Calcium Supplement Guidelines. Retrieved 2011, from The University of Arizona: http://ag.arizona.edu/pubs/health/az1042.pdf

Hurrell RF, Reddy MB, Juillerat MA, Cook JD. Degradation of phytic acid in cereal porridges improves iron absorption by human subjects. *American Journal of Clinical Nutrition* 2003. May;77(5):1213-19. Retrieved 2010, from *The American Journal of Clinical Nutrition:* http://www.ajcn.org/content/77/5/1213.full?sid=ca49577b-64e1-43da-b8a6-0f8860fdceff

In the Drink: When it Comes to Calories, Solid is Better than Liquid. Nutrition Action Healthletter, November 2000, pg. 7-9. Retrieved 2011, from Human Physiology and Diagnosis: http://www.maximivanov.com/nutrition3.pdf

Jacobson MF. Liquid Candy: How Soft Drinks Are Harming Americans' Health. Retrieved 2011, from the Center for Science in the Public Interest: http://www.cspinet.org/new/pdf/liquid_candy_final_w_new_supplement.pdf

Johnson LA. Drug prices to plummet in wave of expiring patents. *ABC 12 News* July 25, 2011. Retrieved 2011, from *ABC 12 News:* http://www.abc12.com/story/15138834/drug-prices-to-plummet-in-wave-of-expiring-patents

June Russell's Health Facts: Antacids. Dr. Jeffery Blumberg, Tufts University, one of the world's authorities on vitamins and antioxidant. People's Pharmacy, Public Radio, Nov. 7, 1998. Retrieved 2011, from June Russell's Health Facts: http://www.jrussellshealth.org/antacids.html

Koebnick C, Garcia AL, Dagnelie PC, Strassner C, Lindemans J, Katz N, Leitzmann C, Hoffmann I. Long-term consumption of a raw food diet is associated with favorable serum LDL cholesterol and triglycerides, but also with elevated plasma homocysteine and low serum HDL cholesterol in humans. *J Nutr.* 2005. Oct;135(10):2372-8. PMID: 16177198

Kozlovsky A., et al. Effects of Diets High in Simple Sugars on Urinary Chromium Losses. *Metabolism* 1986. June;35(6):515_518. PMID: 3713513

Lemann J Jr, Lennon Ej, Piering WR, Prien EL Jr, Ricanati ES. Evidence that Glucose Ingestion Inhibits Net Renal Tubular Reabsorption of Calcium and Magnesium. *The Journal of Laboratory and Clinical Medicine* 1970. April;75(4):578-85. PMID: 5444345

Li T., et al. Vitamin A Depletion Induced by Cigarette Smoke Is Associated with the Development of Emphysema in Rats. *The Journal of Nutrition* 2003. August;133(8): 2629-34. Retrieved 2010, from *The Journal of Nutrition:* http://jn.nutrition.org/content/133/8/2629.abstract

Lukaski HC. Magnesium, Zinc, and chromium nutriture and physical activity. *American Journal of Clinical Nutrition* 2000. Aug;72(2):585s-93S. Retrieved 2010, from *The American Journal of Clinical Nutrition:* http://www.ajcn.org/content/72/2/585S.full?maxtoshow=&HITS=1...=1035710067874_336&stored_search=&FIRSTINDEX=0&journalcode=ajcn

Macfarlane BJ, et. al. Inhibitory effect of nuts on iron absorption *Am J Clin Nutr* February 1988/47(2): 270-274. Retrieved 2011, from *American Journal of Clinical Nutrition:* http://www.ajcn.org/content/47/2/270.full.pdf+html?sid=5cfe7f4d-40ad-4419-b09f-1cff5cde019f

Mariani P, Viti MG, Montuori M, La Vecchia A, Cipolletta E, Calvani L, Bonamico M. The gluten-free diet: a nutritional risk factor for adolescents with celiac disease? *J Pediatr Gastroenterol Nutr.* 1998. Nov;27(5):519-23. PMID: 9822315.

Melia AT, Koss-Twardy SG, Zhi J. The effect of orlistat, an inhibitor of dietary fat absorption, on the absorption of vitamins A and E in healthy volunteers. *Journal of Clinical Pharmacology* 1996. Jul;36(7):647-53. PMID: 8844448.

Micronutrient Information: Coenzyme Q10. Retrieved 2011, from the Linus Pauling Institute, Oregon State University: http://lpi.oregonstate.edu/infocenter/othernuts/coq10/

Mosher WD., et al. Use of Contraception and Use of Family Planning Services in the United States: 1982-2002. Advance Data: From Vital and Health Statistics 2004. December No. 350. Retrieved 2011, from Centers for Disease Control and Prevention, National Center for Health Statistics: http://www.cdc.gov/ nchs/data/ad/ad350.pdf

Nagel R. Living With Phytic Acid. *Wise Traditions*, March 2010. Retrieved 2010, from The Weston A. Price Foundation: http://www.westonaprice.org/food-features/living-with-phytic-acid

Nutrient Depletion Checker. Reference Database. Retrieved 2011, from Natural Medicines Comprehensive Database: http://naturaldatabase.therapeuticresearch.com/(X(1S(iixaos45tyktianfrgmtqeym))/nd/Search.aspx?cs=&s=ND&pt=14&spt=5&sh=&AspxAutoDetectCookieSupport=1

Nutrition: Explore Our Menu, Starbucks. Retrieved 2011, from Starbucks: http://www.starbucks.com/menu/catalog/nutrition?drink=all#view_control=nutrition

The Nutrition Source: How to Spot Added Sugar on Food Labels. Healthy Drinks. Retrieved 2011, from Harvard School of Public Health: http://www.hsph.harvard.edu/nutritionsource/healthy-drinks/added-sugar-on-food-labels/

O'Donnell K. Small but Mighty: Selected Micronutrient Issues in Gastric Bypass Patients. *Practical Gastroenterology* May 2008. Nutrition Issues In Gastroenterology, Series #62. Retrieved 2011, from the University of Virginia School of Medicine: http://www.medicine.virginia.edu/clinical/departments/medicine/divisions/digestive-health/nutrition-support-team/nutrition-articles/ODonnellArticle.pdf

Optimizing Your Diet: Best Foods for Specific Minerals. MIT Sports Medicine. Retrieved 2011, from Massachusetts Institute of Technology: http://web.mit.edu/athletics/sportsmedicine/wcrminerals.html

Pasquel FJ. Hyperglycemia During Total Parenteral Nutrition: An important marker of poor outcome and mortality in hospitalized patients. *Diabetes Care* 2010. April;33(4):739-41. Retrieved 2011, from American Diabetes Association: *Diabetes Care:* http://care.diabetesjournals.org/content/33/4/739.full

Rokitzki L, Logemann E, Huber G, Keck E, Keul J. alpha-Tocopherol supplementation in racing cyclists during extreme endurance training. *International Journal of Sports Nutrition* 1994. Sep;4(3):253-64. PMID: 7987360.

Ruxton CHS. Nutritional implications of obesity and dieting. Review. *Nutrition Bulletin* 2011. 36:199-211. Retrieved 2011, from Wiley online library: http://onlinelibrary.wiley.com/doi/10.1111/j.1467-3010.2011 .01890.x/abstract

Sanchez A., et al. Role of Sugars in Human Neutrophilic Phagocytosis, *American Journal of Clinical Nutrition* 1971. Nov;261:1180_1184. Retrieved 2011, from The American Journal of Clinical Nutrition: http://www.ajcn.org/content/26/11/1180.abstract

Schectman G, Byrd JC, Gruchow HW. The influence of smoking on vitamin C status in adults. *American Journal of Public Health* 1989. 79(2):158-62. Retrieved 2010, from *American Journal of Public Health*: http://ajph.aphapublications.org/ cgi/content/abstract/79/2/158.pdf

Sensa Weight-Loss System: How It Works, Feel Full Faster, Lose Weight. Retrieved 2011, from Try Sensa: http://www.trysensa.com/how-sensa-works.htm

Silverman R. Hey Sugar, Sugar! How much sugar is in my child's juice? February 23, 2008. Retrieved 2011, from Dr. Robyn Silverman, *Parenting:* http://www.drrobynsilverman.com/parenting-tips/hey-sugar-sugar-how-much-sugar-is-in-my-childs-juice/

Sports Drinks: Winners and Losers. *Good Morning America* 2005. Retrieved 2010, from *ABC News:* http://abcnews.go.com/GMA/OnCall/story?id=969246

Sternberg S. Study links birth control pill to artery-clogging plaque. *Health and Behavior* November 7, 2007. Retrieved 2010, from *USA Today:* http://www.usatoday.com/news/health/2007-11-06-birth-control-heart_N.htm

Take the Stairs. Stairwell messages. Retrieved 2011, from the Centers for Disease Control and Prevention, Healthier Worksite Initiative: http://www.cdc.gov/ nccdphp/dnpao/hwi/downloads/stairwell_messages.pdf

Taylor DS. Stress can cause nutrient deficiencies; enough of the right nutrients can prevent stress, and controlling stress can, in turn, prevent nutrient deficiencies. *Better Nutrition* 1989-90. Retrieved 2011, from CBS Interactive Business Network, BNET: http://findarticles.com/p/articles/mi_m0860/is_n11_ v51/ai_8097915/?tag=content;col1 quote%20magazine%20itself

Vegetarian Diet. Retrieved 2010, from The George Mateljan Foundation, The Worlds Healthiest Foods: http://www.whfoods.com/genpage.php?tname=diet &dbid=6

Venditti P, Di Meo S. Effect of training on antioxidant capacity, tissue damage, and endurance of adult male rats. *International Journal of Sports Medicine* 1997. Oct;18(7):497-502. PMID: 9414071

Ventura EE, Davis JN, Goran MI. Sugar Content of Popular Sweetened Beverages Based on Objective Laboratory Analysis: Focus on Fructose Content. *Obesity* 2011. April;19(4):868-74. Epub 2010 Oct 14. PMID: 20948525

Vitamin B Deficiency And Poor Athletic Performance Linked. *Sports Medicine/Fitness News* 2006. Retrieved 2010, from Medical News Today: http://www.medicalnewstoday.com/releases/56869.php

Watzl B, Watson RR. Role of Alcohol Abuse in Nutritional Immunosuppression. *The Journal of Nutrition.* Symposium: Nutrition, Immunomodulation and AIDs April 25, 1991, 733-37. Retrieved 2010, from Breit Links: http://breitlinks.com/alcoholawareness/AlcAwarePDFs/AlcAbuseNutrionalImunosuppression.pdf

Wenk C, Kuhnt M, Kunz P, Steiner G. Methodological studies of the estimation of loss of sodium, potassium, calcium and magnesium through the skin during a 10 km run. *Z Ernahrungswiss* 1993. Dec;32 (4):301-7. PMID: 8128751

What's New and Beneficial About Spinach. Retrieved 2010, from The George Mateljan Foundation, The Worlds Healthiest Foods: http://www.whfoods.com/ genpage.php?tname=foodspice&dbid=43

Wright ME., et al. Higher baseline serum concentrations of vitamin E are associated with lower total and cause-specific mortality in the Alpha- Tocopherol, Beta-Carotene Cancer Prevention Study. *American Journal of Clinical Nutrition* 2006. Nov;84(5):1200-1207. Retrieved 2011, from *The American Journal of Clinical Nutrition:* http://www.ajcn.org/content/84/5/1200.full.pdf+html?sid=c2f064db-db25-450f-9422-8fcea0517e77

Chapter 7. The Balanced Diet—Fact or Fiction? Four Popular Diet Plans Examined

Appel LJ., et al. A Clinical Trial of the Effects of Dietary Patterns on Blood Pressure. *The New England Journal of Medicine* 1997. April;336:1117-24. Retrieved 2010, from *The New England Journal of Medicine:* http://www.nejm.org/doi/full/10.1056/NEJM199704173361601

Atkins RC. *Atkins for Life: The Complete Controlled Carb Program for Permanent Weight Loss and Good Health.* St. Martin's Press, NY 2003. ISBN 0-312-32522-8. Pg. 161

Calton JB. Prevalence of micronutrient deficiency in popular diet plans. *Journal of the International Society of Sports Nutrition* 2010. Jun;7:24. doi: 10.1186/1550-2783-7-24. PMID: 20537171. Retrieved 2010, from the National Center for Biotechnology Information: http://www.ncbi.nlm.nih.gov/pmc/articles/ PMC2905334/

The DASH Diet Eating Plan. Retrieved 2011, from Dash Diet: http://www.dashdiet.org/

Sample menus for the DASH eating plan, Nutrition and healthy eating. Retrieved 2010, from the Mayo Clinic: http://www.mayoclinic.com/health/dash-diet/HI00046/NSECTIONGROUP=2

Dollahite J, Franklin D, McNew R. Problems encountered in meeting the Recommended Dietary Allowances for menus designed according to the Dietary Guidelines for Americans. *J Am Diet Assoc.* 1995. Mar;95(3):341-4, 347; quiz 345-6. PMID: 7860947

Greene B. *The Best Life Diet.* Simon & Schuster Paperbacks, NY 2006. ISBN-10: 1-4165-4069-5 (pbk). Pg. 180

McDonald's USA Nutrition Facts for Popular Menu Items: Nutrition Info. Retrieved 2011, from McDonald's: http://nutrition.mcdonalds.com/nutritionexchange/nutritionfacts.pdf

Misner B. Food alone may not provide sufficient micronutrients for preventing deficiency. *Journal of the International Society of Sports Nutrition* 2006, 3:51-55. Retrieved 2010, from the *Journal of the International Society of Sports Nutrition:* http://www.jissn.com/content/3/1/51

Nutrition Information: Veggie Delite. Retrieved 2011, from Subway: http://www.subway.com/Menu/ Product.aspx ?CC=USA&LC=ENG&ProductId=16&MenuId=35&MenuTypeId=1

Pachocka L, Klosiewicz-Latoszek L. [Changes in vitamins intake in overweight and obese adults after low-energy diets]. *Rocz. Panstw. Zakl. Hig.* 2002. 53(3):243-52. PMID: 12621879. Retrieved 2011, from National Center for Biotechnology Information: http://www.ncbi.nlm.nih.gov/pubmed/12621879

Prevention Guide, The South Beach Diet 2-Week Quickstart Plan, Issue 3 2008. Pg. 29

Truby H et al. Commercial weight loss diets meet nutrient requirements in free living adults over 8 weeks: A randomized controlled weight loss trial. *Nutrition Journal* 2008. 7:25. doi:10.1186/1475-2891-7-25. Retrieved 2011, from Nutrition Journal: http://www.nutritionj.com/content/7/1/25

USDA national nutrient database for standard reference (Release 20). Retrieved 2009, from United States Department Of Agriculture, Agricultural Research

Wang X., et al. Weight Regain is Related to Decreases in Physical Activity During Weight Loss. *Med Sci Sports Exerc.* 2008. Oct;40(10):1781-88. doi: 10.1249/MSS.0b013e31817d8176. Retrieved 2010, from National Center for Biotechnology Information: http://www.ncbi.nlm.nih.gov/pmc/articles/ PMC2797708/

World's Healthiest Foods Database, Food Processor for Windows nutrition analysis software, version 7.60. Salem/ ESHA Research, Retrieved 2010, from The George Mateljan Foundation, The Worlds Healthiest Foods: http://www. whfoods.com/genpage.php?tname=nutrientprofile&dbid=62

Chapter 8. The Obesity Puzzle: Micronutrient Sufficiency—The Missing Piece

Ames BN. The Metabolic tune-up: metabolic harmony and disease prevention. *Journal of Nutrition* 2003. May;133(5 Suppl 1):1544s-8S. PMID: 12730462.

Asfaw A. Micronutrient deficiency and the prevalence of mothers' overweight/obesity in Egypt. *Econ Hum Biol.* 2007. Dec;5(3):471-483. PMID: 17449338.

Associated Press. Health experts: Obesity pandemic looms. Diet and nutrition 2006. Retrieved 2011, from MSNBC: http://www.msnbc.msn.com/id/14657885/ns/health-diet_and_nutrition/t/health-experts-obesity-pandemic -looms/#.TlFsYM3UCeZ

Associated Press. Obesity Bigger Threat Than Terrorism? Healthwatch 2010. Retrieved 2010, from *CBS News:* http://www.cbsnews.com/stories/2006/03/01/ health/main1361849.shtml

Biocare P. Recent Study Reinforces the Benefits of Omega-3 for Weight Control. NPI Center 2005. Retrieved 2010, from New Hope 360: http://newhope360.com/ recent-study-reinforces-benefits-omega-3-weight-control

Bottomley J. Economic costs of diabetes in the US in 2007—Implications for Europe. *Journal of Diabetes & Vascular Disease* 2008. March;8(2):96–100. Retrieved 2010, from Sage Journals online: http://dvd .sagepub.com/ content/8/2/ 96.refs

Can Foods Forestall Aging? News & Events. Retrieved 2011, from USDA, Agricultural Research Service: http://www. ars.usda.gov/is/AR/archive/feb99/ aging0299.htm

Catalanotto FA. The trace metal zinc and taste. *The American Journal of Clinical Nutrition* 1978. June;31:1098-1103. Retrieved 2010, from *American Journal of Clinical Nutrition:* http://www.ajcn.org/content/ 31/6/1098.full.pdf

Decorde K, Teissedre PL, Sutra T, Ventura E, Cristol JP, Rouanet JM. Chardonnay grape seed procyanidin extract supplementation prevents high-fat diet-induced obesity in hamsters by improving adipokine imbalance and oxidative stress markers. *Mol Nutr Food Res.* 2009. May;53(5):659-66. PMID: 19035554.

Mervyn Deitel M.D., editor of *Obesity Surgery,* puts it this way, "The commonest form of malnutrition in the western world is obesity." Retrieved 2010, from the National Center for Biotechnology Information: http://www.ncbi.nlm. nih.gov/pmc/articles/PMC2082679/

The developing world's new burden: obesity. Focus. Retrieved 2010, from the Food And Agriculture Organization of the United Nations: http://www.fao.org/FOCUS/E/obesity/obes3.htm

Dr. Oz's Cure For Stubborn Belly Fat. First for Women, March 14, 2011. Pg. 32-37.

Dzieniszewski J. Nutritional status of patients hospitalized in Poland. *European Journal of Clinical Nutrition* 2005. 59:552-60. doi:10.1038/sj.ejcn.1602117. Retrieved 2011, from *European Journal of Clinical Nutrition:* http://www. nature.com/ejcn/journal/v59/n4/abs/1602117a.html

Feinstein A. *Prevention's Healing with Vitamins: The Most Effective Vitamin And Mineral Treatments For Everyday Health Problems And Serious Disease.* Rodale 1996. ISBN 1-57954-018-X, Pg. 441.

Garemo M, Lenner RA, Strandvik B. Swedish pre-school children eat too much junk food and sucrose. *Acta Paediatr.* 2007. Feb;96(2):266-72. PMID: 17429918.

Gilsanz V, Kremer A, Mo AO, Wren TA, Kremer R. Vitamin D Status and Its Relation to Muscle Mass and Muscle Fat in Young Women. *J Clin Endocrinol Metab.* 2010. April;95(4):1595-1601. PMCID: PMC2853984.

Hill JO, Trowbridge FL. Childhood obesity: Future directions and research priorities. *Pediatrics* 1998. Mar;101(3 pt 2):570-4. PMID: 12224663.

Johnston CS. Strategies for Healthy Weight Loss: From Vitamin C to the Glycemic Response. *Journal of the American College of Nutrition* 2005. June;24(3):158-65. Retrieved 2010, from the *Journal of the American College of Nutrition*: http://www.jacn.org/content/24/3/158.full

Kotz D. Time in the Sun: How Much Is Needed for Vitamin D? *Family Health* 2008. Retrieved 2010, from *U.S. News and World Report*: http://health.usnews.com/healthnews/familyhealth/heart/articles/2008/06/23/time-in-the-sun-how-much-is-needed-for-vitamin-d

Kremer R, Campbell PP, Reinhardt T, Gilsanz V. Vitamin D status and its relationship to body fat, final height, and peak bone mass in young women. *J Clin Endocrinol Metab.* 2009. Jan;94(1):67-73. Epub 2008 Nov 4. PMID: 18984659.

Kumar J, Muntner P, Kaskel FJ, Hailpern SM, Melamed ML. Prevalence and associations of 25-hydroxyvitamin D deficiency in US children: NHANES 2001-2004. *Pediatrics* 2009. Sep;124(3):e362-70. Epub 2009 Aug 3. PMID:19661054.

Major GC, Doucet E, Jacqmain M, St-Onge M, Bouchard C, Tremblay A. Multivitamin and dietary supplements, body weight and appetite: results from a cross-sectional and randomized double-blind placebo-controlled study. *British Journal of Nutrition* 2008. May;99:1157-67. doi: 10.1017/S0007114507853335. PMID: 17977472. Retrieved 2010, from Faculte de medecine de l'Universite Laval: http://w3.fmed.ulaval.ca/chaireobesite/education/docs/AT_Rev3_Major_Vitamines.pdf

Mann D. Vitamin D deficiency common in U.S. children. *Health* 2009. Retrieved 2010, from CNN Health: http://articles.cnn.com/2009-08-03/health/vitamin.d.children_1_vitamin-d-levels-low-vitamin-d-levels-vitamin-d-deficiency?_s=PM:HEALTH

Mercola J. Shocking Update—Sunshine Can Actually Decrease Your Vitamin D Levels. Health Blog 2009. Retrieved 2009, from Mercola: http://articles.mercola.com/sites/articles/archive/2009/05/12/shocking-update-sunshine-can-actually-decrease-your-vitamin-d-levels.aspx

Moor de Burgos A, Wartanowicz M, Zienlanski S. Blood vitamin and lipid levels in overweight and obese women. *European Journal of Clinical Nutrition* 1992. Nov;46(11):803-8. PMID: 1425534.

Noreen EE, Sass MJ, Crowe ML, Pabon VA, Brandauer J, Averill LK. Effects of supplemental fish oil on resting metabolic rate, body composition, and salivary cortisol in healthy adults. *Journal of the International Society of Sports Medicine* 2010. Oct;7:31. PMID: 20932294.

Not enough vitamin D in the diet could mean too much fat on adolescents. Research 2009. Retrieved 2010, from Physorg: http://www.physorg.com/news156088325.html

Obesity Contributes to Vitamin D Deficiency. HealthBloggers 2008. Retrieved 2010, from Wellsphere: http://www.wellsphere.com/exercise-article/obesity-contributes-to-vitamin-d-deficiency/237074

"The Obesity Crisis in America" Statement of Richard H. Carmona, M.D., M.P.H., F.A. C.S., Surgeon General 2003. Retrieved 2010, from U.S. Department of Health & Human Services, Office of the Surgeon General: http://www.surgeongeneral.gov/news/testimony/obesity07162003.htm

Obesity Rates Continue to Climb in the United States. Public Health News Center 2007. Retrieved 2010, from Johns Hopkins Bloomberg School of Public Health: http://www.jhsph.edu/publichealthnews/press_releases/2007/wang_adult_obesity.html

Overweight and Obesity: Causes and Consequences. Retrieved 2011, from the Centers for Disease Control and Prevention: http://www.cdc.gov/obesity/causes/ economics.html

Pinhas-Hamiel O, Newfield RS, Koren I, Agmon A, Lilos P, Phillip M. Greater prevalence of iron deficiency in overweight and obese children and adolescents. *International Journal of Obesity* 2003. 27:416-18. doi:10.1038/sj.ijo.0802224. Retrieved 2010, from *International Journal of Obesity*: http://www.nature .com/ijo/journal/v27/n3/full/0802224a.html

Pollan M. *In Defense of Food: An Eater's Manifesto*. Penguin Press 2008. ISBN-10: 1594201455. Pg. 122.

Ruzickova J, Rossmeisl M, Prazak T, Flachs P, Sponarova J, Veck M, Tvrzicka E, Bryhn M, Kopecky J. Omega-3 PUFA of marine origin limit diet-induced obesity in mice by reducing cellularity of adipose tissue. *Lipids* 2004, Dec;39(12):1177-85. PMID: 15736913.

Simontacchi C. Mineral Deficiencies And Food Cravings. Retrieved 2011, from the Diabetes Information Library: http://www.diabetesinfocenter.org/View.aspx?url=Article819

The spectrum of malnutrition. Factsheet. Retrieved 2011, from the Food and Agriculture Organization of the United Nations: http://www.fao.org/worldfoodsummit/english/fsheets/malnutrition.pdf

Streib L. World's Fattest Countries. *Forbes,* Lifestyle/Health 2007. Retrieved 2010, from Forbes: http://www.forbes.com/2007/02/07/worlds-fattest-countries-forbeslife-cx_ls_0208worldfat.html

Tordoff MG, Bachmanov AA, Reed DR. Forty mouse strain survey of voluntary calcium intake, blood calcium, and bone mineral content. *Physiol Behav.* 2007. Aug;91(5):632-43. PMCID: PMC2085359.

U.S. Obesity Trends: Trends by State 1985-2010. Retrieved 2010, from the Centers for Disease Control and Prevention: http://www.cdc.gov/obesity/data/trends.html

Van Gaal L, DeLeeuw I, Vadhanavikit S, Folkers K. Exploratory Study of Coenzyme Q10 in Obesity. Biomedical and Clinical Aspects of Coenzyme Q. Vol. 4, pp. 369-73, Elsevier Science Publishers B.V., 1984. Reference to study Retrieved 2011, from *ABC MoneyWatch*: http://findarticles.com/p/articles/mi_mOFKA/is_n8_v58/ai_18549482/

Weight Reduction with VLDC and N-3 PUFA Leads to Higher Decrease of Weight and BMI in Severely Obese Women. NAASO's 2004 Annual Meeting, Volume 12, October 2004, Supplement, Program Abstracts. No 249-P. Retrieved 2010, from New Hope 360: http://newhope360.com/www.npicenter.com/anm/templates/newsATemp.aspx?articleid=11527&zoneid=22

White E., et al. VITamins And Lifestyle Cohort Study: Study Design and Characteristics of Supplement Users. *American Journal of Epidemiology* 2004. 159(1):83-93. doi: 10.1093/aje/kwh010. Retrieved 2010, from *Oxford Journals:* http://aje.oxfordjournals.org/content/159/1/83.full

Zhang W., et al. Dietary a-Lipoic Acid Supplementation Inhibits Atherosclerotic Lesion Development in Apolipoprotein E-Deficient and Apolipoprotein E/Low-Density Lipoprotein Receptor-Deficient Mice. *Circulation* 2008. Dec;117:421-28. Retrieved 2010, from American Heart Association: http://circ.ahajournals.org/content/117/3/421short

Chapter 9. The ABCs of Optimal Supplementation: A Recipe for Success

Ames BN. Low micronutrient intake may accelerate the degenerative diseases of aging through allocation of scarce micronutrients by triage. *Proceedings of the National Academy of Sciences* 2006. Nov; 103(47):17589-94. Retrieved 2010, from *Proceedings of the National Academy of Sciences of the United States of America*: http://www.pnas.org/content/103/47/17589.full.pdf

Beating Egg Whites. Cooking & Recipes/Preparation/Eggs. Retrieved 2011. From *Dummies*: http://www.dummies.com/how-to/content/beating-egg-whites0.html

Carter KC. The germ theory, beriberi, and the deficiency theory of disease. *Med Hist.* 1977. April:21(2):119-36. PMCID: PMC1081945. . Retrieved 2010, from National Center for Biotechnology Information: http://www.ncbi.nlm.nih.gov/pmc/articles/PMC1081945/?pageindex=15

Dietary Reference Intake (DRI) & Recommended Dietary Allowance (RDA). Ask the Dietitian. Retrieved 2011, from Ask the Dietitian: http://www.dietitian.com/rda.html

Dietary Supplement Fact Sheet: Vitamin B_{12}. Health Professional. Retrieved 2010, from the Office of Dietary Supplements, National Institutes of Health: http://ods.od.nih.gov/factsheets/vitaminb12/

Dr. Oz's Anti-Aging Checklist. *The Oprah Winfrey Show* 2008. Retrieved 2010, from Oprah: http://www .oprah.com/health/Dr-Ozs-Ultimate-Anti-Aging-Checklist/19

Evans JL, Brar BS. Tissue Cytochrome Oxidase Activity and Copper, Iron, and Pantothenic Acid Nutrition in the Growing Rat. *The Journal of Nutrition* 1974. 104:1285-91. Retrieved 2010, from *The Journal of Nutrition*: http://jn.nutrition.org/content/104/10/1285.full.pdf

40% of American Adults Report Experiencing Difficulty Swallowing Pills; National Survey Shows Many Failed to Take medication as Directed Because of Difficulty Swallowing Pills. PRNewswire 2004. Retrieved 2010, from The Free Library: http://www.thefreelibrary.com/40%25+of+American+Adults+Report+Experiencing+Difficulty+Swallowing...-a0112187875

Gourley DR. APhA Complete Review For Pharmacy. *American Pharmaceutical Association,* 7 Pap/Cdr edition, January 2010. ISBN-10: 1582121451. Pg. 51

The History of Vitamins (and a short history of scurvy, beriberi, and pellagra). Retrieved 2011, from Wellness Directory of Minnesota: http://www.mnwelldir.org/docs/history/vitamins.htm

Lieberman S, Bruning NP. *The Real Vitamin and Mineral Book.* Avery 2003. ISBN-10: 1583331522. Pg. 30.

Löbenberg R, Steinke W. Investigation of vitamin and mineral tablets and capsules on the Canadian market. *J Pharm Pharmaceut Sci* 2006. Feb;9(1):40-49. Retrieved 2010, from University of Alberta: http://www.ualberta.ca/~csps/ JPPS9(1)/Loebenberg.R/tablets.htm

Mahato RI. Chapter 3: Dosage Forms and Drug Delivery Systems. Textbook: *APhA'S Complete Review For Pharmacy.* Castle Connolly Graduate Medical Publishing, Ltd. New York, NY 2004. Pg. 37-63.

Major GC, Doucet E, Jacqmain M, St-Onge M, Bouchard C, Tremblay A. Multivitamin and dietary supplements, body weight and appetite: results from a cross-sectional and randomized double-blind plecebo-controlled study. *British Journal of Nutrition* 2008. May;99:1157-67. doi: 10.1017/S0007114507853335. PMID: 17977472. Retrieved 2010, from Faculte de medecine de l'Universite Laval: http://w3.fmed.ulaval.ca/chaireobesite/education/docs/AT_Rev3_Major_Vitamines.pdf

Mann D. Post-Bariatric Surgery Supplement Savvy. Nutrition. Retrieved 2010, from Consumer Guide To Bariatric Surgery: http://www.yourbariatricsurgeryguide.com/nutrition/

Moser LR, Ordman AB. Design from a study to determine optimal dosage of ascorbic acid and alpha- tocopherol in humans. AGE 2006. 28(1): 77-84, DOI: 10.1007/s11357-006-9000-1.

One Man, Carl F. Rehnborb. History. Retrieved 2011, from Nutrilite: http://www.nutrilite.com/en-us/Nature/whyNutrilite/our-history.aspx

Ordman A. Key to Protection from Age-associated Disease: AM/PM. Retrieved 2011, from Medical Doctors Research: http://www.mdri.com/healthy_living/staying_healthy/ampmvitamins.php

Physicians' Desk Reference 54th edition, 2000. Medical Economics Company. ISBN: 1-56363-330-2. Pg. 1674.

Sen CK, Khanna S, Roy S. Tocotrienols: Vitamin E Beyond Tocopherols. *Life Science* 2006. March;78 (18):2088-89. doi: 10.1016/j.lfs.2005.12.001. Retrieved 2010, from National Center for Biotechnology Information: http://www.ncbi.nlm. nih.gov/pmc/articles/PMC1790869/

Stevens LM. Vitamins A to K. *JAMA* Patient Page. *The Journal of the American Medical Association* 2002. June;287(23):3166. Retrieved 2011, from the *Journal of the American Medical Association*: http://jama.ama-assn.org/content/287/23/ 3166.full.pdf

Stewart M. *The Martha Stewart Living Cookbook.* Clarkson Potter: New York, 2000. ISBN-10: 0609607502. Pg. 591.

Stone I. *The Healing Factor. Vitamin C Against Disease.* New York: Grosset & Dunlap, 1972. ISBN 0-448-11693-6. Foreword by Albert Szent-Gyorgyi, M.D., Ph.D. Pg. xi-xii. Retrieved 2010, from University of Washington: http://faculty.washington.edu/ely/stoneforewords.html

Turner N. Six tips to get the most out of your vitamins. Chatelaine: Health/Diet 2011. Retrieved 2011, from Chatelaine: http://www.chatelaine.com/en/article/23626—six-tips-to-get-the-most-out-of-your-vitamins

What are excipients? Retrieved 2011, from HealthLine: http://healthline.cc/ images/Excipient.pdf

What Vitamins Should You Take? America's Health 2006. Retrieved 2010, from *ABC Good Morning America:* http://abcnews.go.com/GMA/OnCall/story?id=1580193&page=1

Chapter 10. The Web of Competition and the Dynamic Duos of Synergy: The ABCs Continued

Barrett J. The Gurus' Guide to Daily Nutrition. *Newsweek Magazine* 2006. Retrieved 2010, from Juvenon: http://juvenon.com/news/nw-guru1.htm

Bauman WA., et al. Increased Intake of Calcium Reverses Vitamin B12

Malabsorption Induced by Metformin. *Diabetes Care* 2000. Sept:23(9):1227-31. Retrieved 2011, from Victor Herbert: http://victorherbert.com/cv800.pdf

Brink S, Solovitch S. Daily Vitamin: Is It Really Necessary? *Los Angeles Times,* Health. Retrieved 2011, from *Los Angeles Times:* http://articles.latimes.com/2006/dec/04/health/he-vitamins4

Cangemi FE. TOZAL Study: An open case control study of an oral antioxidant and omega-3 supplement for dry AMD. *BMC Ophthalmology* 2007. Feb;7:3. doi:10.1186/1471-2415-7-3. Retrieved 2010, from Preventive Health Solutions: http://www.preventivehealthsolutions.com/documents/TOZAL_study.pdf

Dr. Oz's Ultimate Supplement Checklist. Videos. Retrieved 2010, from *The Dr. Oz Show:* http://www.doctoroz.com/videos/dr-ozs-ultimate-supplement-checklist

Fletcher RH, Fairfield KM. Vitamins for chronic disease prevention in adults: Clinical Applications. *Journal of the American Medical Association* 2002. Jun 19;287(23):3127-29. doi:10.1001/jama.287.23.3127 PMID: 12069676

Ghishan FK, Said HM, Wilson PC, Murrell JE, Greene GL. Intestinal transport of zinc and folic acid: a mutual inhibitory effect. *American Journal of Clinical Nutrition* 1986. February;43:258-62. Retrieved 2010, from *The American Journal of Clinical Nutrition:* http://www.ajcn.org/content/43/2/258.full.pdf

Hyman M. How Dietary Supplements Reduce Health Care Costs. Retrieved 2011, from Dr. Hyman: http://drhyman.com/how-dietary-supplements-reduce-health-care-costs-3250/

Jenab M., et al. Association between pre-diagnostic circulating vitamin D concentration and risk of colorectal cancer in European populations: a nested case-control study. *BMJ* 2010. 340:b5500. doi: 10.1136/bmj.b5500. Retrieved 2010, from BMJ: http://www.bmj.com/content/340/bmj.b5500.full? maxto show=&HITS=10&hits=10&RESULTFORMAT=&fulltext=jenab&searchid=1&FIRSTINDEX=0&sortspec=date&resourcetype=HWCIT

Kotulak R. Vitamin a day just what doctors order. *Chicago Tribune* 2002. Retrieved 2010, from *Chicago Tribune:* http://articles.chicagotribune.com/2002-06-19/news/0206190305_1_vitamins-rdas-pellagra

Mercola J. Read This Shocking Vitamin D Report or You'll Kick Yourself for the Next Decade. Health Blog 2010. Retrieved 2010, from Mercola: http://articles.mercola.com/sites/articles/archive/2010/03/16/warning-new-proof-confirms-if-you-take-this-supplement-vitamin-d-will-not-work as-well.aspx

Most multivitamin extras don't add up. Tuffs University Health & Nutrition Letter Feb 1st 2010. Retrieved 2010, from Goliath: http://goliath.ecnext.com/coms2/gi_0199-12432585/Most-multivitamin-extras-don-t.html

Multivitamins: Your Insurance Policy for an Imperfect Diet. Be Well eNews 2009. Retrieved 2011, from Cleveland Clinic Health: http://cchealth.cleveland clinic.org/be-well-enews/multivitamins-your-insurance-policy-imperfect-diet

Nutrition's dynamic dues. Harvard Health Letter. Retrieved 2010, from Harvard Health Publications: http://www.health.harvard.edu/newsletters/Harvard_ Health_Letter/2009/July/Nutritions-dynamic-duos

The Nutrition Source. Nutrition Insurance Policy: A Daily Multivitamin. What should you eat" Retrieved 2011, from Harvard School of Public Health: http://www.hsph.harvard.edu/nutritionsource/what-should-you-eat?/multivitamin/index.html

The Nutrition Source: Three of the B Vitamins: Folate, Vitamin B6, and Vitamin B12. What should you eat? Retrieved 2011, from Harvard School of Public Health: http://www.hsph.harvard.edu/nutrition source/what-should-you-eat/vitamin-b/

The Nutrition Source, Vitamins: The Bottom Line, A daily multivitamin is a great nutrition insurance policy. Some extra vitamin D may add an extra health boost. What should you eat? Retrieved 2011, from Harvard School of Public Health: http://www.hsph.harvard.edu/nutritionsource/what-should-you-eat/vitamins/index.html

Sharonova IN, Vorobjev VS, Hass HL. Interaction between copper and zinc at GABA(A) receptors in acutely isolated cerebellar Purkinje cells of the rat. *Br J Pharmacol.* 2000. June;130(4):851-56. Retrieved 2010, from the National Center for Biotechnology Information: http://www.ncbi.nlm.nih.gov/pmc/articles/PMC1572144/

Shrimpton D.H. Pharmacy Practice: Chemical reaction—Dr Derek H Shrimpton, scientific advisor to the European Federation of Health Product Manufacturers (EHPM) considers the nutritional implications of micronutrient interactions. *Chemist & Druggist* 2004. Retrieved 2010, form Highbeam Business: http://business.highbeam.com/409991/article-1G1-116778433/pharmacy-practice-chemical-reaction

Van den Berg H, Van Vliet T. Effect of simultaneous, single oral doses of ß-carotene with lutein or lycopene on the ß-carotene and retinyl ester responses in the triacylglycerol-rich lipoprotein fraction of men. *American Journal of Clinical Nutrition* 1998. July;68(1):82-89. Retrieved 2010, from *American Journal of Clinical Nutrition:* http://www.ajcn.org/content/68/1/82.long

Vitamin B2 (Riboflavin): Overview. Retrieved 2010, from the University of Maryland Medical Center: http://www.umm.edu/altmed/articles/vitamin-b2-000334.htm

Warnock S. Researchers continue to find nutrition's value in preventing—even treating—AMD. *Ocular Surgery* news U.S. edition 2001. Retrieved 2010, from ONS super site: http://www.osnsupersite.com/view.aspx?rid=13762

Wasserman RH. Vitamin D and the Dual Processes of Intestinal Calcium Absorption. *The Journal Of Nutrition* 2004. Nov;134(11):3137-39. Retrieved 2010, from *The Journal of Nutrition*: http://jn.nutrition.org/content/134/11/ 3137.full

Willett WC, Skerrett PJ. Eat Drink and Be Healthy. Simon & Schuster 2005. ISBN-10: 0-7432-6642-0. Pg. 24.

Chapter 11. The Hypothesis of Health: Using the Naked Facts to Conquer Naked Calories

Ames BN. The Metabolic Tune-Up: Metabolic Harmony and Disease Prevention. *The Journal of Nutrition* 2003. May;133:1544S-1548S. Retrieved 2010, from *The Journal of Nutrition:* http://jn.nutrition.org/content/133/5/1544S.full

Barel A., et al. Effect of oral intake of choline-stabilized orthosilicic acid on skin, nails and hair in women with photodamaged skin. *Archives of Dermatological Research.* 297(4):147-53. DOI: 10.1007/s00403-005-0584-6. Retrieved 2011, from Springer Link: http://www.springerlink.com/content/f50xw4669778468j/

Carlton RM, Ente G, Blum L, Heyman N, Davis W, Ambrosino S. Rational dosages of nutrients have a prolonged effect on learning disabilities. *Altern Ther Health Med.* 2000. May:6(3):85-91. PMID: 10802909

Cawthon RM, Smith KR, O'Brien E, Sivatchenko A, Kerber RA. Association between telomere length in blood and mortality in people aged 60 years or older. *The Lancet* 2003. Feb;361(9355):393-5. doi:10.1016/S0140-6736(03)12384-7. Retrieved 2010, from *The Lancet*: http://www.thelancet.com/journals/lancet/article/PIIS0140-6736(03)12384-7/fulltext#article_upsell

Chronic Disease Prevention and Health Promotion. Chronic Disease. Retrieved 2010, from Centers for Disease Control and Prevention: http://www.cdc.gov/chronicdisease/overview/index.htm

Clark LC. Decreased incidence of Prostate cancer with selenium supplementation: results of a double-blind cancer prevention trial. *Br J Urol.*1998. May:81(5):730-4. PMID: 9634050.

Da Vanzo JE., et al. An Evidence?Based Study of the Role of Dietary Supplements in Helping Seniors Maintain their Independence. Dietary Supplement Education Alliance 2006. Retrieved 2010, from The Lewin Group Inc.: http://www.lewin.com/content/publications/3393.pdf

DaVanzo J., et al. A Study of the Health and Cost Effects of Five Dietary Supplements. Dietary Supplement Education Alliance. Retrieved 2010, from Natural Products Foundation: http://www.naturalproducts info.org/clientuploads/healthimpact1.pdf

Friso S., et al. Low plasma vitamin B-6 concentrations and modulation of coronary artery disease risk. *American Journal of Clinical Nutrition* 2004. June;79(6):992-98. Retrieved 2010, from *The American Journal of Clinical Nutriton:* http://www.ajcn.org/content/79/6/992.long

Geleijnse JM., et al. Dietary intake of menaquinone is associated with a reduced risk of coronary heart disease: the Rotterdam Study. *The Journal of Nutrition* 2004. Nov; 134(11):3100-5. Retrieved 2013, from the National Center for Biotechnology Information: http://www.ncbi

Hyman M. How Dietary Supplements Reduce Health Care Costs. Retrieved 2010, from Dr. Hyman: http://drhyman.com/how-dietary-supplements-reduce-health-care-costs-3250/

Kanellakis S., et al. Changes in parameters of bone metabolism in postmenopausal women following a 12-month intervention period using dairy products enriched with calcium, vitamin D, and phylloquinone (vitamin K(1)) or menaquinone-7 (vitamin K (2)): the Postmenopausal Health Study II. *Calcified Tissue International* 2012. Apr;90(4):251-62. doi: 10.1007/s00223-012-9571-z. Epub 2012 Mar 4. Retrieved 2013, from the National Center for Biotechnology Information: http://www.ncbi.nlm.nih.gov/pubmed/22392526

Life Extension Update Exclusive. "Longer telomeres associated with multivitamin use." *Life Extension.* 3/17/09. Retrieved 2010, from Life Extension: http://www.lef.org/newsletter/2009/ 0317_Longer-Telomeres-Associated-with-Multivitamin-Use.htm

Melamed ML, Michos ED, Post W, Astor B.. 25-hydroxyvitamin D levels and the risk of mortality in the general population. *Arch Intern Med.* 2008. Aug;168(15):1629-1637. Retrieved 2010, from *Archives of Internal Medicine:* http://archinte.ama-assn.org/cgi/content/full/168/15/1629

National Health Care Expenditures Data. Centers for Medicare and Medicaid Services, Office of the Actuary, National Health Statistics Group January 2010. Retrieved 2011, from U.S. Department of Health & Human Services: https://www.cms.gov/NationalHealthExpendData/02_NationalHealthAccountsHistorical.asp#TopOfPage

Popper PA. *Forks over knives.* Video. Retrieved 2011, from *Forks over Knives:* http://forksoverknives.com/

Schoenthaler SJ, Bier ID. The effect of vitamin-mineral supplementation on juvenile delinquency among American schoolchildren: a randomized, double-blind placebo-controlled trial. *J Altern Complement Med.* 2000. Feb;6(1):7-17. PMID: 10706231.

Showell MG, Brown J, Yazdani A, Stankiewicz MT, Hart RJ. Antioxidants for male subfertility. Cochrane Database of Systematic Reviews 2011, Issue 1. Art. No.: CD007411. DOI: 10.1002/14651858.CD007411.pub2. Retrieved 2011, from Wiley Online Library: http://onlinelibrary.wiley.com/doi/10.1002/14651858 .CD007411.pub2/full

Voutilainen S., et al. Low serum folate concentrations are associated with an excess incidence of acute coronary events: the Kuopio Ischemic Heart Disease Risk Factor Study. *Eur J Clin Nutr.* 2000. May;54(5): 424–8. PMID: 10822291.

Urberg M, Zemel MB. Evidence for synergism between chromium and nicotinic acid in the control of glucose tolerance in elderly humans. *Metabolism* 1987. September;36(9):896-9. doi:10.1016/0026-0495(87)90100-4. Retrieved 2010, from Science Direct: http://www.sciencedirect.com/science/article/pii/ 0026049587901004

Xu Q, Parks CG, DeRoo LA, Cawthon RM, Sandler DP, Chen H. Multivitamin use and telomere length in women. *American Journal of Clinical Nutrition* 2009. June;89(6):1857-63. PMID: 19279081.

Index

Beta-blocking drugs, 117

Beta-carotene, 37, 40, 76, 78, 80, 81, 87, 95, 117, 118, 121, 123, 187, 198, 199, 200, 205, 208. *See also* Vitamin A.

Beydoun, May, 160

Binge eating, 57

Biochemical competition of micronutrients, 198

Biochemical synergy of micronutrients, 203

Bioflavonoids. *See* Accessory micronutrients.

Biological age, 225

Biotin. *See* Vitamin B7 (biotin).

Bison, grass-fed, 81

Bisphosphonate, micronutrient depletions and, 117

Blanching process, 84

Blood clotting, 33, 56, 126, 207

Blood pressure, 11, 15, 30, 52, 54, 56, 57, 110, 117, 118, 120, 125, 140, 141, 159, 160, 162, 163, 206, 207

Blumberg, Jeffrey, 119, 120, 209

Bone deformities, 52,

Bone pain, 57, 119, 120

Boston University School of Medicine, 54, 163

Brain damage, 57

Brigham and Women's Hospital, 139

British Journal of Nutrition, 81, 173, 174, 181, 196, 208

British Medical Journal, 197

Bronchitis, 52

Brown sugar, 108

Bruising, easy, 56

C

Caffeine, 11, 105, 106, 107, 112, 131

Calciferol, 40

Calcium, 15, 17, 18, 19. 31. 40, 49, 50, 51, 57, 59, 62, 65, 66, 79, 82, 87, 90, 91, 102, 103, 104, 105, 106, 107, 108, 117, 118, 120, 121, 124, 132, 133, 138, 140, 141, 151, 152, 165, 166, 170, 180, 190, 191, 192, 203, 207, 214, 215, 216, 216, 224, 227

  salt craving and deficiency of, 165

  side effects of deficiency, 120

  U.S. population and intake of, 62

Calcium channel blocking drugs, 118

California Vitamins, 180

Caloric value, 31

Calories. *See* Naked calories.

Calton, Jayson and Mira, about, 1–2

Calton Project, the, 3–12, 44, 45, 48, 72, 158, 180, 223, 232

Cancer, 8, 10, 11, 15, 17, 18, 33, 52, 53, 54, 55, 56, 57, 59, 61, 66, 78, 79, 80, 81, 83, 125, 126, 140, 159, 160, 163, 183, 184, 206, 214, 223, 224, 232

Cane crystals, 108

Cane sugar, 108

Canned food. *See* Food packaging, as an EMD.

Caramel, 108

Carbohydrates. *See* Macronutrients.

Cardiac glycoside, 118

Cardiovascular disease, 17, 53, 56, 57, 59, 61, 78, 126, 132, 163, 183, 232

Carmona, Richard H., 159

Carnitine, 132, 168

Carnosine, 132

Carotenoids, 215

Carrington Research Extension Center, 81

Cass, Hyla, 113

Cataracts, 52, 56, 57, 61, 83, 126

Celiac disease, 132

Centers for Disease Control and Prevention. *See* U.S. Centers for Disease Control and Prevention (CDC).

Chemical competition, of micronutrients, 197

Chemical synergy, of micronutrients, 203

Chemicals, toxic. *See* Toxic chemicals.

Chicken(s), 78, 81, 83

  experiment on, 178

  micronutrient content of, 49

Childhood Obesity Research Center, 110

Children's Hospital, 163

Children's Nutrition Research Centre of the Royal Children's Hospital, 152

Chloride, 40

Cholesterol levels, 11, 30, 52, 57, 102, 104, 117, 132, 136, 206

Cholesterol-lowering drugs, 114, 115

Choline, 40, 57, 140

Chromium, 18, 41, 58, 102, 104, 108, 109, 117, 121, 132, 140, 151, 169, 170, 199, 205, 225

Clinical competition of micronutrients, 198

Clinical synergy of micronutrients, 203–204

Cobalamin, 40

Coenzyme Q10. *See* CoQ10 (coenzyme Q10).

Coffee consumption. *See* Caffeine.

Coke Classic, sugar content comparison, 111

Cold pasteurization. *See* Irradiation.

Colgate, 180

Colorectal cancer, 54, 57, 224

Columbus, Christopher, 177

Competition of micronutrients, 181, 194, 196–198, 200, 202

  web of, 199

Congestive heart failure, 54, 56, 114

Conjugated estrogen, 118

Conjugated linoleic acid (CLA),79

M

Macrominerals, 32, 40, 57

Macronutrients, 35, 36, 70
  as building blocks, 36
  defined, 31

Magnesium, 17, 31, 40, 49, 50,
  51, 59, 62, 66, 79, 87, 90, 102,
  103, 104, 106, 107, 108, 109,
  117, 118, 120, 121, 124, 128,
  132, 133, 138, 140, 141, 152,
  165, 170, 180, 187, 191, 199,
  205, 213, 215, 216
  side effects of deficiency, 54,
    57, 120
  sugar craving and, 165
  U.S. population and intake of,
    59, 62

Malnourishment, 173, 174, 222

Malnutrition, 14, 49, 172

Malt syrup, 108

Maltose, 108

Mangan, Dennis, 55

Manganese, 41, 57, 102, 104, 132,
  140, 199, 205

Manson, JoAnn, 55

Marler, John B., 48

Mayo Clinic, 122, 140

Mccollum, Elmer, 179

Medications, as EMDs, 113–121

*Medicine & Science in Sports &
  Exercise,* 156

Megaloblastic anemia, 57, 126

Melamed, Michal, 163

Melatonin, 117, 118, 121

Mellanby, Edward, 102

Mercola, Joseph, 83, 197

Mercury, 92, 124, 125

Meridia, 131

Mertz, Walter, 46, 47

Metabolism, 225

Micronutrient absorption. *See*
  Absorption.

Micronutrient competition, 36,
  37, 196–202, 212, 218, 222,
  228, 231
  domino effect, 206–207

Micronutrient deficiency, 3, 11,
  14, 15, 16, 17, 19, 30, 38, 39,
  50, 52, 53, 54, 56, 66, 67, 72,
  97, 102, 116, 129, 136, 141,
  142, 143, 156, 160, 161, 162,
  164, 166, 170, 171, 172, 173,
  174, 177, 178, 184, 189, 208,
  220, 221, 222, 223, 226, 228,
  229, 232

Micronutrient Deficiency Challenge, 22
  quiz, 23–26
  discussion, 27–28

Micronutrient deficiencies, drugs
  and. *See* Medications, as
  EMDs.

Micronutrient density, food
  preparation and, 14

Micronutrient depleters. *See*
  Everyday Micronutrient
  Depleters (EMDs).

Micronutrient depletion as a
  state of emergency, 183–184
  cooking methods and, 88

Micronutrient sufficiency, 17, 18,
  19, 22, 27, 30, 41, 45, 71, 72,
  74, 85, 94, 96, 97, 98, 101,
  102, 104, 105, 106, 112, 113,
  120, 121, 127, 130, 131, 134,
  137, 141, 142, 143, 151, 152,
  167, 179, 208, 209, 211, 215,
  216, 217, 221, 223, 226, 227,
  228, 229, 231, 232

Micronutrient Sufficiency
  Hypothesis of Health, 223,
  226, 227

Micronutrient synergy, 37,
  203–206, 212, 218, 222

Micronutrients, 32
  absorption of. *See* Absorbtion.
  aging and, 53
  beneficial quantities. *See* Ben-
    eficial quantities of micronu-
    trients.
  breakdown of, 34
  cancer prevention and, 53
  categorization of, 31

defined, 14, 31
  effect on macronutrients, 35
  essential, 31–32
  nonessential, 31–32
  RDI requirements, 40–41
    *See also individual micronutri-
    ents.*

Micronutrient-sufficiency level
  determining, quiz for, 23–26
  quiz discussion, 27–28

Milk, 78, 132, 164
  unpasteurized (raw) versus
    pasteurized, 82

Mineral deficiency, soil and, 46
  historical timeline of, 47

Minerals. 32. *See also individal
  minerals.*

Mintel International Group, 112,
  130

Minute Maid Cran-Grape Juice,
  111

Mira's osteoporosis, 17, 30

Misner, William, 136, 137

Modernization, 72, 232
  physical activity and, 9
  See also Calton Project.

Molasses, 108

Molybdenum, 41, 57, 140, 199,
  205

Moore, Thomas, 139

Mother Earth News magazine, 81

Mt. Sinai Hospital, 54

Multiple sclerosis, 52

Multivitamin(s)
  as a weight-loss supplement,
    173–174
  fillers in, 187
  invention of, 180–181
  liquid form, 131, 185, 186, 187,
    188, 191, 194, 196, 211, 212,
    213, 218, 222
  powdered, 187, 188, 194, 196,
    211, 212, 213, 218, 222, 231
  recommendations for choosing,
    213–214
  sugars in, 187

Vitamin B2. *See* Riboflavin (vitamin B2).

Vitamin B3. *See* Niacin (vitamin B3).

Vitamin B5. *See* Pantothenic acid (vitamin B5).

Vitamin B6 (pyridoxine), 40, 57, 62, 87, 95, 132, 139, 140, 169, 170, 199, 205, 207, 224

Vitamin B7 (biotin), 40, 57, 140, 199, 205, 207

Vitamin B9. *See* Folate/folic acid (vitamin B9).

Vitamin C (ascorbic acid), 40, 56, 62, 73, 76, 86, 87, 88, 94, 95, 108, 117, 118, 119, 121, 122, 123, 126, 140, 167, 168, 177, 179, 183, 189, 192, 199, 204, 205, 223

Vitamin D, 17, 18, 40, 54, 55, 56, 59, 81, 91, 102, 104, 117, 118, 119, 120, 121, 124, 125, 132, 140, 162, 163, 164, 165, 169, 179, 197, 199, 203, 205, 207, 209, 211, 212, 213, 214, 215, 225, 227

Vitamin D Solution, The (Holick), 163

Vitamin E, 40, 56, 59, 60, 61, 62, 73, 78, 79, 80, 81, 90, 126, 127, 131, 140, 167, 179, 199, 205

Vitamin Hypothesis of Disease, 179, 223

Vitamin K, 17, 40, 56, 119, 140, 199, 203, 205. *See also* Phylloquinone.

Vitamin K$_2$, 224

Vitamins, discovery of, 177–180

W

Walli, Jeanne R., 48

Wallinga, David, 92

Water-soluble vitamins, 32

Web of competition, The, 199

Weight Watchers, 152

Weight-loss aids, 130–131

Weight-Loss diets, micronutrient depletion and, 129–131

Western influence on society, 11

Weston A. Price Foundation, 102

White sugar. *See* Refined sugar.

Willett, Walter, 44, 210

Wise Traditions, 102

Wood, Richard J., 214

World Health Organization (WHO), 67, 160, 161, 172

Z

Zeaxanthin, 78, 199, 205

Zinc, 31, 41, 104, 107, 109, 115, 128, 197, 199, 203, 205, 224
 deficiency, 62, 66, 115, 121, 166
 prescription medication and, 117–118
 side effects of deficiency, 53, 54, 57, 120, 166, 170